Clinical Management of Shock - The Science and Art of Physiological Restoration

Edited by Stanislaw P. Stawicki and Mamta Swaroop

Published in London, United Kingdom

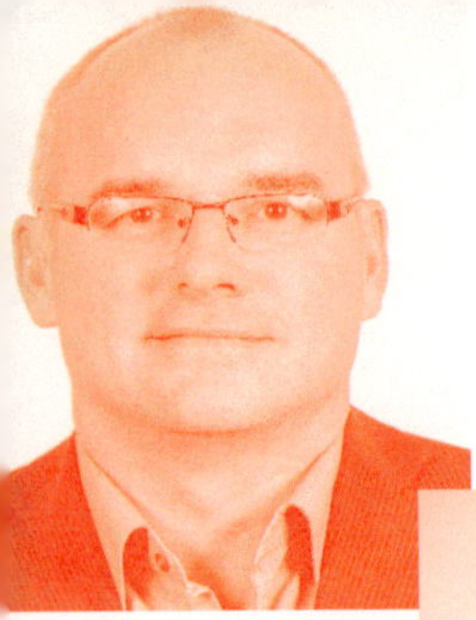
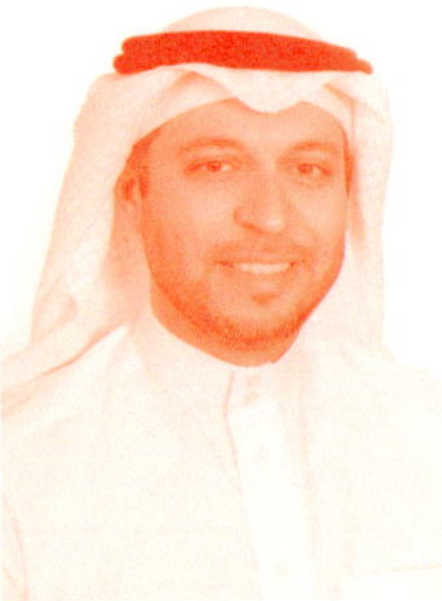
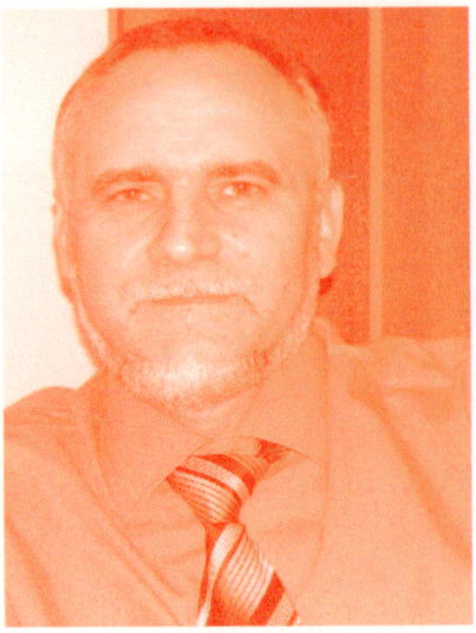
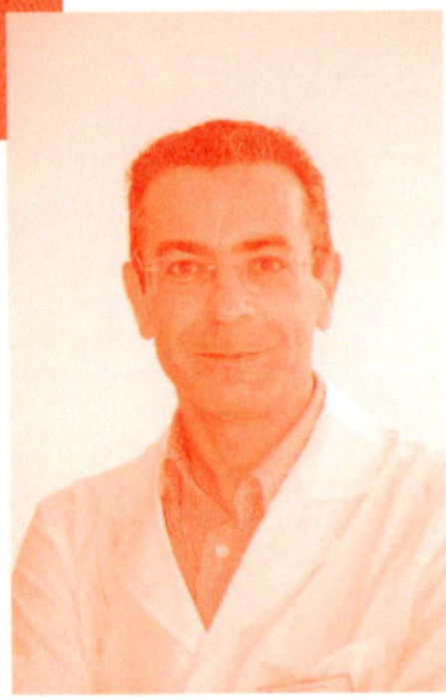
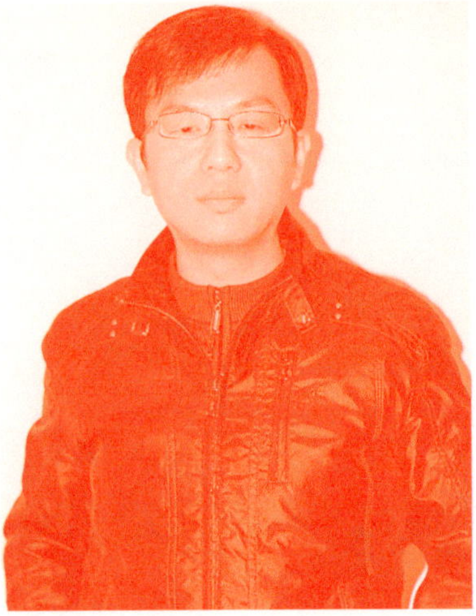
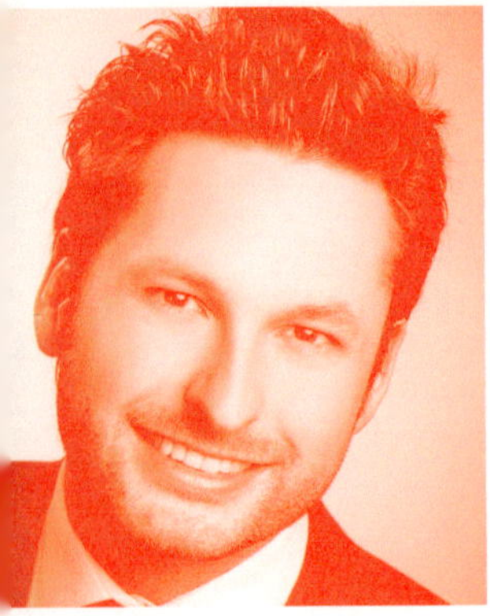
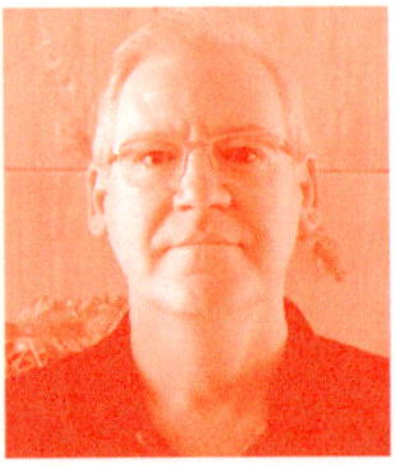

IntechOpen

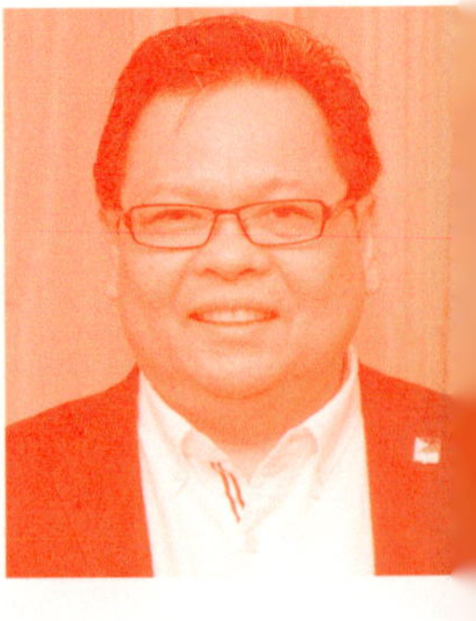
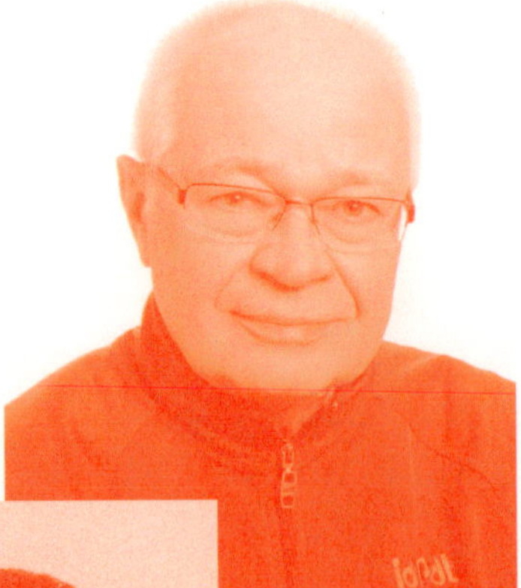
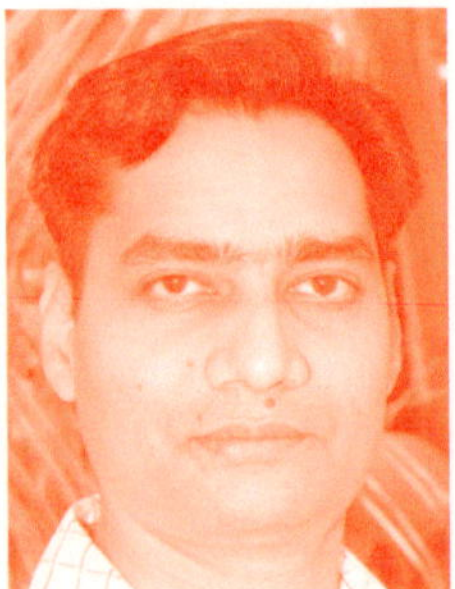
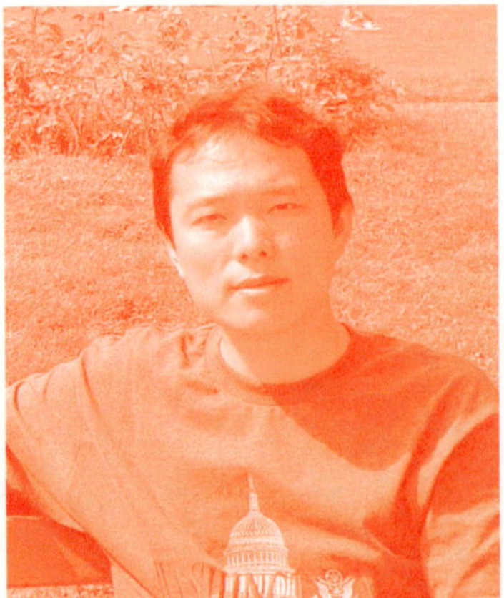
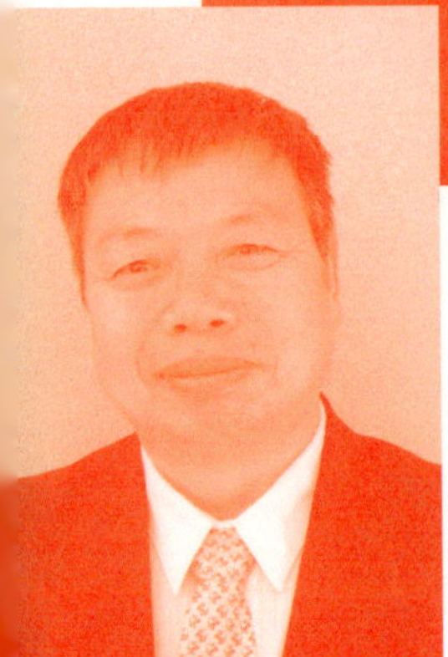
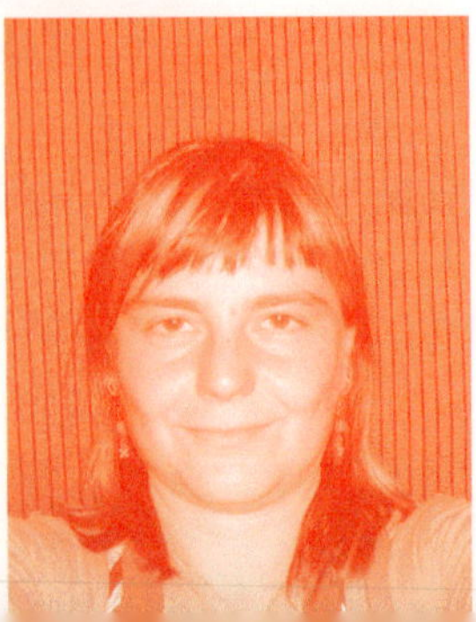

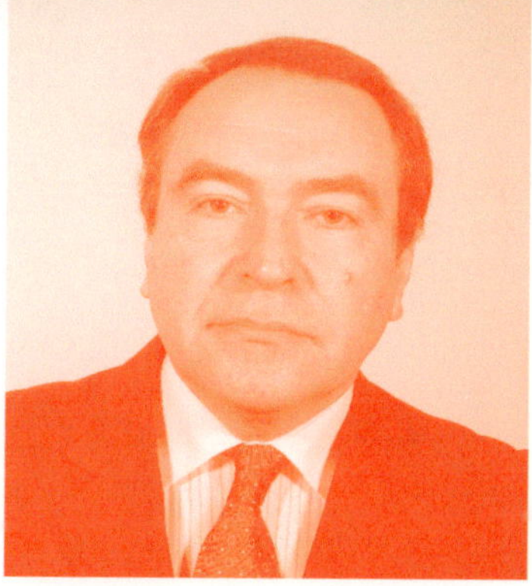
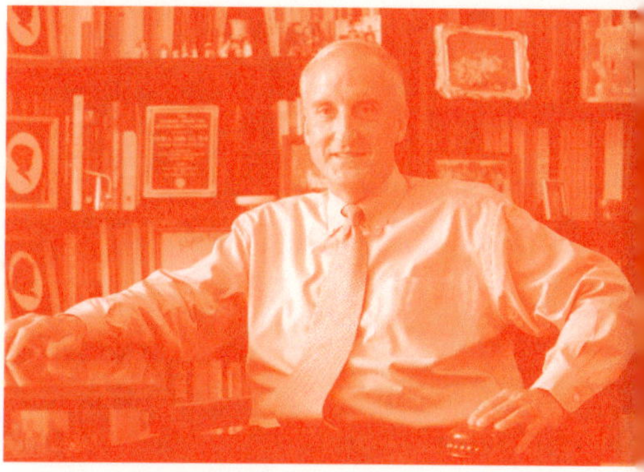
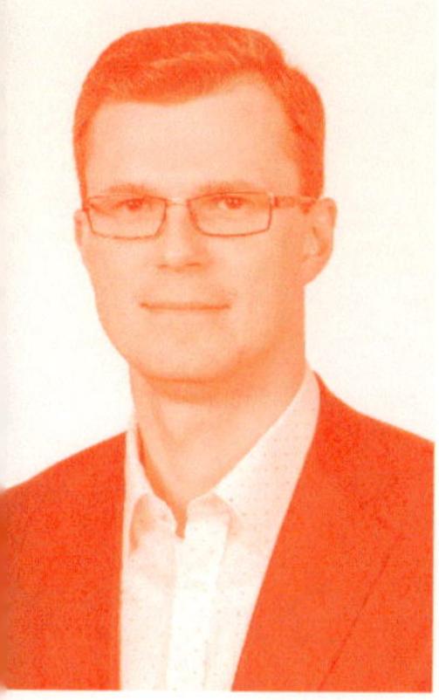
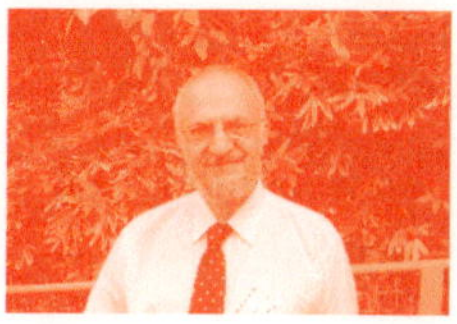
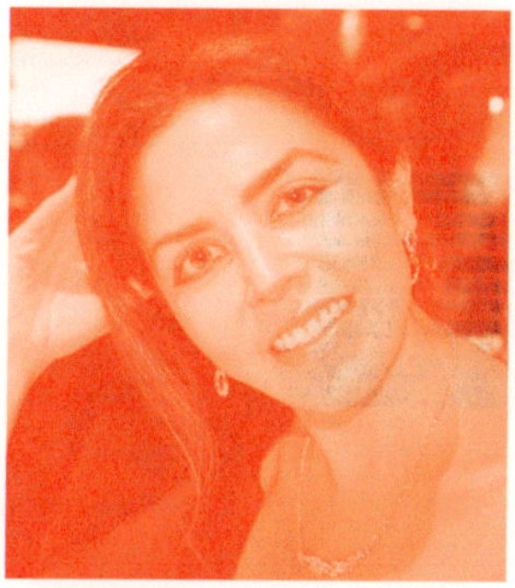

Supporting open minds since 2005

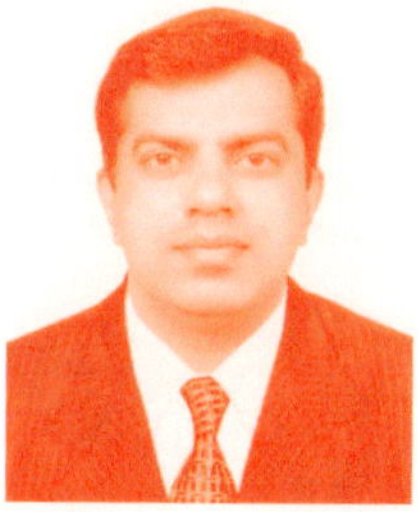
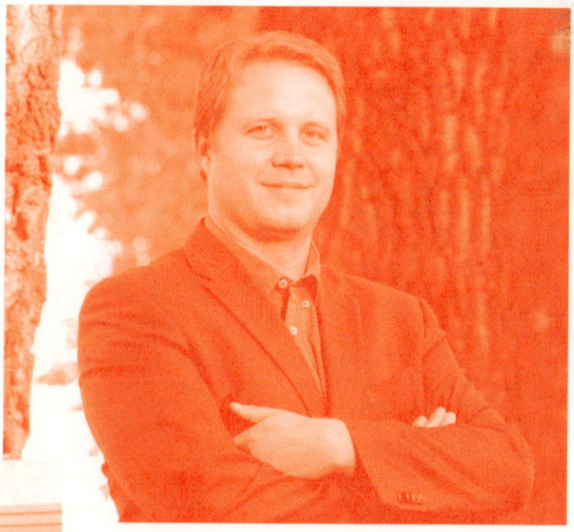
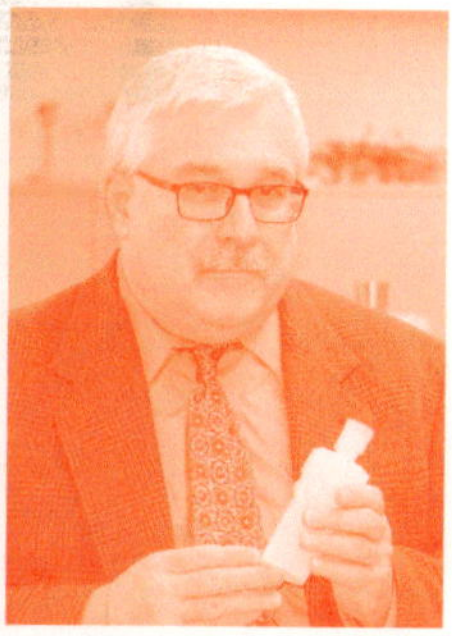
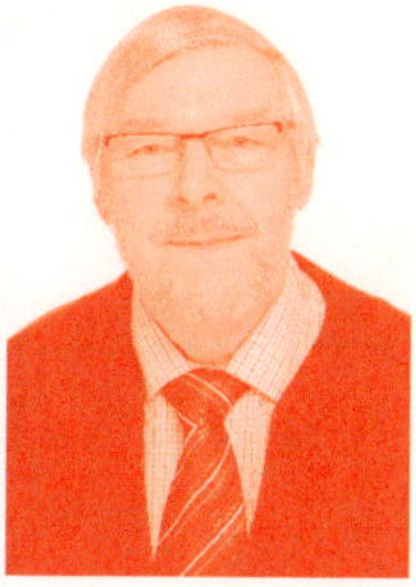
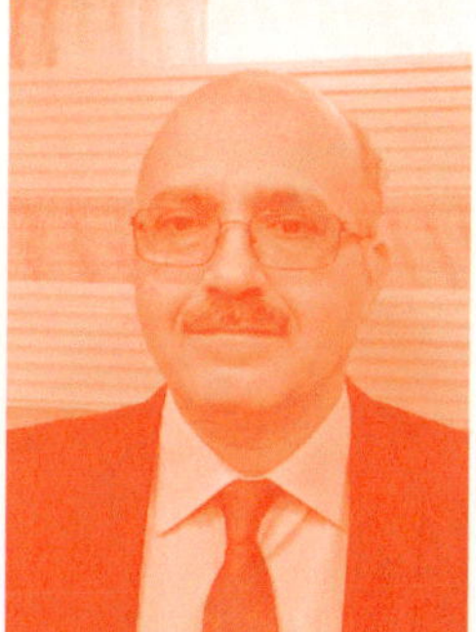
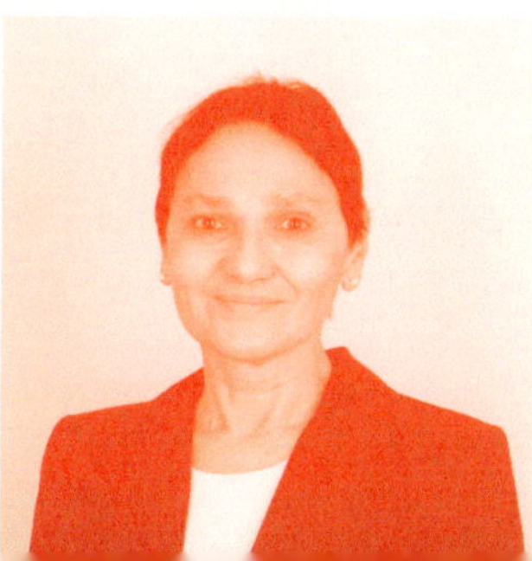
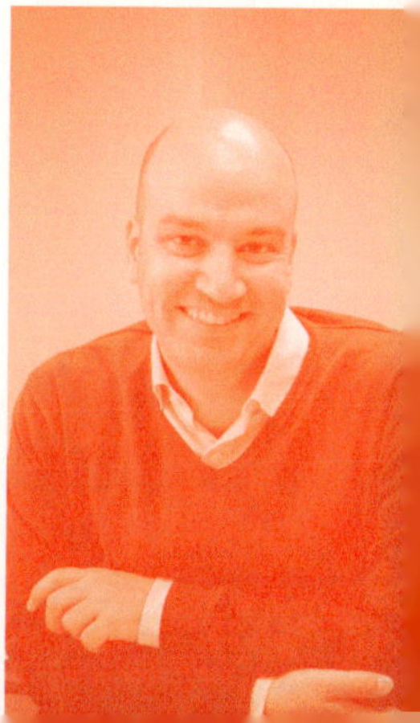

Clinical Management of Shock - The Science and Art of Physiological Restoration
http://dx.doi.org/10.5772/intechopen.73805
Edited by Stanislaw P. Stawicki and Mamta Swaroop

Contributors
Nissar Shaikh, Fevzi Sarper Türker, Alaap Mehta, Ali Khalid, Mamta Swaroop, Mike Hamasaki, Daniel Ackerman, Anna Volski, Steven Falowski, Vikas Yellapu, Keith Conti, Joan Sweeney, Stanislaw P. Stawicki, Jorge E. Tolosa, Neesaytee Boulden, Joseph Bell, Jose Rojas-Suarez, Stephen DeTurk, Anna Pellegrino, Shravan Reddy, John Wilson, Stanislaw Stawicki, Thomas J. Papadimos, Mamta Swaroop, Débora Maria da Gomes Cunha, Guilherme Galdino da Silva, Kathryn C. Kelley, Kyle Dammann, Alex Alers, Thomas B. Zanders, Charles Bendas, John Sojka, Andrew C. Krakowski, Umm-E-Amara, Jazib Hassan, Zeeshan Qazi, Arshad Chanda, Zia Mahemood, Mahommad Zubair, AR Raju Vegensa, Abdul Gafoor M. Tharayil, Adel Ganaw, Ranjan Matthias, Muna Al Musalmani

First published in London, United Kingdom, 2020 by IntechOpen
IntechOpen is the global imprint of INTECHOPEN LIMITED, registered in England and Wales, registration number: 11086078, 7th floor, 10 Lower Thames Street, London, EC3R 6AF, United Kingdom
Printed in Croatia

British Library Cataloguing-in-Publication Data
A catalogue record for this book is available from the British Library

Additional hard and PDF copies can be obtained from orders@intechopen.com

Clinical Management of Shock - The Science and Art of Physiological Restoration
Edited by Stanislaw P. Stawicki and Mamta Swaroop
p. cm.
Print ISBN 978-1-83881-170-9
Online ISBN 978-1-83881-171-6
eBook (PDF) ISBN 978-1-83881-172-3

For EU product safety concerns:
IN TECH d.o.o., Prolaz Marije Krucifikse Kozulić 3, 51000 Rijeka, Croatia, info@intechopen.com or visit our website at intechopen.com.

Meet the editors

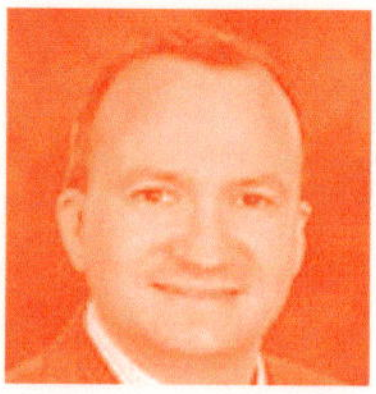

Stanislaw P. Stawicki, MD, MBA, FACS, FAIM, is Chair of the Department of Research of Innovation, St. Luke's University Health Network, Bethlehem, Pennsylvania. He is Professor of Surgery at Temple University School of Medicine, Philadelphia, Pennsylvania. Dr. Stawicki has edited more than sixteen books on the topics of clinical research, graduate medical education, medical leadership, critical care, and patient safety. He is a member of multiple editorial boards and has coauthored nearly 600 publications. He has given multiple scientific presentations on four continents and is board certified in general surgery, surgical critical care, and neurocritical care.

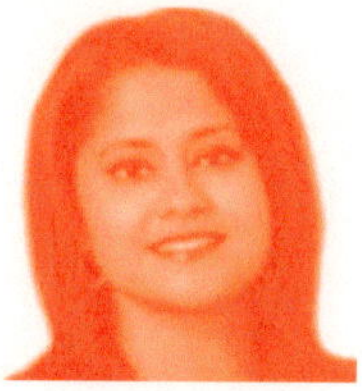

Mamta Swaroop, MD, FACS FICS FAIM, is Associate Professor of Surgery in the Division of Trauma and Critical Care, the Director for the Center for Global Surgery in the Institute for Global Health, and the Global Surgery Program Director at Northwestern University Feinberg School of Medicine. Her lab, the Northwestern Trauma and Surgical Initiative (www.ntsi.global), aims to build sustainable access to surgical care through education and research in low-resource settings. The NTSI conducts community-directed research and programmatic I development in Southeast Asia, South America, and Chicago, Illinois, USA. To honor her family's legacy, she founded a 501(c)(3) NGO, the Sadanah Foundation (www.sadanah.org), to build sustainable access to health care and education in low-resource settings.

Contents

Foreword on Shock

Shock, defined as a state of insufficient perfusion and impaired tissue oxygen delivery, is a life-threatening condition of varied etiologies that requires prompt recognition, diagnosis, and resuscitation [1, 2]. Prehospital shock is associated with a 33–52% in-hospital mortality rate [1]. While trends in frequency and mortality of undifferentiated shock in the emergency department (ED) are under-explored, in-hospital mortality rates of 23–24% have been reported in Danish [1] and US ED settings [3, 4], with 90-day mortality approaching 41% [1]. Moreover, mortality rates for some subtypes of shock may be higher (e.g., trauma patients with hemorrhagic shock) [5]. Mortality further increases with any associated end-organ dysfunction or failure [6], as well as with increased comorbidity burden as measured by the Charlson comorbidity index [1].

Despite technical improvement in diagnostics and advances in treatment, shock remains a critical finding in acute medical care. Reducing time to recognition and targeted treatment are critical aspects of patient care. Shock's clinical recognition is traditionally based on vital sign abnormalities (blood pressure, heart rate), and it may be defined as the presence of hypotension (systolic blood pressure ≤ 100 mmHg) and ≥ 1 organ failures [1]. The Shock Index (SI; systolic blood pressure/heart rate) may further be used as a measure of cardiovascular failure (≥ 1) [7].

Traditionally shock has been classified into four categories: cardiogenic, distributive, hypovolemic, and obstructive. However, although the circulatory system is complex and depends on a multitude of variables, some find it helpful to simplify it to three main components: cardiac function ("the pump"), intravascular volume ("the tank"), and systemic vascular resistance ("the pipes") [2]. In shock, dysfunction occurs within one or more of the three components – the pump, tank, or pipes – such that tissue perfusion and oxygen delivery are impaired [2]. Acute pump malfunction can be caused by arrhythmias, conditions that result in a sudden decrease in cardiac contractility (e.g., myocardial infarction, myocarditis, valvular insufficiency) or by extracardiac conditions that obstruct cardiac output (e.g., pericardial tamponade, pulmonary embolus). Acute tank malfunction primarily results from a decrease in intravascular volume due to hemorrhage, volume loss, or impaired venous return and impaired left ventricular preload (e.g., tension pneumothorax). Pipe malfunction may be observed with processes that alter vascular tone including anaphylaxis, neurogenic (e,g., spinal cord injury), sepsis, and processes that disrupt pipe integrity (e.g., aortic dissection, abdominal aortic aneurysm). Importantly, some entities (e.g., burns, trauma, etc.) may compromise more than one system (pump, tank, pipes). Regardless of the underlying mechanism of shock, if impaired perfusion and oxygen delivery are not recognized and reversed, organ dysfunction, tissue necrosis, and death may ensue.

Significant regional disparities in evidence-based care have been reported, and in-hospital mortality remains high. This book goes beyond the basics of epidemiology, pathophysiology, and recognition, and targets the difficult, and at times confusing, management decisions that clinicians treating shock are faced with including resuscitation fluid (or blood product) selection, mechanical ventilation, vasopressor use, and decisions on surgical intervention. A thorough understanding of these topics is crucial for acute care providers and by studying this book you have taken the important first steps on this journey.

Competing interests

The author has no conflicts of interest to disclose.

Funding

No funding was received for this work

Andrew C. Miller, MD
Department of Emergency Medicine,
Brody School of Medicine,
East Carolina University,
Greenville, NC, USA

References

[1] Holler JG, Henriksen DP, Mikkelsen S, et al. Shock in the emergency department; a 12 year population based cohort study. Scandinavian Journal of Trauma, Resuscitation and Emergency Medicine. 2016;**24**:87

[2] Wacker DA, Winters ME. Shock. Emergency Medicine Clinics of North America. 2014;**32**:747-758

[3] Jones AE, Tayal VS, Sullivan DM, et al. Randomized, controlled trial of immediate versus delayed goal-directed ultrasound to identify the cause of nontraumatic hypotension in emergency department patients. Critical Care Medicine. 2004;**32**:1703-1708

[4] Moore CL. Determination of left ventricular function by emergency physician echocardiography of hypotensive patients. Academic Emergency Medicine. 2002;**9**:186-193

[5] Heckbert SR, Vedder NB, Hoffman W, et al. Outcome after hemorrhagic shock in trauma patients. The Journal of Trauma. 1998;**45**:545-549

[6] Peres Bota D, Melot C, Lopes Ferreira F, et al. The Multiple Organ Dysfunction Score (MODS) versus the Sequential Organ Failure Assessment (SOFA) score in outcome prediction. Intensive Care Medicine. 2002;**28**:1619-1624

[7] Rady MY, Smithline HA, Blake H, et al. A comparison of the shock index and conventional vital signs to identify acute, critical illness in the emergency department. Annals of Emergency Medicine. 1994;**24**:685-690

Preface

From the healthcare provider perspective, the word "shock" is associated with a mixed array of feelings, including dread, well-founded fear, and deep respect. The physiological state of shock is well recognized for the associated destructive consequences, and its successful management requires prompt identification, immediate action, and sustained effort by all members of the healthcare team [1–4]. Taking after the notion of "sudden violent blow or impact [5]," the physiological state of shock is conceptually similar to the human "fear response" in face of the unexpected of unknown. Putting it all together with the relevant clinical construct of shock, as eloquently stated by Mary Renault, "There is only one kind of shock worse than the totally unexpected: the expected for which one has refused to prepare [6]." This mindset of advanced preparation and constant readiness constitutes the foundation of the modern approach toward shock – early detection and prompt treatment for optimal outcomes.

Despite the heterogeneity of "shock" as a clinico-pathological entity, there are some common threads that permeate all forms and manifestations of shock, with apparent increase in observed commonalities in the more advanced (and often irreversible) stages of the systemic syndrome. Whether hemorrhagic, septic, or anaphylactic, the state of shock is felt similarly at the tissue level – there is an acute decrease in vital supplies to tissues, resulting in system-wide cellular distress. The body and its systems do their best to compensate for the maldistribution of oxygen and nutrients, up to a certain point [7–9]. This is commonly recognized as so-called compensated shock. Beyond that, the body loses its ability to adjust any further, thus descending into a state of "uncompensated shock," with a refractory state characterized by vasoplegia and irreversible cardiovascular failure [10, 11].

As the reader journeys through the chapters of the book, he or she will read about various biomarkers and endpoints of resuscitation, explore different types of shock (e.g., septic, hemorrhagic, anaphylactic), and learn about some of the less often discussed topics such as neurogenic and spinal shock as well as amniotic fluid embolism. Although not specifically discussed as a focus of a dedicated chapter, cardiogenic shock and cardiac dysfunction will be discussed throughout this collective work, especially as it relates to the various stages and manifestations of different shock states. Our other goals were to keep things clinically relevant and practically oriented, thus enabling the reader to apply the newly acquired knowledge in their everyday clinical routines.

This book is a collection of unique chapters, each dedicated to a different area within the expansive and heterogeneous subject of shock. As the reader progresses through the book, we hope to help stimulate further discourse and innovative thinking about the topic. We also hope to shed light on various other dimensions of a clinical problem that all too often becomes reduced to protocolized management approaches without much reflection on its true mechanistic and energetic implications and impact. While the authors hope that this textbook will enlighten healthcare providers as to diagnosis and treatment of shock, it must be acknowledged that the currently available guidelines regarding the treatment of this malady do not provide guidance on post-hospital care or recovery [12–14]. In the latter context, an entire unexplored area of long-term complications of critical care awaits much needed research [15, 16]. It is also critical that basic, translational and clinical research on shock is sufficiently balanced between different types of shock to improve our understanding of all pertinent pathophysiologic states, whether due to infection, amniotic fluid emboli, myocardial infarction, or neurological injury. In this way, scientific progress will help improve outcomes for patients with both rare and common forms of shock.

Stanislaw P. Stawicki, MD, MBA, FACS, FAIM
Department of Research and Innovation,
St. Luke's University Health Network,
Bethlehem, Pennsylvania, USA

Mamta Swaroop, MD, FACS
Department of Surgery,
Institute for Global Health,
Center for Global Surgery,
Northwestern University School of Medicine,
Chicago, Illinois, USA

References

[1] Cocchi MN et al. Identification and resuscitation of the trauma patient in shock. Emergency Medicine Clinics of North America. 2007;**25**(3):623-642

[2] Hasdai D et al. Cardiogenic shock complicating acute coronary syndromes. The Lancet. 2000;**356**(9231):749-756

[3] Costa AJ. Anaphylactic shock: Guidelines for immediate diagnosis and treatment. Postgraduate Medicine. 1988;**83**(4):368-373

[4] Summers RL et al. Characterization of the spectrum of hemodynamic profiles in trauma patients with acute neurogenic shock. Journal of Critical Care. 2013;**28**(4):531.e1-531.e5

[5] Oxford_Lexico_Dictionary. Main definitions of 'shock' in English. 2020. Available from: https://www.lexico.com/en/definition/shock [Accessed: 25 March 2020]

[6] Good_Reads. Shock Quotes. 2020. Available from: https://www.goodreads.com/quotes/tag/shock [Accessed: 25 March 2020]

[7] Balk RA. Pathogenesis and management of multiple organ dysfunction or failure in severe sepsis and septic shock. Critical Care Clinics. 2000;**16**(2):337-352

[8] Amundson B, Jennische E, Haljamäe H. Correlative analysis of microcirculatory and cellular metabolic events in skeletal muscle during hemorrhagic shock. Acta Physiologica Scandinavica. 1980;**108**(2):147-158

[9] Menger M, Vollmar B, Messmer K. Sepsis and nutritional blood flow. In: Sepsis. Springer; 1994. pp. 163-173

[10] Gamcrlidze M et al. Vasoplegia in septic shock. Georgian Medical News. 2015;**239**:56-62

[11] Stawicki SP et al. Methylene blue and vasoplegia: Who, when, and how? Mini Reviews in Medicinal Chemistry. 2008;**8**(5):472-490

[12] Chen AX, Simpson SQ, Pallin DJ. Sepsis guidelines. New England Journal of Medicine. 2019;**380**(14):1369-1371

[13] Herran-Monge R et al. Epidemiology and changes in mortality of sepsis after the implementation of Surviving Sepsis Campaign guidelines. Journal of Intensive Care Medicine. 2019;**34**(9):740-750

[14] Butler FK et al. Fluid resuscitation for hemorrhagic shock in tactical combat casualty care: TCCC guidelines change . Fort Sam, Houston, TX: Army Institute of Surgical Research; 2014 [14-01-2 June 2014]

[15] Desai SV, Law TJ, Needham DM. Long-term complications of critical care. Critical Care Medicine. 2011;**39**(2):371-379

[16] Quartin AA et al. Magnitude and duration of the effect of sepsis on survival. Jama. 1997;**277**(13):1058-1063

Chapter 1

Introductory Chapter: Shock is a Physiological State of War

Stanislaw P. Stawicki, Thomas J. Papadimos and Mamta Swaroop

1. Introduction

Among specialists in critical care medicine, emergency medicine, infectious diseases, and trauma surgery, shock elicits a sense of impending immediacy and sets off a cascade of clinical interventions designed to support systemic circulation. This includes urgent focus on ensuring end-organ perfusion, definitive treatment of the underlying cause (from anaphylaxis to sepsis), and providing subsequent physiological restoration. Despite the apparent heterogeneity of "shock" as a clinico-pathological entity, there are some common threads that permeate all forms and manifestations of shock, with apparent increase in observed commonalities in the more advanced (and often irreversible) stages of the systemic syndrome [1–7].

Let us take a closer look at septic shock as an excellent example of the above concepts. More than 19 million people annually develop sepsis, which is defined as a "life-threatening acute organ dysfunction secondary to infection [8]." Approximately 14 million survive to hospital discharge, 50% recover, 33% die in the following year, and about 15% experience continuing problems and ailments [8]. Patients who survive hospitalization develop, on average, one to two new functional problems (such as challenges with simple tasks like dressing or other daily functions one may otherwise take for granted); a significant increase in cognitive difficulties; as well as various behavioral sequelae such as anxiety, depression, and post-traumatic stress disorder (PTSD) [8]. Survival of sepsis, septic shock, and other forms of shock (e.g., hemorrhagic, anaphylactic, cardiogenic, neurogenic) has improved in recent years [9–13]. Yet our understanding of the war-like ravages the state of shock creates remains limited, especially in the context of the cumulative impact of the initial physiologic insult, its duration and severity and the subsequent recovery. This book aims to highlight commonly encountered forms of shock by focusing on contemporary diagnostic and treatment approaches. For the purposes of this introductory chapter, the authors will focus on one of the best understood models of shock—the septic shock. References to other types of shock will also be made when appropriate.

2. Gearing for wartime

In the acute setting, it is easy to become mesmerized by the superficial manifestations of the physiological devastation inflicted by shock as it affects the human body—elevated (or depressed) temperature, low blood pressure, diaphoresis,

IntechOpen

tachycardia, etc. [14–16]. For most providers, these signs, combined with laboratory markers, such as leukocytosis, specifically bandemia [17–19], an elevated C-reactive protein [19, 20], or perhaps alterations in procalcitonin [20], send out an alert, prompting aggressive and largely protocolized clinical management. Yet, an in-depth understanding of what is mechanistically occurring throughout the body, as well as the magnitude and scale of the events that are taking place, tends to be lacking.

When examining the hematologic system during sepsis and septic shock, the body undergoes a shift, readily comparable to a transition to a *war economy* [21]. In effect, the contingencies in time of war require that a "system of producing, mobilizing and allocating resources to defend and sustain" is put in place to ensure the means necessary for survival [22]. This rapid, often "violent" change is bidirectional; the host's invader attacks the patient physiologically, and the host, in return, mounts a vigorous defense. The sudden physiological retooling, including massive changes in resource allocation are difficult to grasp. Consider the effect of sepsis and the associated doubling of the white blood cell (WBC) count. More specifically, it has been estimated that approximately 4.4% of the entire body mass of a healthy, 70 kg man is allocated to blood cells [23]. This translates to approximately 3.1 kg! Assuming about 2.2 kg of the totality of all blood cells are erythrocytes or red blood cells (RBCs), it is reasonable to also assume the approximate normal WBC mass would be in the range of 0.9–1.0 kg [24]. It has also been estimated that the human body produces, on average, approximately 100 Watts (Joules/sec) of energy [25, 26]. Consequently, the hypothetical doubling of the WBC count within a 24–48-hour period during sepsis is thus representative of a net gain of approximately 0.9–1.0 kg of new WBCs—an amazing feat of energy and power, in that it takes anywhere between 5 and 50 Joules/sec to form these new cells [27–29] and about 0.9–1.0 Joules/sec/kg to effectively power this freshly conceived army of defenders [26].

Similar to the preparation for and the conduct of war, the body experiences an acute and massive elevation in its baseline metabolic needs as it is actively fighting for its survival. Vast energetic surge is allocated to sustaining various forms of synthetic activity and enabling multiple, synergistic defense mechanisms, including immune cell metabolism, the production and release of innumerable cytokines, hormones, and the on-demand creation of other complex molecules and processes [30–36]. While we discuss these microbiological, immunological, and energetic "frontlines," we must not forget the active resistance that our pathologic foes are putting up. The medical community must apply proper stewardship of its antibiotic assets, only using our limited resources (e.g., "therapeutic bullets") when needed and only rarely resorting to the "nuclear option" of widest available spectrum of agents in our antibiotic armamentarium [37]. In fact, the emergence of antibiotic resistance is a worldwide concern, and it is highly reflective and typical of warfare-like conflict and combat. Effects of this phenomenon are far-reaching, including patients, physicians, pharmacists, administrative actions, and broadly understood public health infrastructure. Antibiotic resistance adds $1383 to the cost of caring for a patient with a bacterial infection. Using the estimates of Thorpe et al. [37], the number of such resistant infections in 2014 alone amounted to a national cost of $2.2 billion annually [37].

It is important to note that other forms of shock, such as hemorrhagic shock, also trigger a variety of similarly extensive metabolic responses [38]. Although the inciting mechanism may be different, there are certain "end pathway" similarities and parallelisms. For example, the post-hemorrhage state can be characterized as having the following stages: "ischemia-reperfusion," "leukocytic," and "angiogenic" [39]. Likewise, new erythrocytes must be produced in large quantities to replace those lost during the hemorrhagic injury. Not unexpectedly, energy depletion is one of the key determinants of tissue (and systemic) recovery following shock [38].

From more philosophical (and also structural) perspective, when the human body is exposed to near-lethal state of shock, a large number of individual cells will die, regardless of whether the organism survives or not. Perhaps one might call this "compensated" versus "uncompensated" shock, depending on the extent of damage that is difficult to "see or quantify." Thus, the question arises—at any particular organ system or tissue level—"how many cells can die before the organ (or the entire organism) can no longer function, cope, and/or survive?"

3. Finding new equilibrium

As the body gains the upper hand over the tectonic shifts brought upon it by this state of shock, a temporary new equilibrium is achieved, whereby the state of heightened physiologic alert continues, but some signs of normalization and stabilization return. The so-called systemic inflammatory response syndrome (SIRS) starts to resolve [40]. For example, the WBC count begins to trend back toward normal (or baseline) range, constant fevers are interrupted by increasingly frequent afebrile periods, and the patient's intravenous fluid and vasopressor requirement begins to decrease [40, 41]. In more sophisticated terms, objectified measurement of this re-equilibration and normalization process can be seen by down-trending of various physiologic acuity indices, such as the sepsis-related organ failure assessment (SOFA) score [42]; different iterations of the acute physiology and chronic health evaluation (APACHE) score [43, 44]; as well as the simplified acute physiology (SAPS) score [45].

Although this particular state does not yet represent a "truce," because such an ebb and flow of physiological parameters is not conducive to the well-being of the host, it is a general signal that "hostilities" are subsiding. From the perspective of medical care, there has to be an end to hostilities, with the pendulum shifting in favor of the host. Sometimes it is an outright win, but most times the successes of care are negotiated with the "invaders" over time. Importantly, the quicker the end of hostilities, the better it is for the patient. Nonetheless, as the new equilibrium is reached, there is a price to pay for fighting off an invader. Usually, it is the use and liquidation of valuable assets (e.g., muscle wasting, cellular death). In financial terms, there is a large "physiologic" loan with a lot of interest to be paid on the way to recovery. Achieving equilibrium requires a strategy that incorporates effective interventions, in addition to quality care in early shock, such as the management of delirium, pain, and agitation, as well as early mobilization to attenuate atrophy of the patient's musculature and nervous system [8, 46]. The next step in the patient's recovery, as outlined in the subsequent section, is the re-tooling of the "war economy" back into "peacetime economy" of everyday functioning.

4. Return to peace

As discussed and logically outlined in previous sections of this chapter, the all-out effort of the human body to initially react, then more formally respond to the shock state, eventually leads to a binary outcome. For the most acutely ill patients, it is mortality versus survival. Once the probability of mortality decreases and the likelihood of survival rises sufficiently, the human physiological machine must at some point transition out of *war economy* mode and return to the baseline *peace economy* [47]. In economic terms, this translates into a gradual metamorphosis from war-related activities, or catabolism, into peace-related ones, or anabolism, whereby factories producing armored vehicles, machine guns, bombs and missiles in wartime, now re-tool to make civilian vehicles, refrigerators, or perhaps personal computers [47, 48]. Essentially, this is a fairly well-structured "recovery plan." It is very much akin to the Marshall Plan (a 1948 American initiative to aid post-World War II Europe) [49]. Wherein, not only physiological and psychological assistance and recovery are necessary, but also an expenditure of resources to help one overcome any morbidities in order to restore function and enable the patient to become a contributing member of the society. This process occurs both on the short-term and long-term scales. Acute physiological problems are solved early, the solutions providing for life, i.e., survival. Nonetheless, there are long-term problems also, such as PTSD, and the "aftershocks" of functional and cognitive decline which create high costs to the patient and society [50, 51]. The recovery costs are not only biological and psychological, but also financial. For example, hospital-associated cost of sepsis increased from $58,000 USD per patient in 2015 to $70,000 USD per patient in 2018 with patients who developed sepsis being 10% more likely to have septic shock on hospital admission. This represents an estimated increase of $1.5 billion USD over a 3-year period [52].

The processes and difficulties involved in the physiological transition from *war economy* to *peace economy* are exceedingly complex and poorly understood. The ravages of the war, no matter the final victory, leave the patient with long-term disability, cognitive decline, pressure-related wounds, end-organ damage and dysfunction, and signs of accelerated physiological aging [53–63]. A patient suffering from chronic post-sepsis state should receive ample support, including close medical follow-up, physical therapy, occupational therapy, and speech therapy. Previously compared to the "Marshall Plan," such post-sepsis intensive recovery should focus on restoring the patient to optimal functioning, including activities of daily living (ADL); good exercise capacity; rebuilding of muscle strength (skeletal, respiratory and otherwise); and other key areas of independent living [64, 65]. In a more philosophical way, the "price of survival" (and recovery to the point of fully resuming ADLs) is measured through some form of a complex mathematical relationship where chronological age becomes modified (e.g., advanced) according to the totality of physiological stress, the total amount of energy expended, as well as the rate of that energetic expenditure while fighting to survive the shock state. Similar observations can be made about post-traumatic and other forms of shock discussed in this book, as evidenced by the increasing amount of literature documenting post-critical care disability and complications [66–70]. Finally, there seems to be a relationship between the "time to treatment" and patient outcomes across all types of shock, including short-, mid-, and long-term considerations.

In essentially all forms of shock (septic, cardiogenic, hypovolemic, anaphylactic, and neurogenic), there are highly impactful transformations of energy, or bioenergetics. Such alterations in the production and utilization occur through cellular and metabolic processes and result in mitochondrial dysfunction and oxidative stress that influence patient outcomes [71]. In shock states, despite hemodynamic recovery and recovery of oxygen-related variables, there seems to be a persistent oxygen extraction deficit. Dysfunction of oxygen transport pathways during the critical illness of the patient underlies the events resulting in organ failure. We have a limited technical ability to measure tissue oxygenation bioenergetics. Consequently, it is imperative that we develop effective, easily applied, novel techniques that allow a quantitative approach into the determinants of microcirculatory and mitochondrial oxygenation [72, 73].

5. Conclusions

This book is a collection of unique chapters, each dedicated to a different area within the expansive and heterogeneous subject of shock. As the reader progresses through the book, we hope to help stimulate further discourse and innovative thinking about the topic and to shed light on a clinical problem that all too often becomes reduced to protocolized management approaches without much reflection into its true mechanistic and energetic implications and impact. While the authors hope that this textbook will enlighten practitioners as to diagnosis and treatment of shock, it must be acknowledged that the current sepsis guidelines regarding the treatment of this malady do not provide sufficient guidance on post-hospital care or recovery. It is also critical that basic, translational, and clinical research on shock is well balanced between different types of shock to improve our understanding of all pertinent pathophysiologic states. In this way, scientific progress will help improve outcomes for patients with both rare and common forms of shock.

Author details

Stanislaw P. Stawicki[1]*, Thomas J. Papadimos[2] and Mamta Swaroop[3]

1 Department of Research and Innovation, St. Luke's University Health Network, Bethlehem, Pennsylvania, USA

2 Department of Anesthesiology, The Ohio State University College of Medicine, Columbus, Ohio, USA

3 Department of Surgery, Northwestern University School of Medicine, Chicago, Illinois, USA

*Address all correspondence to: stawicki.ace@gmail.com

References

[1] Conway EE, Singer LP. Hemorrhagic shock and encephalopathy: An entity similar to heatstroke. American Journal of Diseases of Children. 1991;**145**(7):719-719

[2] Parrillo JE et al. Septic shock in humans: Advances in the understanding of pathogenesis, cardiovascular dysfunction, and therapy. Annals of Internal Medicine. 1990;**113**(3):227-242

[3] Natanson C et al. Role of endotoxemia in cardiovascular dysfunction and mortality. *Escherichia coli* and *Staphylococcus aureus* challenges in a canine model of human septic shock. The Journal of Clinical Investigation. 1989;**83**(1):243-251

[4] Kissoon N et al. Sepsis—The final common pathway to death from multiple organ failure in infection. Critical Care Medicine. 2016;**44**(6):e446

[5] Robin JK, Oliver JA, Landry DW. Vasopressin deficiency in the syndrome of irreversible shock. Journal of Trauma and Acute Care Surgery. 2003;**54**(5):S149-S154

[6] Morgenthaler NG et al. Copeptin, a stable peptide of the arginine vasopressin precursor, is elevated in hemorrhagic and septic shock. Shock. 2007;**28**(2):219-226

[7] Blair E et al. Clinical physiology of late (refractory) gram-negative bacteremic shock. The American Journal of Surgery. 1969;**117**(4):573-586

[8] Prescott HC, Angus DC. Enhancing recovery from sepsis: A review. JAMA. 2018;**319**(1):62-75

[9] Kumar A, Tremblay V. Sepsis and septic shock. In: Adult Critical Care Medicine. Cham, Switzerland: Springer; 2019. pp. 147-165

[10] Arias J, Levy B, De Backer D. Fifty years of management of vasodilatory shock. International Anesthesiology Clinics. 2019;**57**(2):31-47

[11] Levy B et al. Vasoplegia treatments: The past, the present, and the future. Critical Care. 2018;**22**(1):52

[12] Puymirat E et al. Cardiogenic shock in intensive care units: Evolution of prevalence, patient profile, management and outcomes, 1997-2012. European Journal of Heart Failure. 2017;**19**(2):192-200

[13] Commins SP. Outpatient emergencies: Anaphylaxis. Medical Clinics. 2017;**101**(3):521-536

[14] Dellinger RP et al. Surviving sepsis campaign: International guidelines for management of severe sepsis and septic shock: 2008. Intensive Care Medicine. 2008;**34**(1):17-60

[15] Sung E, George J, Porter M. Sepsis in pregnancy. Fetal and Maternal Medicine Review. 2011;**22**(4):287-305

[16] O'Grady NP et al. Guidelines for evaluation of new fever in critically ill adult patients: 2008 update from the American College of Critical Care Medicine and the Infectious Diseases Society of America. Critical Care Medicine. 2008;**36**(4):1330-1349

[17] Aird WC. The hematologic system as a marker of organ dysfunction in sepsis. In: Mayo Clinic Proceedings; Elsevier; 2003

[18] Ward MJ et al. The degree of bandemia in septic ED patients does not predict inpatient mortality. The American Journal of Emergency Medicine. 2012;**30**(1):181-183

[19] Da OS, Ohlsson A, Kenyon C. Accuracy of leukocyte indices and C-reactive protein for diagnosis of neonatal sepsis: A critical review. The

Pediatric Infectious Disease Journal. 1995;**14**(5):362-366

[20] Castelli GP et al. Procalcitonin and C-reactive protein during systemic inflammatory response syndrome, sepsis and organ dysfunction. Critical Care. 2004;**8**(4):R234

[21] Hancock WK, Gowing MM. British War Economy. London: His Majesty's Stationery Office; 1949

[22] Le Billon P. Wars of Plunder: Conflicts, Profits and the Politics of Resources. New York, NY: Columbia University Press; 2012

[23] Bianconi E et al. An estimation of the number of cells in the human body. Annals of Human Biology. 2013;**40**(6):463-471

[24] Quora. What is The Mass of Red Blood Cells in Humans? [Internet]. 2017. Available from: https://www.quora.com/What-is-the-mass-of-red-blood-cells-in-humans [Accessed: 05 January 2018

[25] Anthony S. Will Your Body Be the Battery of the Future? [Internet]. 2012. Available from: https://www.extremetech.com/extreme/135481-will-your-body-be-the-battery-of-the-future [Accessed: 05 January 2018]

[26] BioNumbers. Cell Biology by The Numbers: What is the Power Consumption of a Cell? [Internet]. Available from: http://book.bionumbers.org/what-is-the-power-consumption-of-a-cell/ [Accessed: 05 January 2018]

[27] Flamholz A, Phillips R, Milo R. The quantified cell. Molecular Biology of the Cell. 2014;**25**(22):3497-3500

[28] Barth U. How Many Cells Are in Your Body? Probably More Than You Think! [Internet]. 2017. Available from: https://handling-solutions.eppendorf.com/cell-handling/about-cells-and-culture/detailview/news/how-many-cells-are-in-your-body-probably-more-than-you-think/ [Accessed: 05 January 2018]

[29] Iqbal A. The Physics Factbook: Energy in ATP [Internet]. 2000. Available from: https://hypertextbook.com/facts/2000/AmberIqbal.shtml [Accessed: 05 January 2018]

[30] Selye H et al. On the therapeutic value of adrenal cortical hormones in traumatic shock and allied conditions. Canadian Medical Association Journal. 1940;**43**(1):1

[31] Witthaut R et al. Plasma atrial natriuretic peptide and brain natriuretic peptide are increased in septic shock: Impact of interleukin-6 and sepsis-associated left ventricular dysfunction. Intensive Care Medicine. 2003;**29**(10):1696-1702

[32] Waage A et al. The complex pattern of cytokines in serum from patients with meningococcal septic shock. Association between interleukin 6, interleukin 1, and fatal outcome. Journal of Experimental Medicine. 1989;**169**(1):333-338

[33] Dinarello CA. Proinflammatory and anti-inflammatory cytokines as mediators in the pathogenesis of septic shock. Chest. 1997;**112**(6):321S

[34] Fourrier F et al. Septic shock, multiple organ failure, and disseminated intravascular coagulation: Compared patterns of antithrombin III, protein C, and protein S deficiencies. Chest. 1992;**101**(3):816-823

[35] Filkins J. Monokines and the metabolic pathophysiology of septic shock. In: Federation proceedings; 1985

[36] Park DW, Zmijewski JW. Mitochondrial dysfunction and immune cell metabolism in sepsis. Infection & Chemotherapy. 2017;**49**(1):10-21

[37] Thorpe KE, Joski P, Johnston KJ. Antibiotic-resistant infection treatment costs have doubled since 2002, now exceeding $2 billion annually. Health Affairs. 2018;**37**(4):662-669

[38] D'Alessandro A et al. Early hemorrhage triggers metabolic responses that build up during prolonged shock. American Journal of Physiology. Regulatory, Integrative and Comparative Physiology. 2015;**308**(12):R1034-R1044

[39] Aller M-A et al. A review of metabolic staging in severely injured patients. Scandinavian Journal of Trauma, Resuscitation and Emergency Medicine. 2010;**18**(1):27

[40] Rangel-Frausto MS et al. The natural history of the systemic inflammatory response syndrome (SIRS): A prospective study. JAMA. 1995;**273**(2):117-123

[41] Frausto MSR et al. The dynamics of disease progression in sepsis: Markov modeling describing the natural history and the likely impact of effective antisepsis agents. Clinical Infectious Diseases. 1998;**27**(1):185-190

[42] Vincent J-L et al. The SOFA (sepsis-related organ failure assessment) score to describe organ dysfunction/failure. Intensive Care Medicine. 1996;**22**(7):707-710

[43] Knaus WA et al. The APACHE III prognostic system: Risk prediction of hospital mortality for critically III hospitalized adults. Chest. 1991;**100**(6):1619-1636

[44] Chatzicostas C et al. Comparison of Ranson, APACHE II and APACHE III scoring systems in acute pancreatitis. Pancreas. 2002;**25**(4):331-335

[45] Le Gall J-R, Lemeshow S, Saulnier F. A new simplified acute physiology score (SAPS II) based on a European/North American multicenter study. JAMA. 1993;**270**(24):2957-2963

[46] Rachoin J-S, Dellinger RP. Recommendations for sepsis management. In: Critical Care Nephrology. Philadelphia, Pennsylvania: Elsevier; 2019. pp. 534-539

[47] Goodhand J. From war economy to peace economy? Reconstruction and state building in Afghanistan. Journal of International Affairs. 2004;**58**(1):155-174

[48] Del Castillo G. Rebuilding war-torn states: The challenge of post-conflict economic reconstruction. OUP Oxford; 2008

[49] De Long JB, Eichengreen B. The Marshall plan: History's most successful structural adjustment program. National Bureau of Economic Research. 1991; NBER Working Paper No. 3899

[50] Heyland DK et al. Long-term health-related quality of life in survivors of sepsis. Short form 36: A valid and reliable measure of health-related quality of life. Critical Care Medicine. 2000;**28**(11):3599-3605

[51] Paladino L et al. Reflections on the ebola public health emergency of international concern, part 2: The unseen epidemic of posttraumatic stress among health-care personnel and survivors of the 2014-2016 Ebola outbreak. Journal of Global Infectious Diseases. 2017;**9**(2):45

[52] Castellucci M. Sepsis Treatment Costs Shoot Up $1.5 Billion for Hospitals Over Three Years [Internet]. 2019. Available from: https://www.modernhealthcare.com/safety-quality/sepsis-treatment-costs-shoot-up-15-billion-hospitals-over-three-years [Accessed: 11 June 2019]

[53] Sharshar T et al. Brain lesions in septic shock: A magnetic resonance imaging study. Intensive Care Medicine. 2007;**33**(5):798-806

[54] Dalton R et al. Polyneuropathy and myopathy in the elderly. HSR Proceedings in Intensive Care & Cardiovascular Anesthesia. 2012;**4**(1):15

[55] Reilly EF et al. Pressure ulcers in the intensive care unit: The "forgotten" enemy. Opus. 2007;**12**:17-30

[56] Needham DM, Feldman DR, Kho ME. The functional costs of ICU survivorship: Collaborating to improve post-ICU disability. American Thoracic Society. American Journal of Respiratory and Critical Care Medicine. 2011;**183**(8):962

[57] Vest MT et al. Disability in activities of daily living, depression, and quality of life among older medical ICU survivors: A prospective cohort study. Health and Quality of Life Outcomes. 2011;**9**(1):9

[58] Liu C et al. Acute kidney injury and inflammatory response of sepsis following cecal ligation and puncture in d-galactose-induced aging rats. Clinical Interventions in Aging. 2017;**12**:593

[59] Spurney RF, Fulkerson WJ, Schwab SJ. Acute renal failure in critically ill patients: Prognosis for recovery of kidney function after prolonged dialysis support. Critical Care Medicine. 1991;**19**(1):8-11

[60] Milbrandt EB et al. Toward an integrated research agenda for critical illness in aging. American Journal of Respiratory and Critical Care Medicine. 2010;**182**(8):995-1003

[61] Hotchkiss RS et al. Sepsis and septic shock. Nature Reviews. Disease Primers. 2016;**2**:16045

[62] Annane D, Sharshar T. Cognitive decline after sepsis. The Lancet Respiratory Medicine. 2015;**3**(1):61-69

[63] Cohen MS et al. Patient frailty: Key considerations, definitions, and practical implications. Challenges in Elder Care. London, United Kingdom: IntechOpen; 2016. pp. 9-36

[64] Major M et al. Surviving critical illness: What is next? An expert consensus statement on physical rehabilitation after hospital discharge. Critical Care. 2016;**20**(1):354

[65] Iwashyna TJ et al. Population burden of long-term survivorship after severe sepsis in older Americans. Journal of the American Geriatrics Society. 2012;**60**(6):1070-1077

[66] Desai SV, Law TJ, Needham DM. Long-term complications of critical care. Critical Care Medicine. 2011;**39**(2):371-379

[67] Winters BD et al. Long-term mortality and quality of life in sepsis: A systematic review. Critical Care Medicine. 2010;**38**(5):1276-1283

[68] Hochman JS et al. Early revascularization and long-term survival in cardiogenic shock complicating acute myocardial infarction. JAMA. 2006;**295**(21):2511-2515

[69] Williams T et al. Data linkage enables evaluation of long-term survival after intensive care. Anaesthesia and Intensive Care. 2006;**34**(3):307-315

[70] Cannon JW. Hemorrhagic shock. New England Journal of Medicine. 2018;**378**(4):370-379

[71] Bozza FA et al. Bioenergetics, mitochondrial dysfunction, and oxidative stress in the pathophysiology of septic encephalopathy. Shock. 2013;**39**:10-16

[72] Ince C, Mik EG. Microcirculatory and mitochondrial hypoxia in sepsis, shock, and resuscitation. Journal of Applied Physiology. 2015;**120**(2):226-235

[73] Dolin HH et al. A novel combination of biomarkers to herald the onset of sepsis prior to the manifestation of symptoms. Shock (Augusta, Ga.). 2018;**49**(4):364

Chapter 2

New Biomarkers of Sepsis with Clinical Relevance

Débora Maria da Gomes Cunha, Guilherme Galdino da Silva and Mike Yoshio Hamasaki

Abstract

A 2016 task force convened by multiple societies proposed a new definition of sepsis, termed Sepsis 3. The new clinical diagnosis of sepsis is based on variation points in the Sequential (Sepsis-related) Organ Assessment Score (SOFA) and excluded Systemic Inflammatory Response Syndrome (SIRS) as a criterion for defining the diagnosis. Although the new definitions have provided improvements in understanding the disease, the main concern generated by Sepsis 3 is the reduced sensitivity to detect cases that might have an unfavorable course, mainly in early conditions. By limiting the diagnosis to organic dysfunction, the new concept tends to select a more severely ill population. In this way, biomarkers to diagnose sepsis may allow early intervention, which can reduce the risk of death. Although lactate is currently the most commonly used biomarker to identify sepsis, other biomarkers may help to enhance lactate's effectiveness and may be used as a tool for staging the disease, prognosis, and response to intervention. The objective of this chapter is to present possible new biomarkers that are clinically relevant.

Keywords: biomarkers, cytokines, haptoglobin, lactate, sRAGE, sepsis

1. Introduction

The first definition of sepsis was described in a consensus conference in 1991. Known as Sepsis 1, it advocated the hypothesis that infection was directly proportional to the systemic inflammatory response syndrome (SIRS). Ten years later, in a new conference (Sepsis 2), the SIRS diagnostic method was already questioned by the scientific community about its low specificity. However, in the current situation, Sepsis 2 did not offer many alternatives because of the lack of evidence to substantiate the above arguments [1, 2].

Although SIRS criteria have been described for more than three decades as a host's clinical expression to systemic infection and have contributed greatly to the understanding of sepsis in various pathophysiological areas, the need for a new conference in 2016 was recognized, where the sepsis' concepts were reviewed again [2, 3].

Sepsis 3 was proposed by the Society of Critical Care Medicine (SCCM) together with the European Society of Intensive Care Medicine (ESICM), which established that the disease is linked to life-threatening organic dysfunction that is secondary to the body's unregulated responses to the infection. This new definition extinguished the term of severe sepsis and completely abandoned the use of SIRS in the diagnosis of sepsis [4].

In order to promote a new and more sensitive diagnostic method than the previous one, the score of sequential organ failure assessment (SOFA) was instituted. Due to the complexity of the SOFA's rapid completion and the concern of the impossibility of a fast and early disease identification, "quick SOFA" (qSOFA) was also established in Sepsis 3 [3].

Despite the improvements obtained through Sepsis 3, in the same year of the new guidelines, Williams et al. [4] demonstrated in 2016 that the new diagnostic model is not very sensitive in the early stages of disease. These observations are of great clinical relevance because the treatment of sepsis is more effective in early stages.

One of the alternatives used for the early diagnosis of patients in several diseases is the Point-of-Care Testing (POCT), a laboratory test carried out in the places where the intensive treatment is done. POCT has become popular among physicians because its agility in the patients' diagnosis has been shown to be effective, including requiring fewer samples collected from the patient [5].

Unlike traditional laboratory tests, POCT does not require a permanent dedicated space, since it has kits and instruments that can be transported to where the patient is, thus immediately allowing the dosage of several substances, not only in hospital or professional environments, and can be operated by patients in their home [6].

Currently, POCT is used to test a range of pathological conditions, including diabetes, hypertension, hyperlipidemia, and asthma, as well as monitoring of bone density, body composition, and anticoagulation, and these tests are expanding rapidly (from 12 to 15% annually) [6].

Despite the great validity of the POCT test, this method presents operational and environmental instability and is difficult to standardize in intensive care settings [7, 8]. In addition, the clinical status of patients with sepsis is very unstable and the disease severity usually changes abruptly [1]. Thus, it is necessary to recognize new specific and sensitive biological markers for the sepsis diagnosis.

Biomarkers were defined by the National Institute of Health as a characteristic that should be measured and served as an indicator of a normal, pathological state or a response to a pharmacological agent. They shall be characterized by accuracy and reproducibility and may be used as important tools for diagnosis, as well as promoting early diagnosis, indicating the stage of the disease, prognosis, and mechanisms of intervention.

More than 100 biomarkers have already been described and proposed for sepsis; combinations between them have also been demonstrated. However, due to the different stages of severity observed in sepsis in the most diverse populations, it has been complicated to define which marker can be used as a parameter to improve therapeutic strategies. Therefore, for sepsis, a good biomarker has to be able to identify early alterations in order to prevent multiple organ dysfunction and consequently reduce the mortality of patients with this pathology.

New biomarkers could promote better monitoring of the patient's condition and, possibly, a more accurate definition of the disease prognosis. This chapter aims to describe the biological markers already established for sepsis, as well as to cite those that in our opinion show promising results.

2. Established biological markers

2.1 Lactate

Lactate (or lactic acid) is the anaerobic glycolysis end product, and its blood levels increase significantly in the hypoperfusion or hypoxia cases. Due to an imbalance between lactate production and lactate clearance in patients with sepsis, hyperlactatemia is a common condition in these patients [9, 10].

The first study that connected the production of lactate with sepsis was performed by Bakker et al. [11] in 1991. In this study, they demonstrated that the tissues of patients with sepsis or septic shock did not adequately use the O_2 molecule and that survivors of the disease had lower blood lactate levels than those who died from the disease.

Five years after this finding, Bernardin et al. [12] demonstrated that the changes in the blood lactate level occur within the first 24 hours of treatment, and in addition to blood pressure fluctuation, may be strong indicators of short-term survival prognosis in patients diagnosed with septic shock.

In a paper published in 2013, a Brazilian clinical care research group has demonstrated that hyperlactatemia can be caused by mitochondrial dysfunction and the use of adrenergic drugs in the condition of septic shock [13]. Léguillier et al. [14] demonstrated in 2018 that the lactate dosage, associated with POCT, bring a possible new strategy for the early treatment of patients with suspicion of sepsis [14].

As predicted in Sepsis 3, the most common use of lactate dosage is in the differentiation between sepsis and septic shock in intensive care units (ICUs), and this information is very important and useful for medical professionals.

However, Guo et al. [15] demonstrated in their study that an isolated and simple dosage of arterial lactate is not satisfactory in recognizing the sepsis prognosis. Therefore, they suggest that such dosages need to be supported by results from other biological markers, such as C-reactive protein (CRP), B-type natriuretic peptide (BNP), and N-terminal proBNP (NT-proBNP).

2.2 C-reactive protein

C-reactive protein (CRP) is an acute inflammatory phase protein produced in the liver, currently believed to be a reliable indicator of inflammation and tissue damage, as it is elevated in cases of infection, inflammatory response, damage, and necrosis of the tissue [16]. Among its actions are platelet activation, chemotaxis acceleration, and enhancement of cell-mediated immunity by promoting phagocytosis [17].

One of the first studies to correlate CRP with sepsis was conducted in 1987 by Mustard et al. In this study, it was observed that postoperative CRP levels can predict septic complications even before its clinical manifestation [18].

This protein is also used to differentiate the sepsis of a noninfectious systemic inflammatory response syndrome in trauma patients, in which the high level of this protein in the first 4 days after injury is a reliable indication of infection [19].

In 2013, a study conducted at the Department of Pediatrics at Yonsei University of Medicine showed that high levels of CRP in the mother may indicate a risk of infection of the newborn and that these values would be related to the severity of the disease presented by these babies [16].

Also, in 2013, Oliveira et al. [20] compared CRP with another established biomarker, procalcitonin (PCT). In this study, it was observed that the protein is as effective as PCT to guide antibiotic therapy in patients with sepsis, showing that the group guided by CRP levels required less treatment time when compared to the control groups.

In a study published in 2017, Wang et al. [21] once again correlated CRP with sepsis when comparing the CRP's serum level with those of other proinflammatory cytokines, suggesting that this would be a potential target for the treatment of patients with sepsis.

However, although there is considerable sensitivity in the CRP oscillation to describe the disease intensity in already diagnosed patients, this biomarker has low specificity in determining sepsis, which prevents CRP from being alone an indicator for the diagnosis of the pathology [15].

2.3 B-type natriuretic peptide

B-type natriuretic peptide (BNP) is a cardiac hormone with natriuretic, diuretic, and vasodilatory properties. It is produced by the ventricular myocardium in response to the stretching of the cardiac muscle, having as its main role the cardiac pressure regulation and homeostasis of the intravascular volume [22]. In this sense, septic shock is recognized as a condition that causes severe changes in blood pressure.

BNP or its inactive N-terminal proBNP cleavage product (NT-proBNP) is mainly used as a biomarker for congestive heart failure [23]. However, Papanikolaou et al. [24] demonstrated in 2014 that the severity of sepsis is the major determinant of BNP increase in the disease-induced myocardial depression in patients with a septic shock. In addition, the same study suggests that the increase in BNP serum levels on the second day of the condition is a strong indication of a poor prognosis.

However, due to the inconsistency of results and the specificity limitations, harsh criticism of this biomarker use has recently arisen, demonstrating the need for further studies to validate the use of this as a biomarker in the sepsis condition [25].

It is currently believed that BNP and NT-proBNP have moderate potential to assess the diseased patients' prognosis. As Bai demonstrated in his meta-analysis published in 2018, the peptide can be used as a tool for defining how the condition will evolve, but further studies are needed to assess the real importance of BNP in the clinic [26].

2.4 Procalcitonin

Procalcitonin (PCT) is a prohormone precursor of calcitonin produced by thyroid C cells. Under normal conditions, PCT is not detected in the circulation; however, in situations of great stress, such as sepsis, it is possible to observe a high extrathyroidal production of PCT. PCT is currently used as a tool to differentiate bactericidal infection from other inflammatory and infectious processes [27].

PCT is correlated with sepsis since 1993 when Assicot et al. [28] demonstrated that this protein was detectable in the plasma of diseased patients and with other types of infection. Since then, studies have demonstrated the efficacy of this tool in the prognosis of patients with sepsis, as demonstrated in the review published in 2001 by Meisner [29], in which it was observed that the PCT's concentration during the sepsis and SIRS stages is high and is directly proportional to the severity of the condition.

This method provides additional information to the diagnosis by other parameters of an inflammatory response; such additional information is not provided by conventional parameters of systemic inflammation. Mustafić et al. [30] also demonstrated in 2018 that it is possible to use PCT to reveal the disease severity and prevent a fatal outcome for the patient with sepsis.

In the same year, Bilgili et al. [31] demonstrated that PCT can differentiate even gram-negative bacteremia from a Gram-positive one, noting that protein values are higher in patients infected with Gram-negative bacteria. However, in these cases, PCT should be used only as a support tool for predictive purposes in diagnostic tests.

Biomarker	Sensitivity (%)	Specificity (%)	AUC	NPV	PPV	References
Lactate	58.3	88.1	0.66	78.7	73.7	[33]
CRP	66	80	0.81	88	51	[34]
Pro-BNP	70.8	47.6	0.66	74.1	43.6	[33]
PCT	88	80	0.87	95	57	[33, 34]
sRAGE	75	85	—	—	—	[35, 36]

Table 1.
Biomarkers and their predictive parameters in sepsis.

Several studies have shown that PCT's serum levels may be a guide in antibiotic therapy and can also be used to safely reduce the excessive exposure of these patients to drugs, thus reducing the adverse effects of sepsis treatment and avoiding the development of multiresistant bacteria [20].

Considering several studies cited in this chapter, the sepsis survival campaign published in 2017 suggested that the PCT monitoring should be used to verify the dosage and duration of antimicrobial treatment in patients with sepsis [32].

In **Table 1**, we summarize some parameters that reveal the predictive potential of the biomarkers mentioned above. Among them, we emphasize the sensitivity and specificity of each biomarker demonstrated by the ROC curve. The area under the ROC curve (AUC) represents the performance of the biomarker. We also specified in the table the positive and negative predictive values for each marker.

3. Promising biomarkers

3.1 Receptor for advanced glycation end products

The receptor for advanced glycation end products (RAGE) recipient is a standard recognition receptor that participates in a wide variety of physiological and pathological processes, such as diabetic complications, cancer, atherosclerosis, and inflammation.

The studies that relate soluble RAGE (sRAGE), the extracellular domain of RAGE, to the sepsis are very recent since even the discovery of this receptor's soluble form occurred in 2009 [37]. It has been reported that an increase in the level of sRAGE would be a protective mechanism since its presence in plasma contributes to the removal or neutralization of ligands for RAGE, thus acting as a "false" receptor [38]. However, Wang et al. [39] reported a deletion effect of sRAGE in the inflammatory process, since it would bind to CD11b receptors of leukocytes, thus propagating inflammation.

Based on these contradictory results in scientific literature, in 2014, our group published a study demonstrating a positive correlation between serum levels of sRAGE with IFN-γ in patients with sepsis. We also observed significant correlations between levels of IL-1α, IL-6, IL-8, IL-10, and IP-10 and sRAGE in patients with septic shock. We concluded that sRAGE blood levels may be associated with the mortality of patients with septic shock [35].

Further studies support this assertion, such as the study by Matsumoto et al. [40] demonstrated that the sRAGE serum level of patients with sepsis increases directly proportional to the severity of the disease, suggesting that sRAGE reflects on the RAGE's signaling pathway inducing an excessive inflammatory response involved in endothelial injury and coagulopathy.

In the same year, Wang et al. [41] demonstrated that the decrease in sRAGE levels in mice results in improved sepsis-induced lung damage, thus decreasing mortality in this condition. Another study by Narvaez-Rivera et al. [36] demonstrated in 2015 that sRAGE's level in the plasma is high in patients with community-acquired pneumonia associated with sepsis and is also an independent factor for the likelihood of a fatal outcome.

Further studies are still needed to elucidate the mechanism of action of sRAGE in sepsis and septic shock; however, this receptor appears to be a promising biological marker for sepsis.

3.2 Nitric oxide

Nitric oxide (NO) is a highly reactive soluble gas that is endogenously synthesized by the three isoforms of the nitric oxide synthase enzyme (NOS), neuronal NOS (nNOS or NOS1), inducible NOS (iNOS or NOS2), and endothelial NOS (eNOS or NOS3). These molecules are known to be highly involved in cardiovascular homeostasis, so recent research has focused on its action on sepsis-induced heart disease [42].

In 2014, Nardi et al. [43] showed an increased NOS1 expression in vascular tissues in the sepsis condition, suggesting that this molecule could be a way to justify vascular dysfunction induced by the disease. This study suggests that the inhibition of this isoform may be an alternative to restore the effectiveness of vasopressors in later cases of sepsis.

In the same year, Martin et al. reported an association between NOS2 and NOS3 with sepsis. In the study, the authors suggest that this association could be related to the high level of NO in the blood plasma, which could consequently induce a failure of hemodynamics and increase the mortality of septic patients [44].

More recently, the critical care department of the First People's Hospital in Chun'an (China) demonstrated that monitoring changes in NO serum and amyloid A levels can be an efficient tool for defining patient prognosis and, when compared with CRP, would present better clinical results [45]. Despite the positive results on the use of nitric oxide as a biological marker for sepsis, many studies are still needed to fully understand its role in this condition.

3.3 Haptoglobin

Haptoglobin (Hp) is a protein whose main biological function is to bind free hemoglobin (Hb) and to prevent the loss of iron and subsequent kidney damage following intravascular hemolysis. When red cells are lysed, Hb binds to circulating Hp forming the Hp-Hb complex, which is then degraded by the reticuloendothelial system [46].

Although it is recognized that Hp is predominantly synthesized in the liver, studies reveal the expression of this protein also in other parts of the body, such as the lung, kidneys, heart, spleen, thymus, and brain [47–49]. There are reports that Hp levels are influenced by the acute inflammatory process and that such protein exerts an important antimicrobial and antioxidant function [50–52].

It is known that some patients with sepsis present deformity of hemoglobins, thus causing lysis of these cells and releasing them into the circulation [53]. In this context, the decrease in blood levels of Hp has already been described as a factor linked to increased mortality in patients diagnosed with sepsis, and, in animal models of sepsis, Hp supplementation has been shown to be able to decrease biomarkers of acute systemic inflammation [54, 55].

Even with this result, prospective and randomized studies are still needed to better elucidate the potential protective effects of endogenous and exogenous haptoglobin against the deleterious effects of free hemoglobin in septic patients.

3.4 Cytokines as biomarkers

Sepsis is characterized by two phases: a period of hyperinflammation, where the innate immune system is overactivated leading to production of proinflammatory cytokines such as TNF, IL-1b, IL-6, and IL8, and another period of immunosuppression where both adaptive and innate immunity are acting [56]. Clinical trials in septic patients showed an increase in the above-mentioned pro-inflammatory cytokines [57, 58].

However, contradictory results have been obtained for TNF and IL-1b. For example, the treatment of septic patients with anti-TNF antibodies did not affect the clinical outcome of patients [59]. In addition, these cytokines are not altered only in sepsis, after surgery or in autoimmune disease they are also altered and therefore are not specific.

On the other hand, studies have reported that IL-6 shows great promise as a biomarker [60–63]. Like TNF and IL-1b, IL-6 is not altered only in sepsis; nevertheless, several studies have shown its importance in the prognosis of sepsis presenting strong correlations with patient mortality [62, 63]. These results were also shown in an animal model of acute septic peritonitis (CLP) [61]. In this way, IL6 levels can show which patients may develop severe sepsis, and this reflects on possible interventions. Like IL6, IL8 has also been mentioned as a prognostic biomarker in septic patients especially in the early stages of the disease [64].

In the immunosuppression stage, IL-10 plays a key role in development of CARS trying to reduce hyperinflammation [65]. Therefore, studies have shown that high levels of IL-10 are correlated with a worse outcome and death [65–67]. In neonatal sepsis, IL-10 also proved to be an accurate biomarker. **Figure 1** illustrates the model proposed by van der Poll and van Deventer [68], emphasizing that the development of CARS still occurs in the pro-inflammatory phase of the disease. Thus, the mortality observed in the early stages of sepsis may be related to the hyper-inflammatory phase, and the late-stage deaths are related to the immunosuppressive phase as well as to secondary infections [56].

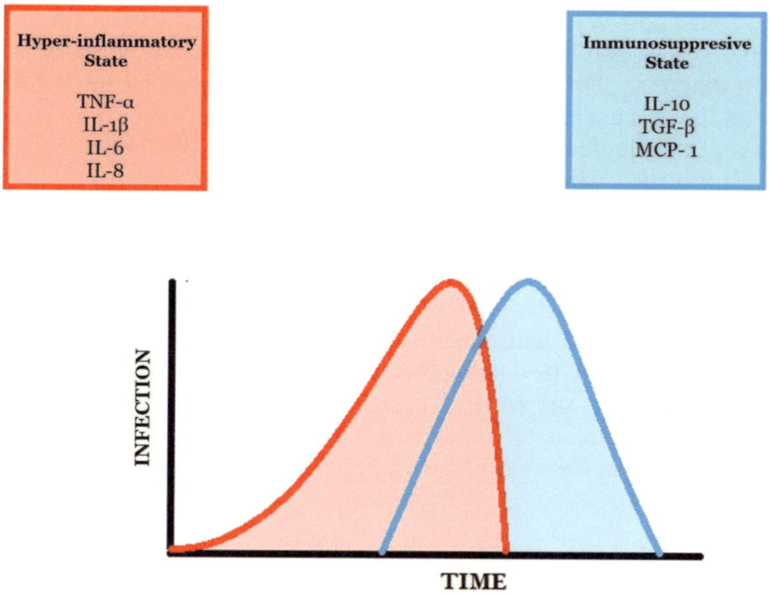

Figure 1.
Stages of sepsis and cytokine profile.

Accordingly, the cytokine profile in the septic patient could provide information about the stage of the disease and the patient's prognosis, contributing to a better intervention. In addition, we currently have a multiplex assay that simultaneously measures multiple cytokines with small plasma samples; however, this information should be interpreted with caution since the dosages of some cytokines in septic patients appear unclear in the literature needing to be standardized. Once standardized, the multiplex assay may be useful in the clinic.

3.5 Biomarker combinations

As previously seen, no biomarker has 100% sensitivity or specificity capable of predicting the clinical outcome for the patient with sepsis. Studies have shown that combining biomarkers may facilitate diagnosis and predict the outcome more faithfully.

As above mentioned, Guo demonstrated that the combination among lactate, CRP and BNP, or NT-proBNP has greater specificity for prognosis than isolated lactate dosage, being 100 and 69.23%, respectively [15]. Yu and colleagues [45] also showed that combining NO with SAA is an important tool to improve the prognosis of septic patients.

Clinical scores are not effective in early identification of infection in critically ill patients; however, combining these scores with biomarkers allows an early and accurate identification of sepsis. For example, Yoo and co-workers found that combining Modified Early Warning Score (MEWS), a tool for monitoring sepsis, with blood lactate levels was efficient for early identification of the disease [69]. The same was found by Bozza et al. [70] and Oberholzer et al. [71] when they combined the levels of MPC-1 or IL-6 with APACHE II, respectively, and found greater accuracy in the prognosis of the patients.

Other biomarkers aforementioned are also more accurate when combined. Han et al. showed that the association with CRP and PCT is an important tool to differentiate bacterial sepsis from other possible types of infection in critically ill patients [72]. Angeletti et al. [73] also showed that the combination among PCT, Tumor Necrosis Factor-α (TNF-α), and the adrenomedullin hormone fragment may help in the prior diagnosis and prognosis of septic patients, thus optimizing treatment of patients.

As mentioned above, IL-6, IL10, and IL-8 cytokines may also be altered in septic patients. In this way, combining cytokine dosage with another biomarker may improve the diagnosis. For example, it has been shown that combining CRP dosage with IL8 and IL2 was useful in the diagnosis of neonatal sepsis [74]. Another study with adult septic patients measured TNF, IL6, and IL10 and demonstrated that combining IL6 (pro-inflammatory) with IL10 (anti-inflammatory) cytokines was useful in establishing the prognosis. Moreover, high levels of IL-6 and IL-10 were related to high patient mortality [75].

Another combination has been demonstrated by Wong and colleagues who showed that interleukin-27 (IL-27) when combined with PCT can improve the diagnostic accuracy in septic patients when compared to each biomarker alone [76]. In 2012, Andaluz-Ojeda et al. [66] using the multiplex assay demonstrated that combining pro—IL-6 and IL-8—and anti-inflammatory cytokine—IL10 and MCP-1—levels was more predictive than analyzing each cytokine separately. Furthermore, high levels of these cytokines were positively correlated with the patient's mortality rate.

4. Conclusion

In this chapter we have outlined some biological markers established in the literature and that have recognized clinical relevance for sepsis, such as CRP [18], lactate [11], BNP [24], and procalcitonin [28]. In addition, we also present some biomarkers that we believe are promising for the disease (sRAGE, NO, and haptoglobin).

The choice of the promising biomarkers cited in this chapter considered the clinical relevance of each of them (demonstrated by several studies) and our experience in the field. However, we recognize that there is a broad spectrum of quality papers published in the area of biomarkers for sepsis and that unfortunately those were not mentioned in this chapter.

Among the new research targets, we believe that sRAGE may be one of the most promising ones in severe sepsis. Our group demonstrated that this soluble receptor can be used as a tool to define the death prognosis of patients with septic shock, presenting a sensitivity of 75% and specificity of 85% [35].

In conclusion, it is noticeable that the currently used methods, even effective ones, require optimization. In this sense, one of the alternatives is combining biological markers, such as those exposed in this chapter, in order to increase the sensitivity and specificity of the diagnosis and prognosis of patients with sepsis, so that the treatment of this disease is increasingly early and efficient.

Author details

Débora Maria da Gomes Cunha, Guilherme Galdino da Silva and Mike Yoshio Hamasaki*
Escola da Saúde do Centro Universitário das Faculdades Metropolitanas Unidas, São Paulo, Brazil

*Address all correspondence to: mike.yoha@gmail.com

References

[1] Marik PE, Taeb AM. SIRS, qSOFA and new sepsis definition. Journal of Thoracic Disease. 2017;**9**(4):943-945

[2] Fang X, Wang Z, Yang J, Cai H, Yao Z, Li K, et al. Clinical evaluation of sepsis-1 and sepsis-3 in the ICU. Chest. 2018;**153**(5):1169-1176. DOI: 10.1016/j.chest.2017.06.037

[3] Singer M, Deutschman CS, Seymour C, Shankar-Hari M, Annane D, Bauer M, et al. The third international consensus definitions for sepsis and septic shock (sepsis-3). Journal of the American Medical Association. 2016;**315**(8):801-810

[4] Williams JM, Greenslade JH, McKenzie JV, Chu K, Brown AFT, Lipman J. Systemic inflammatory response syndrome, quick sequential organ function assessment, and organ dysfunction: Insights from a prospective database of ED patients with infection. Chest. 2017;**151**(3): 586-596. DOI: 10.1016/j.chest.2016.10.057

[5] Wagar EA, Yasin B, Yuan S. Point-of-care testing: Twenty years' experience. Laboratory Medicine. 2008;**39**(9):560-563. Available from: https://academic.oup.com/labmed/article-lookup/doi/10.1309/9R9Y0V68Y3BA0KDN

[6] Gutierres SL, Welty TE. Point-of-care testing: An introduction. The Annals of Pharmacotherapy. 2004;**38**(1):119-125

[7] Nichols JH. Point of care testing. Clinics in Laboratory Medicine. 2007;**27**(4):893-908

[8] Bonini P, Plebani M, Ceriotti F, Rubboli F. Errors in laboratory medicine. Clinical Chemistry. 2002;**48**(5):691-698

[9] Zhang Z, Xu X, Chen K. Lactate clearance as a useful biomarker for the prediction of all-cause mortality in critically ill patients: A systematic review study protocol. BMJ Open. 2014;**4**(5):1-4

[10] Singer AJ, Taylor M, Domingo A, Ghazipura S, Khorasonchi A, Thode HC, et al. Diagnostic characteristics of a clinical screening tool in combination with measuring bedside lactate level in emergency department patients with suspected sepsis. Academic Emergency Medicine. 2014;**21**(8):853-857

[11] Bakker J, Coffernils M, Leon M, Gris P, Vincent JL. Blood lactate levels are superior to oxygen-derived variables in predicting outcome in human septic shock. Chest. 1991;**99**(4):956-962

[12] Bernardin G, Pradier C, Tiger F, Deloffre P, Mattei M. Blood pressure and arterial lactate level are early indicators of short-term survival in human septic shock. Intensive Care Medicine. 1996;**22**(1):17-25

[13] Ranzani OT, Monteiro MB, Ferreira EM, Santos SR, Machado FR, Noritomi DT. Reclassifying the spectrum of septic patients using lactate: Severe sepsis, cryptic shock, vasoplegic shock and dysoxic shock. Revista Brasileira de Terapia Intensiva. 2013;**25**(4):270-278

[14] Léguillier T, Jouffroy R, Boisson M, Boussaroque A, Chenevier-Gobeaux C, Chaabouni T, et al. Lactate POCT in mobile intensive care units for septic patients? A comparison of capillary blood method versus venous blood and plasma-based reference methods. Clinical Biochemistry. 2018;**55**:9-14

[15] Guo Y, Yang H, Gao W, Ma C, Li T. Combination of biomarkers in predicting 28-day mortality for septic patients. Journal of the College of Physicians and Surgeons—Pakistan. 2018;**28**(9):672-676

[16] Jeon JH, Namgung R, Park MS, Park KI, Lee C. Positive maternal C-reactive protein predicts neonatal sepsis. Yonsei Medical Journal. 2014;**55**(1):113-117

[17] Zimmerman MA, Selzman CH, Cothren C, Sorensen AC, Raeburn CD, Harken AH. Diagnostic implications of C-reactive protein. Archives of Surgery. 2003;**138**(2):220-224

[18] Mustard RA. C-Reactive protein levels predict postoperative septic complications. Archives of Surgery. 1987;**122**(1):69. Available from: http://archsurg.jamanetwork.com/article.aspx?doi=10.1001/archsurg.1987.01400130075011

[19] Miller PR, Munn DD, Meredith JW, Chang MC. Systemic inflammatory response syndrome in the trauma intensive care unit: Who is infected? Journal of Trauma and Acute Care Surgery. 1999;**47**(6):1004-1008

[20] Oliveira CF, Botoni FA, Oliveira CRA, Silva CB, Pereira HA, Serufo JC, et al. Procalcitonin versus C-reactive protein for guiding antibiotic therapy in sepsis: A randomized trial. Critical Care Medicine. 2013;**41**(10):2336-2343

[21] Wang L, Zhao H, Wang D. Inflammatory cytokine expression in patients with sepsis at an intensive care unit. Experimental and Therapeutic Medicine. 2018;**16**(3):2126-2131. Available from: http://www.spandidos-publications.com/10.3892/etm.2018.6376

[22] Suttner S, Boldt J. Natriuretic peptide system: Physiology and clinical utility. Current Opinion in Critical Care. 2004;**10**(5):336-341. Available from: http://www.ncbi.nlm.nih.gov/pubmed/15385748%5Cnhttp://graphics.tx.ovid.com/ovftpdfs/FPDDNCGCECKKPO00/fs047/ovft/live/gv031/00075198/00075198-200410000-00006.pdf

[23] Tang WH, Francis GS, Morrow DA, Newby LK, Cannon CP, Jesse RL, et al. National Academy of Clinical Biochemistry Laboratory Medicine Practice Guidelines: Clinical utilization of cardiac biomarker testing in heart failure. Clinical Biochemistry. 2008;**41**(4-5):210-221

[24] Papanikolaou J, Makris D, Mpaka M, Palli E, Zygoulis P, Zakynthinos E. New insights into the mechanisms involved in B-type natriuretic peptide elevation and its prognostic value in septic patients. Critical Care. 2014;**18**(3):R94

[25] McLean AS, Huang SJ. Brain not processing: Is finding a role for BNP in sepsis like fitting a square peg into a round hole? Critical Care. 2014;**18**(4):1-2

[26] Bai YL, Hu BL, Wen HC, Zhang YL, Zhu JJ. Prognostic value of plasma brain natriuretic peptide value for patients with sepsis: A meta-analysis. Journal of Critical Care. 2018;**48**:145-152. DOI: 10.1016/j.jcrc.2018.08.040

[27] Christ-Crain M, Müller B. Procalcitonin in bacterial infections—Hype, hope, more or less? Swiss Medical Weekly. 2005;**135**(31-32):451-460

[28] Assicot M, Bohuon C, Gendrel D, Raymond J, Carsin H, Guilbaud J. High serum procalcitonin concentrations in patients with sepsis and infection. Lancet. 2017;**341**(8844):515-518. DOI: 10.1016/0140-6736(93)90277-N

[29] Meisner M. Pathobiochemistry and clinical use of procalcitonin. Clinica Chimica Acta. 2002;**323**(1-2):17-29

[30] Mustafić S, Brkić S, Prnjavorac B, Sinanović A, Porobić Jahić H, Salkić S. Diagnostic and prognostic value of procalcitonin in patients with sepsis. Medicinski Glasnik. 2018;**15**(2):93-100

[31] Bilgili B, Haliloğlu M, Aslan MS, Sayan İ, Kasapoğlu US, Cinel İ.

Diagnostic accuracy of procalcitonin for differentiating bacteraemic gram-negative sepsis from gram-positive sepsis. Turkish Journal of the Anaesthesiology and Reanimation. 2018;**46**(1):38-43

[32] Rhodes A, Evans LE, Alhazzani W, Levy MM, Antonelli M, Ferrer R, et al. Surviving Sepsis Campaign: International guidelines for management of sepsis and septic shock: 2016. Intensive Care Medicine. 2017;**43**:304-377

[33] Phua J, Koay ESC, Lee KH. Lactate, procalcitonin, and amino-terminal pro-B-type natriuretic peptide versus cytokine measurements and clinical severity scores for prognostication in septic shock. Shock. 2008;**29**(3):328-333

[34] Oberhoffer M et al. Outcome prediction by traditional and new markers of inflammation in patients with sepsis. Clinical Chemistry and Laboratory Medicine. 1999;**37**(3):363-368

[35] Hamasaki MY, Barbeiro HV, De Souza HP, Machado MCC, Da Silva FP. sRAGE in septic shock: A potential biomarker of mortality. Revista Brasileira de Terapia Intensiva. 2014;**26**(4):392-396

[36] Narvaez-Rivera RM, Rendon A, Salinas-Carmona MC, Rosas-Taraco AG. Soluble RAGE as a severity marker in community acquired pneumonia associated sepsis. BMC Infectious Diseases. 2012;**12**(1):15. Available from: http://www.biomedcentral.com/1471-2334/12/15

[37] Maillard-Lefebvre H, Boulanger E, Daroux M, Gaxatte C, Hudson BI, Lambert M. Soluble receptor for advanced glycation end products: A new biomarker in diagnosis and prognosis of chronic inflammatory diseases. Rheumatology (Oxford, England). 2009;**48**(10):1190-1196

[38] Geroldi D, Falcone C, Emanuele E. Soluble receptor for advanced glycation end products: From disease marker to potential therapeutic target. Current Medicinal Chemistry. 2006;**13**(17):1971-1978. Available from: http://www.eurekaselect.com/openurl/content.php?genre=article&issn=0929-8673&volume=13&issue=17&spage=1971

[39] Wang Y, Wang H, Piper MG, McMaken S, Mo X, Opalek J, et al. sRAGE induces human monocyte survival and differentiation. Journal of Immunology. 2013;**185**(3):1822-1835

[40] Matsumoto H, Matsumoto N, Ogura H, Shimazaki J, Yamakawa K, Yamamoto K, et al. The clinical significance of circulating soluble RAGE in patients with severe sepsis. Journal of Trauma and Acute Care Surgery. 2015;**78**(6):1086-1094

[41] Wang Q, Wu X, Tong X, Zhang Z, Xu B, Zhou W. Xuebijing ameliorates sepsis-induced lung injury by downregulating HMGB1 and RAGE expressions in mice. Evidence-based Complementary and Alternative Medicine. 2015;**2015**:860259

[42] Farah C, Michel LYM, BalligandJL. Nitric oxide signalling incardiovascular health and disease. Nature Reviews Cardiology. 2018;**15**(5):292-316

[43] Nardi GM, Scheschowitsch K, Ammar D, De Oliveira SK, Arruda TB, Assreuy J. Neuronal nitric oxide synthase and its interaction with soluble guanylate cyclase is a key factor for the vascular dysfunction of experimental sepsis. Critical Care Medicine. 2014;**42**(6):391-400

[44] Martin G, Asensi V, Montes AH, Collazos J, Alvarez V, Pérez-Is L, et al. Endothelial (NOS3 E298D)

and inducible (NOS2 exon 22) nitric oxide synthase polymorphisms, as well as plasma NOx, influence sepsis development. Nitric Oxide: Biology and Chemistry. 2014;**42**:79-86. DOI: 10.1016/j.niox.2014.09.004

[45] Yu MH, Chen MH, Han F, Li Q, Sun RH, Tu YX. Prognostic value of the biomarkers serum amyloid A and nitric oxide in patients with sepsis. International Immunopharmacology. 2018;**62**:287-292. DOI: 10.1016/j.intimp.2018.07.024

[46] Shih AWY, Mcfarlane A, Verhovsek M. Haptoglobin testing in hemolysis: Measurement and interpretation. American Journal of Hematology. 2014;**89**(4):443-447

[47] Kalmovarin N, Friedrichs WE, O'Brien HV, Linehan LA, Bowman BH, Yang F. Extrahepatic expression of plasma protein genes during inflammation. Inflammation. 1991;**15**(5):369-379

[48] Yang F, Friedrichs WE, Navarijo-Ashbaugh AL, deGraffenried LA, Bowman BH, Coalson JJ. Cell type-specific and inflammatory-induced expression of haptoglobin gene in lung. Laboratory Investigation. 1995;**73**(3):433-440

[49] Sanchez DJ, Armstrong L, Aguilar R, Adrian GS, Haro L, Martinez AO. Haptoglobin gene expression in human glioblastoma cell lines. Neuroscience Letters. 2001;**303**(3):181-184

[50] Wang Y, Kinzie E, Berger FG, Lim SK, Baumann H. Haptoglobin, an inflammation-inducible plasma protein. Redox Report. 2001;**6**(6):379-385

[51] Eaton JW, Brandt P, Mahoney JR, Lee JT Jr. Haptoglobin: A natural bacteriostat. Science. 1982;**215**(4533): 691-693

[52] Theilgaard-Mönch K, Jacobsen LC, Nielsen MJ, Rasmussen T, Udby L, Gharib M, et al. Haptoglobin is synthesized during granulocyte differentiation, stored in specific granules, and released by neutrophils in response to activation. Blood. 2006;**108**(1):353-361

[53] Baskurt OK, Gelmont D, Meiselman HJ. Red blood cell deformability in sepsis. American Journal of Respiratory and Critical Care. 1998;**157**(2):421-427. Available from: http://www.ncbi.nlm.nih.gov/pubmed/9476853

[54] Arredouani MS, Kasran A, Vanoirbeek JA, Berger FG, Baumann H, Ceuppens JL. Haptoglobin dampens endotoxin-induced inflammatory effects both in vitro and in vivo. Immunology. 2005;**114**(2):263-271

[55] Janz DR, Bastarache JA, Sills G, Wickersham N, May AK, Bernard GR, et al. Association between haptoglobin, hemopexin and mortality in adults with sepsis. Critical Care. 2013;**17**(6):2-9

[56] Biron BM, Ayala A, Lomas-Neira JL. Biomarkers for sepsis: What is and what might be? Biomarker Insights. 2015;**10**:BMI-S29519

[57] Tamayo E et al. Pro-and anti-inflammatory responses are regulated simultaneously from the first moments of septic shock. European Cytokine Network. 2011;**22**(2):82-87

[58] Kurt AN, Aygun AD, Godekmerdan A, Kurt A, Dogan Y, Yilmaz E. Serum IL-1β, IL-6, IL-8, and TNF-α levels in early diagnosis and management of neonatal sepsis. Mediators of Inflammation. 2007;**2007**:31397

[59] Qiu P et al. The evolving experience with therapeutic TNF inhibition in sepsis: Considering the potential

influence of risk of death. Expert Opinion on Investigational Drugs. 2011;**20**(11):1555-1564

[60] Pettilä V et al. Predictive value of procalcitonin and interleukin 6 in critically ill patients with suspected sepsis. Intensive Care Medicine. 2002;**28**(9):1220-1225

[61] Osuchowski MF et al. Stratification is the key: Inflammatory biomarkers accurately direct immunomodulatory therapy in experimental sepsis. Critical Care Medicine. 2009;**37**(5):1567

[62] Lusyati S et al. Cytokines patterns in newborn infants with late onset sepsis. Journal of Neonatal-Perinatal Medicine. 2013;**6**(2):153-163

[63] Machado JR, Soave DF, da Silva MV, de Menezes LB, Etchebehere RM, Monteiro ML, et al. Neonatal sepsis and inflammatory mediators. Mediators of Inflammation. 2014;**2014**:269681

[64] Berner R et al. Plasma levels and gene expression of granulocyte colony-stimulating factor, tumor necrosis factor-α, interleukin (IL)-1β, IL-6, IL-8, and soluble intercellular adhesion molecule-1 in neonatal early onset sepsis. Pediatric Research. 1998;**44**(4):469

[65] Adib-Conquy M, Cavaillon J-M. Compensatory anti-inflammatory response syndrome. Thrombosis and Haemostasis. 2009;**102**(01):36-47

[66] Andaluz-Ojeda D et al. A combined score of pro-and anti-inflammatory interleukins improves mortality prediction in severe sepsis. Cytokine. 2012;**57**(3):332-336

[67] Wu H-P et al. Serial cytokine levels in patients with severe sepsis. Inflammation Research. 2009;**58**(7):385-393

[68] van der Poll T, van Deventer SJH. Cytokines and anticytokines in the pathogenesis of sepsis. Infectious Disease Clinics of North America. 1999;**13**(2):413-426

[69] Yoo JW, Lee JR, Jung YK, Choi SH, Son JS, Kang BJ, et al. A combination of early warning score and lactate to predict intensive care unit transfer of inpatients with severe sepsis/septic shock. The Korean Journal of Internal Medicine. 2015;**30**(4):471-477

[70] Bozza FA et al. Cytokine profiles as markers of disease severity in sepsis: A multiplex analysis. Critical care. 2007;**11**(2):R49

[71] Oberholzer A et al. Plasma cytokine measurements augment prognostic scores as indicators of outcome in patients with severe sepsis. Shock. 2005;**23**(6):488-493

[72] Han JH, Nachamkin I, Coffin SE, Gerber JS, Fuchs B, Garrigan C, et al. Use of a combination biomarker algorithm to identify medical intensive care unit patients with suspected sepsis at very low likelihood of bacterial infection. Antimicrobial Agents and Chemotherapy. 2015;**59**(10):6494-6500

[73] Angeletti S, Dicuonzo G, Fioravanti M, De Cesaris M, Fogolari M, Lo Presti A, et al. Procalcitonin, MR-proadrenomedullin, and cytokines measurement in sepsis diagnosis: Advantages from test combination. Disease Markers. 2015;**2015**:9515321

[74] Reyes CS et al. Role of cytokines (interleukin-1β, 6, 8, tumour necrosis factor-α, and soluble receptor of interleukin-2) and C-reactive protein in the diagnosis of neonatal sepsis. Acta Paediatrica. 2003;**92**(2):221-227

[75] Kellum JA et al. Understanding the inflammatory cytokine response

in pneumonia and sepsis: Results of the genetic and inflammatory markers of sepsis (GenIMS) study. Archives of Internal Medicine. 2007;**167**(15):1655-1663

[76] Wong HR, Lindsell CJ, Lahni P, Hart KW, Gibot S. Interleukin-27 as a sepsis diagnostic biomarker in critically ill adults. Shock. 2014;**40**(5):382-386

Chapter 3

Resuscitation Endpoints in Traumatic Shock: A Focused Review with Emphasis on Point-of-Care Approaches

Kathryn C. Kelley, Kyle Dammann, Alex Alers, Thomas B. Zanders, Charles Bendas and Stanislaw P. Stawicki

Abstract

Trauma resuscitation is a blend of art and science, with the traumatologist at the helm of a large, multidisciplinary team, making split-second decisions and overseeing various parallel processes. Despite tremendous progress over the past few decades, the "art" component continues to play a large part in the overall trauma resuscitation process, with the "science" part slowly but steadily increasing its footprint as a determinant of processes and decisions. Thus, it becomes critical for all clinicians to be able to recognize the evidence-based factors which can be most valuable in guiding trauma resuscitations. This chapter serves as an overview of the current clinical findings, resuscitative endpoints, imaging techniques, and physiologic indices that are most helpful in order to promptly recognize and treat traumatic shock as well as projecting forward to look at novel techniques and biomarkers. Though a single universal marker that accurately and consistently identifies traumatic shock has yet to be discovered, certain factors discussed, such as lactate and base deficit, have been proven to be much more reliable than others.

Keywords: traumatic shock, trauma resuscitation, resuscitative endpoints, imaging techniques, biomarkers in shock

1. Introduction

Trauma is among the leading causes of death across the globe [1, 2]. Yet despite the ubiquitous nature of this public health problem [3–5], our understanding of traumatic shock and the associated outcome determinants and markers continues to be incomplete at the increasingly granular, mechanistic level [6, 7]. For the purposes of this chapter, the term "traumatic shock" refers to any of the number of etiologies that would lead to shock in a trauma patient—most commonly seen is acute hemorrhage, but also other types of shock should also be mentioned, including neurogenic shock and possible late manifestations of obstructive shock and septic shock. There is a wealth of literature related to biomarkers and techniques used in identification of shock—including specifically sepsis and neurogenic shock—but there remains a paucity of studies specifically related to trauma patients.

The goal of this chapter is to provide an overview of the most commonly used endpoints of resuscitation in traumatic shock, beginning with clinical bedside assessments then progressing through various laboratory tests, and finally a discussion of other means of evaluation (e.g., sonography, novel biomarkers, and other miscellaneous approaches).

2. Methods

A total of 9152 candidate publications was identified during a comprehensive literature search using PubMed, Google Scholar™, EBSCOHost, and Bioline International. Search terms included various combinations of "resuscitative endpoints," "traumatic shock," "biomarkers in shock," "study," and "clinical trial." Within the larger subset of candidate publications, 70 studies were deemed suitable in the development of this chapter's content.

3. Clinical evaluation

The most important, and still very much essential, component of determining if a patient is in state of shock is the performance of an accurate clinical examination. There is no substitute for the judgment of an experienced clinician who is attuned to the most subtle manifestations of early (or compensated) shock.

The number one cause of death in the first hour after trauma is hemorrhage, and nearly 40% of all trauma related deaths are secondary to bleeding and its complications [8]. As such, hemorrhagic shock, a unique form of hypovolemic shock, has been the main focus of considerable trauma research and management applications, both in civilian and military settings. However, the astute and well-experienced clinician recognizes that trauma patients are not immune to other types of shock and that different types of shock are not mutually exclusive. Clinical manifestations of shock vary broadly and are based on the underlying etiology, the degree of organ perfusion, and previous organ dysfunction [9]. Understanding of the physical exam findings which may help differentiate between types of shock is a skill paramount to any clinician involved in trauma care. Proper attention to physical exam findings may guide initial therapy before other adjuncts such as imaging studies or laboratory measurements are available.

A complete, "head-to-toe" examination, such as is described for the secondary survey for trauma patients, will reveal multiple findings correlating with hypoperfusion of several organs. Altered mental status, manifesting as confusion, delirium, or coma, reveals decreased cerebral blood flow, most often at mean arterial pressures less than 50 mmHg [10, 11]. The differential diagnosis for any trauma patient who is altered must not only include traumatic brain injury or possible toxin ingestion but also take into account that this mental status change could be an initial presentation of shock. The cardiovascular system is one of the main players in the initial evaluation of shock. Sympathoadrenal stimulation typically causes an increase in heart rate. However, "misleading" heart rate might be present when managing high endurance athletes, geriatric patients, pregnant trauma victims, cardiovascular drug users, those with preexisting cardiovascular disease, or those in neurogenic shock [12–15]. Bradycardia, jugular venous distention, and new onset heart murmur might be present in cardiogenic shock [15, 16]. Distant/muffled heart sounds and pulsus paradoxus might be present in obstructive shock from cardiac tamponade [17]. Obstructive shock from tension hemothorax and/or pneumothorax might be evidenced by distant breath sounds, tracheal deviation, and hypotension [18, 19]. Dyspnea and hypoxia might clue the clinician in on a possible pulmonary embolus and obstructive shock.

Classical teaching would presume that shock is associated to arterial hypotension. Although this might be prevalent in patients suffering from any etiology of shock, arterial hypotension may happen without shock, and hypoperfusion and organ ischemia may happen despite normal blood pressure. Increase in systemic vascular resistance, leading to pale or dusky skin, peripheral cyanosis, damage to small capillaries producing petechiae, decrease in temperature, and delayed capillary refill, is present in almost all forms of shock, except for distributive. Patients in "cold" shock almost universally have alterations in peripheral perfusion. Capillary refill, also termed peripheral perfusion status, can be an easy and rapid assessment of resuscitation status. Abnormal peripheral perfusion has been found to identify normotensive patients with more severe organ dysfunction and correlated with high lactate levels [20]. However, basing resuscitation solely on peripheral perfusion status would not be recommended as this was not found to improve mortality compared to lactate-based resuscitation in septic shock patients [21]. Initial respiratory alterations in shock include an increase in minute ventilation leading to hypocapnia and respiratory alkalosis. Increased work of breathing and attempted respiratory correction of metabolic acidosis, coupled with impaired respiratory muscle function from hypoperfusion, lead to respiratory failure. Although acute kidney injury is commonplace in patients suffering from shock, identifying oliguria requires insertion of a urinary catheter and measurement of output for at least 1 hour; both of these interventions are necessary yet time-consuming. In the absence of prompt intervention, global hypoperfusion leads to failure of multiple organ systems and increases the morbidity and mortality associated to shock [22].

Rapid yet thorough physical examination can lead the clinician to institute therapy to alleviate different causes of shock. Cessation of hemorrhage and volume repletion are the most common maneuvers needed in the trauma bay. However, other culprits of shock are alleviated by, for example, prompt decompression of a tension pneumothorax or cardiac tamponade, rapid administration of fibrinolytic in massive pulmonary embolus, quick activation of the catheterization lab for myocardial ischemia, and fast initiation of vasoactive medications in the setting of heart failure, among others. Adjuncts to the physical exam, such as imaging studies and laboratory values, are valuable assets in the race against time during the management of the patient in shock.

4. Serum lactate

In a study of over 2800 patients, a comparison of four different fundamental serum markers of acidosis was conducted (**Figure 1**) [23]. Although not the first published report of lactate being superior to other well-established serum markers, the authors were able to perform a unique side-by-side comparison of serum lactate versus three other common markers of metabolic acidosis—base deficit, anion gap, and serum bicarbonate [23]. The study demonstrated superiority of lactic acid (AUC, 0.75) and base deficit (AUC, 0.72) over the other indicators (bicarbonate AUC, 0.68, and anion gap AUC, 0.66) [23].

At-risk populations, including the geriatric patients and those with elevated comorbidity-polypharmacy scores (CPS), are at elevated risk of poor outcomes, including morbidity, mortality, and readmissions [24–27]. More specific to the context of trauma, patients with end-stage renal disease, severe peripheral vascular disease, and chronic respiratory failure may present with physiologically misleading vital signs, as evidenced by a study of >30,000 patients examining post-injury vital signs across various age groups [14]. In such setting,

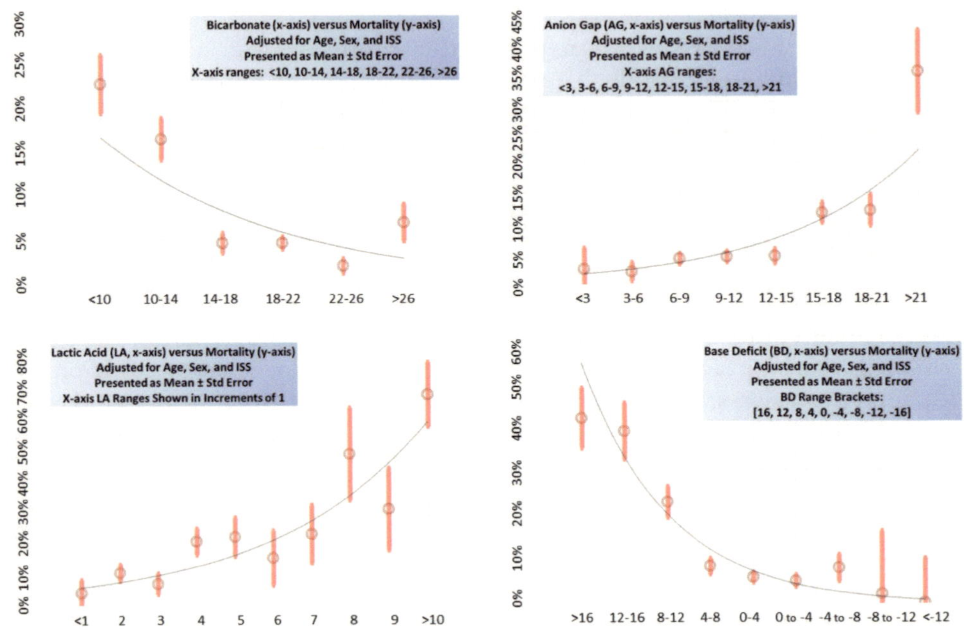

Figure 1.
Traditional serum markers of traumatic shock (clockwise from top left: Bicarbonate, anion gap, base deficit, and lactic acid). Each marker is shown in the context of its associated mortality. If note, all data are adjusted for age, sex, and ISS.

serum lactate may help identify individuals who may be in compensated shock and otherwise exhibit "normal" vital signs [28].

5. Base deficit

Base deficit, calculated directly from pCO_2, HCO_3^-, and pH via blood gas analysis, is often cited among the most reliable predictors of acute metabolic stress following traumatic injury [29, 30]. This particular option may provide enhanced diagnostic utility in at-risk populations, such as the elderly patients who remain normotensive despite significant injury burden [28]. Also, in one study of trauma patients ≤55 years old without head injury, a base deficit ≥8 mmol/L was associated with a 25% mortality rate [30]. However, studies have found that base deficit is less reliable in immediate identification of shock, and more reliable 24 hours after presentation, when irreversible effects of shock have already taken place [30]. Since the numerical value of base deficit is easily influenced by a multitude of other factors related to metabolic acidosis, such as GI losses, diabetic ketoacidosis, and renal dysfunction, serum lactate has been deemed overall more reliable than base deficit [30].

6. Anion gap and other measures of acidosis

In theory, both anion gap and serum bicarbonate should provide a reasonable reflection of systemic acid–base milieu, with clearly established evidence of the correlation between these parameters and increasing metabolic stress [31]. The more recent four-way comparison study shows that although both anion gap and serum bicarbonate fall short of the diagnostic utility of serum lactate or the base deficit, they still provide relevant clinical information for the trauma practitioner. This is especially true in the setting where no other labs may be available [23]. The lethal triad of hemorrhagic shock consists of hypothermia, coagulopathy, and acidosis [32–34]. As such, monitoring of the acid–base status not only assists in guiding further resuscitation, but correction of the acidosis is imperative to improve survival of hemorrhagic shock.

7. Alternative measurements of metabolic stress

Serum pH measurement is yet another option for assessing acute metabolic stress during the immediate post-trauma period, with non-survivor pH ranging between 6.91 and 7.21 across several studies [29]. However, Joynt et al. identified a weakness in using gastric intramucosal pH to distinguish shock survivors from nonsurvivors [35]. At the 48-hour mark, it was found that serum lactate was again a better indicator of survival than serum pH. It is also important to note that improvement in base deficit has been found to be superior to pH in determining improvement in acidotic state [36].

Strong ion gap has additionally been identified as a helpful marker, with one study demonstrating its utility in mortality prediction for victims of major vascular trauma [29]. In that particular study, the strong ion gap ≥5 mEq/L correlated strongly with adverse clinical outcomes (AUC, 0.991) [29]. Other reported experiences suggest that strong ion gap may also offer predictive value in the setting of both adult and pediatric burn injuries [37, 38].

8. Sonography for hemodynamic/shock assessment

Vital signs are key in the initial shock assessment and, however, are often insufficient for evaluating volume status in patients with multiple comorbidities [39]. For this reason, ultrasound has become the standard of care to supplement the initial assessment and gauge resuscitative measures. Although dependent on the user's skillset, both inferior vena cava collapsibility (intravascular volume status surrogate) [40–42] and ventricle contractility (ejection fraction surrogate) can be accurately visualized without needing to record or calculate specific measurements [43]. After volume status is determined, fluid responsiveness (FR) should be assessed. Passive leg raise is a classic way of determining this, as cardiac output or stroke volume is increased by 10% when FR [44]. A more accurate assessment of FR via sonography is measuring variation in stroke volume, from the velocity time integral (VTI) [45]. VTI is the velocity and distance which blood ejects after each contraction, also known as stroke distance [46]. VTI variation more than 14% is highly specific for positive [47]. Finally, significant body of literature exists on the relationship between collapsibility of central veins (e.g., veins peripheral to vena cava) and intravascular volume status. Although less reliable with the more peripheral locations (e.g., subclavian vein more accurate than femoral vein collapsibility), this approach still provides useful clinical information and hemodynamic trends [48–51]. Understanding the above concepts allows one to understand the importance of ultrasound in emergent/trauma settings today.

9. Novel biomarkers in traumatic shock

For most trauma resuscitations involving patients who may be in shock, the use of lactic acid and base deficit as measurements of the overall physiological derangement will be sufficient. However, there is significant room for improvement in terms of diagnostic and predictive accuracy. Many innate similarities exist in the inflammatory responses seen in traumatic shock and sepsis, and many inflammatory signals in tissue injury and end-organ damage are found in responses to both of these conditions. Although not yet extensively studied in the specific subset of trauma patients, novel biomarkers that have been proposed in the diagnosis of shock include sTREM-1 and suPAR [52, 53].

More studied in the setting of sepsis, sTREM1 (a.k.a. soluble triggering receptor expressed on myeloid cells), is a recently discovered immunoglobulin, whose presence has been proven to be greatly upregulated in the presence of bacteria or fungi in cell culture, peritoneal lavage fluid, and tissue samples from patients infected with these microorganisms [52]. Recent studies have shown sTREM1 to be both a diagnostic and prognostic indicator in critically ill patients with shock. sTREM1 has found to be non-inferior to CRP, procalcitonin, IL-6, and TNF-α in identifying postoperative patients with sepsis [52]. suPAR (a.k.a. soluble urokinase-type plasminogen activator system) is found in the blood and organic fluids in all humans and takes part in various immunological functions, such as cell adhesion, migration, chemotaxis, proteolysis, immune activation, tissue remodeling, and signal transduction [52, 53]. suPAR thus reflects the extent of immune activation in a specific individual, serving as a nonspecific prognostic biomarker [53]. It has been associated with hospital length of stay, transfer to the ICU, presence and severity of acute conditions, and risk of death [53]. The TRIAGE III Trial performed in 2018 in Denmark studied suPAR as a prognostic biomarker in patients presenting to the emergency department, finding that suPAR enhanced early risk stratification of patients, but did not lead to any significant changes in short- or long-term all-cause mortality [53].

An increase in extracellular histone levels, which are elevated in response to traumatic injury, correlates with fibrinolysis and activation of anticoagulants [54]. Extracellular histones bind phospholipids, damage cell membranes, and lead to influx of calcium; the sustained intracellular elevation of calcium leads to cell damage and release of cell contents. Circulating histones can lead to distant organ injury, most notably in the lungs, and can ultimately lead to multisystem organ failure [55]. Increases in histone levels from time of admission to 6 hours have been found to be predictive of mortality, paralleling an ongoing release of intracellular antigens that is likewise seen in sepsis [54]. In a 2012 study of 132 critically injured trauma patients, patients within the highest quartile of extracellular histone levels at admission had significantly higher Injury Severity Scores, lower GCS scores, a 1.8-fold higher rate of acute lung injury, a 3.2-fold higher incidence of multisystem organ failure, and 2.1-fold greater mortality [54]. However, further clinical studies on larger scales are needed to confirm whether elevated histones are a reliable indicator of traumatic shock.

Certain biomarkers hold promising potential for rapid early detection of traumatic brain injury (TBI) and neurogenic shock, although no studies with a specific subset of trauma patients have been performed. TBI can often be difficult to assess, as GCS can rapidly decline and standard neurological imaging may poorly characterize minor or occult injuries which could later contribute to clinical decline [56]. S100β is a neurologically derived calcium-binding protein which has increased serum expression following traumatic brain and orthopedic injuries and has also been used to rule out TBI due to its strong negative predictive value [56, 57]. Glial fibrillary acidic protein (GFAP), a cytoskeletal scaffold in astrocytes, is another promising biomarker more specific to TBI than S100β and also has differential expression patterns from low range (3–5) to stable range (13–15) of GCS values [58].

While multiple biomarkers are being investigated for CNS injury, one novel class of regulators, microRNAs (miRNAs), show promise as a potential biomarker for shock. miRNAs are noncoding sequences of genetic material which modulate gene expression in organ development, homeostasis, and disease pathology [59]. For example, miRNAs are associated with the pathogenesis of heart failure through modulation of neurohormonal signaling, and their plasma levels parallel lactate and predict outcomes following cardiac arrest [60–62]. Whether such markers are associated with cardiogenic shock following traumatic injury is unknown and should be investigated. miRNAs have also been implemented as biomarkers for the diagnosis of acute pulmonary embolism [63]. Large pulmonary emboli exhibit similar pathophysiology to acute obstructive shock; therefore, it may be plausible that miRNAs could be a predictor for obstructive shock in a traumatic setting. Additionally, miRNAs have involvement in the pathogenesis of adrenal disease [64]. As the sympathoadrenal axis plays a role in early shock, it may be valuable to investigate adrenal miRNA expression patterns after traumatic injury. One limitation which may limit the future use of miRNAs for the analysis of shock includes the lack of point-of-care testing, requirement of cumbersome miRNA isolation methods, and time-consuming analysis with PCR or microarray technology. However with advancing technology and the importance of miRNA in multiple fields, rapid isolation protocols will soon be on the horizon.

10. Physiological indices

Critical care scoring systems have been well-established to improve care of patients with traumatic shock in the ICU [65]. The following scoring systems give a few examples of how patient prognosis is established. There is no one best scoring system for critical patients, and experts recommend using multiple scores to better risk stratify each patient [65]. Multiple online calculators are readily available to assist in obtaining the score, and typically the most severe values within 24 hours of admission are the figures used for the calculation. The acute physiology and chronic health evaluation (APACHE IV) physiological score was established using more than 110,000 critical care patients and 142 variables to predict mortality and length of stay [65]. Important variables in the calculation include chronic health conditions, admission information and diagnosis, patient age, vital signs, blood gas and ventilation settings, urine output, GCS, and data from CBC and BMP lab work [65]. In comparison to the APACHE, the Simplified Acute Physiology Score (SAPS3) also evaluates how resources are being used between different ICUs based on time spent in ICU [66]. SAPS3 utilizes multiple components, many of which are similar to APACHE scoring system. Important aspects include length of stay before ICU, infections or surgeries while in critical care unit, GCS, vitals, CBC, CMP, blood gases, hospital location prior to ICU admit, and major therapeutic options, such as vasopressors before ICU transfer [66].

Similar to the other scoring systems, sequential organ failure assessment (SOFA) uses multiple organ systems to evaluate patient mortality risk. Variables utilized are the following: cardiovascular, MAP and pressor requirements; CNS, GCS; coagulation, platelet count; hepatic function, bilirubin; renal function, creatinine and urine output; and respiratory function, mechanical ventilation and the PaO2/FiO2 ratio [65]. When viewed as a whole, one can appreciate the similarities and the advantages that each of these scoring systems provides, further emphasizing the importance of using multiple scores in order to improve both clinical awareness and judgment.

11. Miscellaneous topics

Since current laboratory tests do not reliably supply enough diagnostic information about patients that experience acute hemorrhage, which includes trauma patients in hemorrhagic shock, global hemostatic coagulation tests, such as ROTEM/TEG, have emerged as an alternative to traditional coagulation tests such as PT/INR [67]. Though PT/INR can accurately identify the initiation of clotting, these tests do not identify hemostatic capacity in terms of clot formation and maximal thrombin generation [67]. The two semiautomated commercial devices currently on the market for thromboelastography are the ROTEM analyzer and the TEG analyzer; both devices can effectively measure the maximum fibrin clot formation, thus serving as an estimate of the capacity of the coagulation cascade [67]. Thromboelastography has become a valuable asset in identifying coagulopathies and guiding hemostatic therapy and could potentially even prevent unnecessary blood transfusions [67]. These tests are quickly emerging as possible point-of-care devices that can monitor hemorrhage in either the ICU or ED settings [67]. Along with thromboelastography, clot waveform analysis also seems to be a promising resource in monitoring hemorrhagic shock.

In principle, clot waveform analysis (CWA) is based on the aPTT assay and was first described when aPTT and PT were assessed with light transmission [67]. However, the distinct difference with CWA is that the readout from photo-optic registration is prolonged, creating a graph registered over time, whereas aPTT is solely the clotting time [67]. The tracing produced in clot waveform analysis thus reflects the entire process of clot formation and clot lysis [67]. CWA has been used to monitor the course of disseminated intravascular coagulation (DIC) and may be sensitive to even mild deficiencies in Factors II, V, VII, IX, X, and XII, which may prove the test useful in identifying hemophilias A and B [67]. Some studies have even found CWA to be more accurate than CRP and procalcitonin in monitoring the severity and prognosis of sepsis [67]. More clinical data and prospective studies are required, however, to support this evidence. Other emerging technologies that may prove to be highly valuable in the resuscitation of trauma patients are the FloTrac™/Vigileo™ system and the PiCCOplus™ system.

The FloTrac™/Vigileo™ and PiCCOplus™ systems have emerged as dynamic indicators that can accurately predict fluid responsiveness in critically ill patients [68, 69]. By utilizing stroke volume variation (SVV), or the percentage of changes in stroke volume (SV) during the ventilatory cycle, both systems have been shown comparable outcomes in predicting fluid responsiveness [69]. These systems serve as an alternative to static indicators such as central venous pressure (CVP) and pulmonary capillary wedge pressure (PCWP), which have been classically shown to be poor predictors of fluid responsiveness [68].

12. Conclusions

Despite tremendous progress in the management of trauma, universally applicable and highly reliable markers for adequacy of resuscitation remain elusive. For most trauma resuscitations involving patients who may be in shock, the use of lactic acid and base deficit as measurements of the overall physiological derangement will be sufficient.

Author details

Kathryn C. Kelley[1], Kyle Dammann[1], Alex Alers[2], Thomas B. Zanders[3], Charles Bendas[2] and Stanislaw P. Stawicki[4*]

1 Department of Surgery, St. Luke's University Health Network, Bethlehem, Pennsylvania, USA

2 Section of Surgical Critical Care, St. Luke's University Health Network, Bethlehem, Pennsylvania, USA

3 Department of Medicine, Section of Pulmonology and Critical Care, St. Luke's University Health Network, Bethlehem, Pennsylvania, USA

4 Department of Research and Innovation, St. Luke's University Health Network, Bethlehem, Pennsylvania, USA

*Address all correspondence to: stanislaw.stawicki@sluhn.org

References

[1] Krug EG, Sharma GK, Lozano R. The global burden of injuries. American Journal of Public Health. 2000;**90**(4):523

[2] Murray CJ, Lopez AD. Measuring the global burden of disease. New England Journal of Medicine. 2013;**369**(5):448-457

[3] Sharma B. Road traffic injuries: A major global public health crisis. Public Health. 2008;**122**(12):1399-1406

[4] Joshipura M et al. Trauma care systems in India. Injury. 2003;**34**(9):686-692

[5] Baker SP. Injuries: The neglected epidemic: Stone lecture, 1985 America trauma society meeting. The Journal of Trauma. 1987;**27**(4):343-348

[6] Kauvar DS, Lefering R, Wade CE. Impact of hemorrhage on trauma outcome: An overview of epidemiology, clinical presentations, and therapeutic considerations. Journal of Trauma and Acute Care Surgery. 2006;**60**(6):S3-S11

[7] Lui DF et al. Multiorgan failure in trauma: From conception to genomic era. Current Orthopaedic Practice. 2012;**23**(3):235-242

[8] Curry N et al. The acute management of trauma hemorrhage: A systematic review of randomized controlled trials. Critical Care. 2011;**15**(2):R92

[9] Antonelli M et al. Hemodynamic monitoring in shock and implications for management. Intensive Care Medicine. 2007;**33**(4):575-590

[10] Tánczos K, Németh M, Molnár Z. What's new in hemorrhagic shock? Intensive Care Medicine. 2015;**41**(4):712-714

[11] Strehlow MC. Early identification of shock in critically ill patients. Emergency Medicine Clinics. 2010;**28**(1):57-66

[12] Mello PMVC, Sharma VK, Dellinger RP. Shock overview. In: Seminars in Respiratory and Critical Care Medicine. 333 Seventh Avenue, New: Copyright© 2004 by Thieme Medical Publishers, Inc.; 2004

[13] Victorino GP, Battistella FD, Wisner DH. Does tachycardia correlate with hypotension after trauma? Journal of the American College of Surgeons. 2003;**196**(5):679-684

[14] Terzian WTH et al. Admission vital signs in an aging trauma population: How low is too low? International Journal of Academic Medicine. 2017;**3**(2):306-307

[15] Cocchi MN et al. Identification and resuscitation of the trauma patient in shock. Emergency Medicine Clinics of North America. 2007;**25**(3):623-642

[16] Duvernoy CS, Bates ER. Management of cardiogenic shock attributable to acute myocardial infarction in the reperfusion era. Journal of Intensive Care Medicine. 2005;**20**(4):188-198

[17] Forauer AR et al. Pericardial tamponade complicating central venous interventions. Journal of Vascular and Interventional Radiology. 2003;**14**(2):255-259

[18] Sharma A, Jindal P. Principles of diagnosis and management of traumatic pneumothorax. Journal of Emergencies, Trauma, and Shock. 2008;**1**(1):34

[19] Roberts DJ et al. Clinical presentation of patients with tension pneumothorax: A systematic review. Annals of Surgery. 2015;**261**(6):1068-1078

[20] Lima A et al. The prognostic value of the subjective assessment of peripheral perfusion in critically ill patients. Critical Care Medicine. 2009;**37**(3):934-938

[21] Hernández G et al. Effect of a resuscitation strategy targeting peripheral perfusion status vs serum lactate levels on 28-day mortality among patients with septic shock: The ANDROMEDA-SHOCK randomized clinical trial. JAMA. 2019;**321**(7):654-664

[22] Spevetz A, Parillo JE. Shock: Classification, Pathophysiological Characteristics, and Management in Comprehensive Critical Care: Adult. 2nd ed. Philadelphia, PA: Elsevier; 2017. pp. 53-66

[23] Jordan A et al. Mortality predictors in trauma: A single-institution comparison study using a large sample of injured patients. International Journal of Academic Medicine. 2018;**4**(2):192-193

[24] Evans DC et al. Comorbidity-polypharmacy scoring facilitates outcome prediction in older trauma patients. Journal of the American Geriatrics Society. 2012;**60**(8):1465-1470

[25] Justiniano CF et al. Comorbidity-polypharmacy score: A novel adjunct in post–emergency department trauma triage. Journal of Surgical Research. 2013;**181**(1):16-19

[26] Mubang RN et al. Comorbidity–polypharmacy score as predictor of outcomes in older trauma patients: A retrospective validation study. World Journal of Surgery. 2015;**39**(8):2068-2075

[27] Tolentino JC et al. Comorbidity-polypharmacy score predicts readmissions and in-hospital mortality: A six-hospital health network experience. Journal of Basic and Clinical Pharmacy. 2017;**8**(3):98-103

[28] Callaway DW et al. Serum lactate and base deficit as predictors of mortality in normotensive elderly blunt trauma patients. Journal of Trauma and Acute Care Surgery. 2009;**66**(4):1040-1044

[29] Kaplan LJ, Kellum JA. Initial pH, base deficit, lactate, anion gap, strong ion difference, and strong ion gap predict outcome from major vascular injury. Critical Care Medicine. 2004;**32**(5):1120-1124

[30] Husain FA, Martin MJ, Mullenix PS, Steele SR, Elliott DC. Serum lactate and base deficit as predictors of mortality and morbidity. American Journal of Surgery. 2003;**185**:485-491

[31] Leskovan JJ et al. Anion gap as a predictor of trauma outcomes in the older trauma population: Correlations with injury severity and mortality. The American Surgeon. 2013;**79**(11):1203-1206

[32] Smith BP et al. Review of abdominal damage control and open abdomens: Focus on gastrointestinal complications. Journal of Gastrointestinal and Liver Diseases. 2010;**19**(4):425-435

[33] Stawicki SP et al. The concept of damage control: Extending the paradigm to emergency general surgery. Injury. 2008;**39**(1):93-101

[34] Stawicki SP, Cipolla J, Bria C. Comparison of open abdomens in nontrauma and trauma patients: A retrospective study. International Journal of Academic Medicine. 2016;**2**(3):51

[35] Joynt GM, Lipman J. Gastric intramucosal pH and blood lactate in severe sepsis. Anaesthesia. 1997;**52**:726-732

[36] Davis JW, Kaups KL, Parks SN. Base deficit is superior to pH in evaluating clearance of acidosis after traumatic

shock. Journal of Trauma and Acute Care Surgery. 1998;**44**(1):114-118

[37] Berndtson AE et al. Strong ion difference and gap predict outcomes after adult burn injury. Journal of Trauma and Acute Care Surgery. 2013;**75**(4):555-561

[38] Sen S et al. Strong ion gap is associated with mortality in pediatric burn injuries. Journal of Burn Care & Research. 2014;**35**(4):337-341

[39] Cameron J, A C. Current Surgical Therapy. 12th ed. Philadelphia, PA: Elsevier; 2017

[40] Stawicki SP et al. Intensivist use of hand-carried ultrasonography to measure IVC collapsibility in estimating intravascular volume status: Correlations with CVP. Journal of the American College of Surgeons. 2009;**209**(1):55-61

[41] Stawicki SP et al. Prospective evaluation of intravascular volume status in critically ill patients: Does inferior vena cava collapsibility correlate with central venous pressure? Journal of Trauma and Acute Care Surgery. 2014;**76**(4):956-964

[42] Stawicki SP et al. Correlations between pulmonary artery pressures and inferior vena cava collapsibility in critically ill surgical patients: An exploratory study. International Journal of Critical Illness and Injury Science. 2016;**6**(4):194

[43] Ferrada P, Evans D, Wolfe L. Findings of a randomized controlled trial using limited transthoracic echocardiogram (LTTE) as a hemodynamic monitoring tool in the trauma bay. Journal of Trauma and Acute Care Surgery. 2014;**76**:31

[44] Cavallaro F et al. Diagnostic accuracy of passive leg raising for prediction of fluid responsiveness in adults: Systematic review and meta-analysis of clinical studies. Intensive Care Medicine. 2010;**36**:1475-1483

[45] Marik PE et al. Dynamic changes in arterial waveform derived variables and fluid responsiveness in mechanically ventilated patients: A systematic review of the literature. Critical Care Medicine. 2009;**37**:2642-2647

[46] Miller A, Mandeville J. Predicting and measuring fluid responsiveness with echocardiography. Echo Research and Practice. 2016;**3**(2):G1-G12

[47] Marik PE, Baram M, Vahid B. Does central venous pressure predict fluid responsiveness? A systematic review of the literature and the tale of seven mares. Chest. 2008;**134**:172-178

[48] Kent A et al. Sonographic evaluation of intravascular volume status in the surgical intensive care unit: A prospective comparison of subclavian vein and inferior vena cava collapsibility index. Journal of Surgical Research. 2013;**184**(1):561-566

[49] Kent A et al. Sonographic evaluation of intravascular volume status: Can internal jugular or femoral vein collapsibility be used in the absence of IVC visualization? Annals of Thoracic Medicine. 2015;**10**(1):44

[50] Stawicki SP et al. Dynamic behavior of venous collapsibility and central venous pressure during standardized crystalloid bolus: A prospective, observational, pilot study. International Journal of Critical Illness and Injury Science. 2015;**5**(2):80

[51] Patil P et al. Correlations between venous collapsibility and common hemodynamic and ventilatory parameters: A multi-variable assessment. OPUS. 2014;**12**:495-500

[52] Reinhart K et al. New approaches to sepsis: Molecular diagnostics and biomarkers. Clinical Microbiology Reviews. 2012;**25**(4):609-634

[53] Schultz M et al. Use of the prognostic biomarker suPAR in the emergency department improves risk stratification but has no effect on mortality: A cluster-randomized clinical trial (TRIAGE III). Scandinavian Journal of Trauma, Resuscitation and Emergency Medicine. 2018;**26**(1):69

[54] Kutcher ME et al. Extracellular histone release in response to traumatic injury: Implications for a compensatory role of activated protein C. The Journal of Trauma and Acute Care Surgery. 2012;**73**(6):1389-1394

[55] Abrams ST et al. Circulating histones are mediators of trauma-associated lung injury. American Journal of Respiratory and Critical Care Medicine. 2013;**187**(2):160-169

[56] Adrian H et al. Biomarkers of traumatic brain injury: Temporal changes in body fluids. eNeuro. 2016;**3**(6):ENEURO.0294 to 16.2016. Available from: https://search.crossref.org/?q=10.1523%2FENEURO.0294-16.2016

[57] Undén L et al. Validation of the Scandinavian guidelines for initial management of minimal, mild and moderate traumatic brain injury in adults. BMC Medicine. 2015;**13**:292

[58] Lee JY et al. A role of serum-based neuronal and glial markers as potential predictors for distinguishing severity and related outcomes in traumatic brain injury. Journal of Korean Neurosurgical Association. 2015;**58**(2):93-100

[59] Lin S, Gregory RI. MicroRNA biogenesis pathways in cancer. Nature Reviews. Cancer. 2015;**15**:321

[60] Wong LL et al. MicroRNA and heart failure. International Journal of Molecular Sciences. 2016;**17**(4):502

[61] Gilje PLU et al. The association between plasma miR-122-5p release pattern at admission and all-cause mortality or shock after out-of-hospital cardiac arrest. Biomarkers. 2019;**24**(1):29-35

[62] Devaux Y et al. Incremental value of circulating MiR-122-5p to predict outcome after out of hospital cardiac arrest. Theranostics. 2017;**7**(10):2555-2564

[63] Xiao J et al. MicroRNA-134 as a potential plasma biomarker for the diagnosis of acute pulmonary embolism. Journal of Translational Medicine. 2011;**9**:159

[64] Hassan N, Zhao JT, Sidhu SB. The role of microRNAs in the pathophysiology of adrenal tumors. Molecular and Cellular Endocrinology. 2017;**456**:36-43

[65] Vincent JL, Moreno R. Clinical review: Scoring systems in the critically ill. Critical Care. 2010;**14**(2):207

[66] Moreno RP et al. SAPS 3--from evaluation of the patient to evaluation of the intensive care unit. Part 2: Development of a prognostic model for hospital mortality at ICU admission. Intensive Care Medicine. 2005;**31**(10):1345-1355

[67] Lance M. A general review of major global coagulation assays: Thrombelastography, thrombin generation test and clot waveform analysis. Thrombosis Journal. 2015;**13**:1

[68] Cannesson M et al. The ability of stroke volume variations obtained with Vigileo/FloTrac system to monitor fluid responsiveness in mechanically ventilated patients. Anesthesia & Analgesia. 2009;**108**(2):513

[69] Hofer C. Assessment of stroke volume variation for prediction of fluid responsiveness using the modified FloTrac™ and PiCCOplus™ system. Critical Care. 2008;**12**(3):R82

Chapter 4

Hemorrhagic Shock

Fevzi Sarper Türker

Abstract

Hemorrhagic shock is a type of hypovolemic shock, where intravascular blood loss and consequent alterations in the cell due to the hypoxia result in tissue and organ dysfunction, leading to death, once a certain threshold level is exceeded. Inadequate oxygen delivery results with Na/K ATPase pump dysfunction and cell death by this way, but erythrocytes do not use oxygen for their survival. A depolarizing protein can be a reason under in vivo conditions. In severe injury, rapid loss of 25% and more blood volume cause irreversible shock. For blood restoration, crystalloid solutions temporarily provide a practical approach, but they cannot replace the lost erythrocyte mass occurred due to bleeding, and they have no therapeutic value. Excessive use causes several problems, especially coagulopathy and increases the mortality risk. The prompt transfer of patient to an ultimate center for treatment, use of blood and blood products in the treatment, and a swift restoration of hemorrhage source are essential. Tourniquet use in the extremities and balloon occlusion of the aorta can be lifesaving.

Keywords: hemorrhagic shock, hemorrhage, blood restoration, injury

1. Introduction

Hemorrhagic shock develops as a result of intravascular volume loss due to bleeding out of the body or into the anatomical spaces inside, causing insufficient oxygen delivery to the cells. Hemorrhagic shock is a type of hypovolemic shock. If the bleeding does not stop, inadequate oxygen supply may lead to death. Hemorrhagic shock in trauma patients is a predictor of worse outcomes and contributes to early mortality [1]. Intracellular synthesis of anaerobic metabolites impairs hemostasis, resulting in cell death, apoptosis, or necroptosis. Shock may develop due to several reasons including trauma, maternal hemorrhage, gastrointestinal hemorrhage, perioperative hemorrhage, or ruptured aneurysms [2]. Mortality due to bleeding is substantial on a global scale. Annually, 60,000 people in the US and 1.9 million people in the world lose their lives due to hemorrhage and its consequences. Out of them, 1.5 million people die of physical trauma around the world each year [3]. Unexpectedly, trauma affects young people; 1.5 million deaths per year cause an approximate loss of 75 million life year. In addition, functional outcomes are poor, and the long-term mortality rates are high in the hemorrhage survivors [4, 5].

Hemorrhage and hemorrhagic shock treatment is quite difficult and complex procedure as mentioned above. Although our knowledge related to hemorrhagic shock physiopathology has increased, our success in the treatment is limited by failure in injuries and still has high mortality rates. Control of bleeding should be the first priority, but resuscitation should be conducted through crystalloid fluids in the way that it will not form coagulopathy in order to protect hypoxia at the cellular level and so tissues and organs in case where the control cannot be assumed. Crystalloid solutions do not have superiority over each other, and there is not any type of treatment which is absolutely recommended apart from that they are kept limited.

1.1 Brief history

As proposed by the historians, the first written definition of shock is made by Celsus (AD 20) after a penetrating heart injury as "The pulse fades away, the color is extremely pallid, cold and malodorous sweats break out the body as if the body has been wetted by dew, the extremities become cold and death quickly follows" [6]. LeDran, a military surgeon, derived a word from shock as "The bullet thrown from the gunpowder acquires such rapid force that the whole animal participates in the jarring (shock and agitation)" in his article in 1743 [7].

The emergence of biochemistry at the beginning of the twentieth century started serious scientific studies on the pathogenesis of circulatory shock. A number of physiologists agreed on the existence of a toxin released in response to injury, and it was identified to be histamine by Walter Cannon in the US and by Sir Henry Dale in England [8, 9]. However, neither histamine nor other identified vasoactive amines could successively mimic the picture of shock. In the late 1920s and 1930s, Blalock suggested an alternative hypothesis for shock and defined it as direct fluid loss from blood circulation culminating in peripheral vascular failure, a persistence of poor peripheral perfusion. After the proposal of this hypothesis, fluid replacement has become the principal therapy for circulatory shock.

Compilation of Artz and Fitts on that blood and fluids with salt are needed for closing the volume gap occurring after hemorrhage was not commonly appreciated [10]. This concept was supported by highlighting that saline solution should be given in ongoing hemorrhage later [11]. Kinney and Wells criticized the current immediate therapeutic attention to the many problems associated with trauma without regard to the patient's ventilation. Their article established a new objective: therapy in all injured patients should look beyond blood pressure so as to ensure provision and maintenance of effective gas exchange of tissues [12]. While Lansing et al. defended the need for vasoactive medicines for perfusion of vital organs, Nickerson and Gourzis defended the disadvantages of vasoconstriction [13, 14].

The term "golden hour" is widely attributed to R. Adams Cowley, founder of Baltimore's renowned Shock Trauma Institute, who in a 1975 article stated, "the first hour after injury will largely determine a critically injured person's chances for survival"—this was in an era characterized by a lack of an organized trauma system and inadequate prehospital care. The validity of this concept remains controversial. An analogous concept, the "platinum 10 minutes" places a time constraint on the prehospital care of seriously injured patients: no patient should have more than 10 min of scene-time stabilization by the prehospital team prior to transport to definitive care at a trauma center [15].

2. Physiopathology and metabolic alterations

Early theories suggesting that hemorrhagic shock resulted from nervous system dysfunction or from a toxin released from ischemic tissue have been disproved completely. The current view for the underlying mechanism of hemorrhagic shock states that the blood loss leads to an insufficient oxygen delivery to the tissues and consequently activates several homeostatic mechanisms in order to maintain vital organ perfusion [2]. The metabolic changes observed in hemorrhagic shock sustain energy homeostasis to ensure cell vitality [16]. When looking at the cellular and tissue level and if whole organism is taken into consideration, it is observed that the complexity of these events is clarified via the physical trauma-related tissue damage and by the relative effects of hypoperfusion due to hemorrhage. Sufficient oxygen to meet the metabolic requirements of the tissues cannot be supplied due to hemorrhagic shock. Cells switch from aerobic to anaerobic respiration due to hypoperfusion. Lactic acid, inorganic phosphates, and oxygen radicals begin to accumulate as a result of the mounting oxygen debt [17]. In 1877, Claude Bernard discovered that hemorrhage stimulated liver to provide glucose from the lasting glycogen stores [18]. The Second World War enforced the investigators to better understand the pathophysiology of shock. Cuthbertson described the metabolic alterations in two phases: "ebb" phase and "flow" phase. The former representing the reduction in the requirement for both oxygen and temperature followed by the latter is characterized by increase in energy and temperature requirement with consequent elevation of body temperature [19]. With fatal injuries or blood loss, a stage called "necrobiosis" occurs prior to death as defined by Stoner, where the oxygen consumption is reduced and the body temperature decreases [20–22]. Hypoxia due to shock leads to reduction in energy consumption and leads to a hypermetabolic state, where neurohumoral homeostasis increases glucose uptake to supply muscles. If shock persists, glycogen stores are depleted, and glucose is supplied by gluconeogenesis stimulated by hormones. If this process fails, the hyperglycemia turns into hypoglycemia. Pearce and Drucker suggest that glucose infusion during hemorrhagic shock is the cause for extension of life span, since homeostasis uses glucose as an energy substrate for its defense mechanisms [23]. Gann and Foster provided an alternative explanation by defining nonmetabolic role of glucose that is a critical factor. The glucose level is elevated rapidly as a result of hormonal response to injury and this causes the intracellular fluids to move to facilitate restoration of blood volume [24].

The release of damage-associated molecular patterns (DAMPs or alarmins) containing mitochondrial DNA and formyl peptides triggers systemic inflammatory response (SIRS) [25]. Eventually, the cellular homeostasis collapses by depletion of ATP resources, and membrane rupture results in necrosis, apoptosis or necroptosis and cell death [2]. At the tissue level, hypovolemia and vasoconstriction cause hypoperfusion and end organ damage in kidneys, intestines, and skeletal muscles, leading to a multiorgan failure. In the body, pulselessness occurs after a blood loss due to a severe hemorrhage and causes hypoperfusion to the brain and the myocardium, resulting in consequent cerebral anoxia and fatal arrhythmias developing in minutes [26]. Hemorrhage also causes substantial alterations in the vascular endothelium all over the body. Blood and endothelium act together for forming thrombus in the bleeding area [27].

Hemorrhage and shock continue, and both adaptive and maladaptive changes begin to occur in the blood. The coagulation cascade and platelets are activated to form a hemostatic plug in the hemorrhage source [28]. Probably to prevent the development of microvascular thrombosis, fibrinolytic activity increases away from hemorrhage site [29]. The mounting oxygen debt and the elevated catecholamine levels cause a sort of endotheliopathy due to the systemic degradation of the endothelial glycocalyx barrier. Autoheparinization due to increased plasmin activation and glycocalyx degradation result in hyperfibrinolysis and diffuse coagulopathy [27, 29, 30]. A hypercoagulable phenotype is present in almost half of the trauma patients [30]. Reduced platelet activity and margination contribute to hemorrhage and decreased platelet counts, increasing the mortality [31, 32]. Excessive fluid crystalloid resuscitations reduce the coagulation factor levels and decrease oxygen transfer capacity. Cold infusions increase hemorrhagic heat loss, cause energy store depletion, and reduce enzyme functions in the coagulation cascade [33]. Acidosis caused by hypoperfusion becomes more intense due to the excessive administration of the acidic crystalloid solutions. This eventually impairs the functioning of the coagulation factors and results in a vicious cycle, where coagulopathy, hypothermia, and acidosis occur [34].

The valid opinion is that the first response to a serious injury and shock is a robust and innate SIRS followed by a relative immunosuppression state called as compensatory anti-inflammatory response syndrome (CARS), bringing along a period of recovery. If a complication occurs, the cycle will repeat with a newly formed SIRS followed by CARS. While the innate proinflammatory and anti-inflammatory immunity genes are upregulated after the injury, the adaptive immunity genes are downregulated simultaneously. During the recovery period of patients without complications, these responses rapidly decrease to baseline. On the other hand, in patients with complications, the reduction of the excessive response to normal levels occurs more slowly [35].

2.1 Volume restoration

For restoration of impaired energy metabolism, reduced intravascular volume should be replaced immediately. Baue et al. have found out that both colloidal and erythrocyte free fluids meet the requirements for the oxidative metabolism to take place; however, the rapid dilution of hematocrit increases the cardiac output, cardiac workload, and the peripheral circulation [36]. The intravascular circulating volume is more effective in maintaining the energy metabolism compared to the circulating erythrocyte mass [37]. An acute loss in the circulating volume of less than 25% requires an urgent attention since the hematocrit level can be reduced more than 50% before a critical shortage of red blood cells becomes evident. The restoration of the plasma volume after a long duration of hemorrhage has been attributed to the osmotic activity in the capillary bed, induced by the hyperglycemia occurring as a result of hypovolemic shock; however, this has not been proven to be true because a transcapillary osmotic gradient does not develop. Monitoring the cardiac output is a reliable method to evaluate the reduction in the blood flow and to observe the effects of the oxidative metabolism and catecholamine response [38]. Consistent with the observations of Blalock, at the beginning of the shock, blood pressure is an insufficient parameter to demonstrate the status of the circulation. Similarly, no correlations have been found out among the blood glucose levels, hemodynamic changes, and the levels of plasma insulin during hypovolemia [16].

Maintaining the blood volume after the hemorrhage occurs in two phases. The first is initiated by a fall in the capillary of hydrostatic pressure, stopping until when the sum of the capillary hydrostatic pressure and the oncotic pressures equals the sum of interstitial hydrostatic and oncotic pressures. In the second phase, albumin is moved to the capillaries in response to the increase in interstitial pressure. This increase of osmotic pressure in the interstitial space is maintained by the osmotic gradient in the cell membrane caused by the presence of extracellular glucose. While glucose is produced due to the effects of counter-regulatory hormones including cortisol, glucagon, catecholamines, vasopressin, and angiotensin, insulin secretion is inhibited concomitantly. Blockage of any of these hormones will impair the restoration of blood volume. Cortisol is the most critical hormone because the absence of it, the restoration of the blood volume will fail completely [39].

In order for blood volume to be completely restored, all cardiovascular variables, including the cardiac output, are required to be reestablished [40, 41]. In hemorrhage up to a blood loss of 25% of the whole volume, reestablishment of the parameters takes approximately 48 hours. If the hemorrhage-associated blood loss exceeds 26% or more of the blood volume, the restoration of the blood volume will fail [42]. Na/K ATPase pump is essential for the sustainability of the cellular transmembrane potential;

however, the activity of this pump is inhibited in all kinds of circulatory shock. This inhibition is considered to be associated with the impairment in the oxygen delivery. The disturbances in the Na/K ATPase activity cannot only be due to the impairments in the oxygen delivery since erythrocytes do not consume oxygen. The findings of Shire show that intravascular volume loss more than 26% indicates the same threshold value as that of an experimental reduction in the transmembrane potential. This phenomenon is initially observed in the muscle cells followed by the observation in the erythrocytes as well [43, 44].

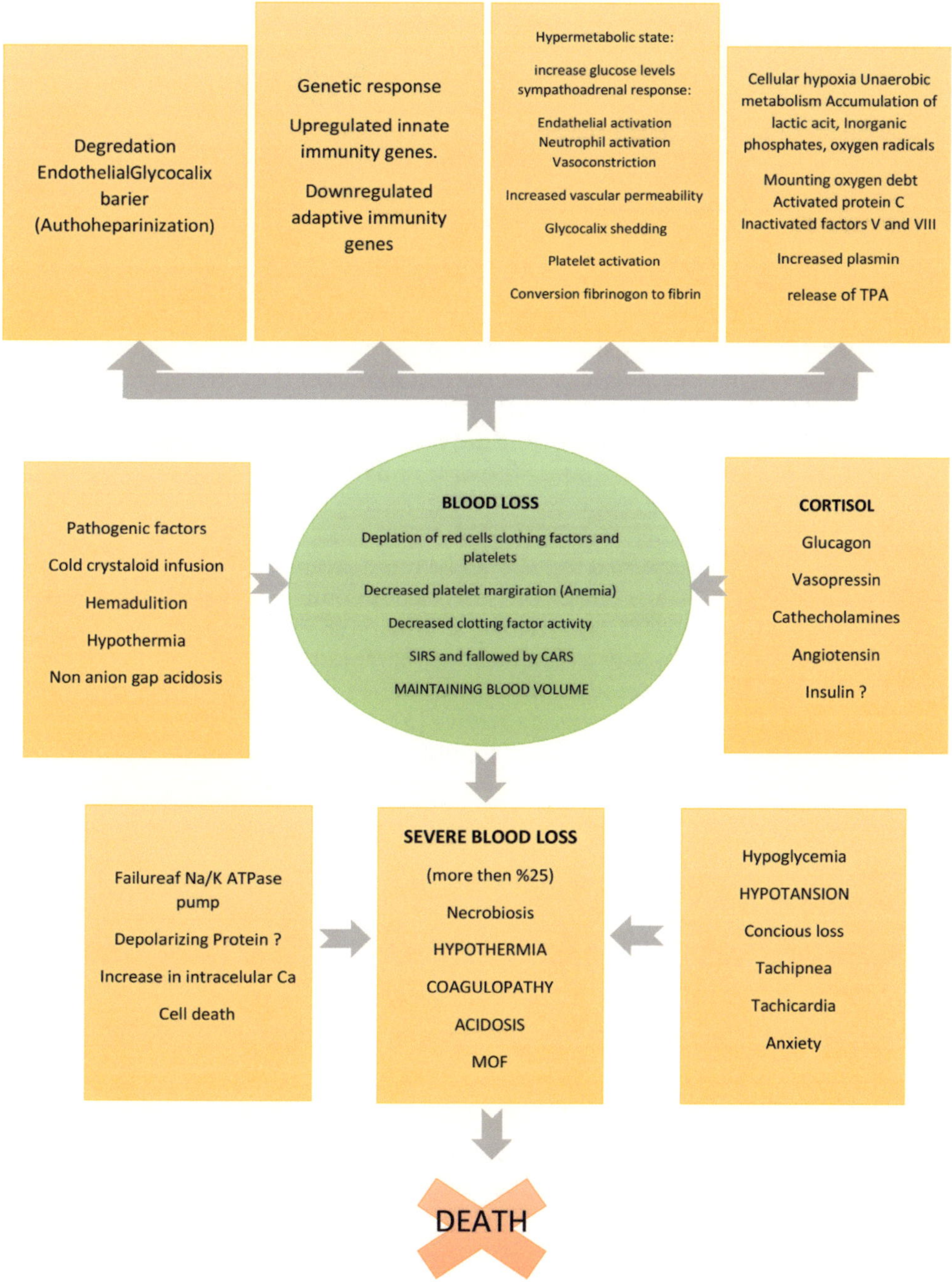

Figure 1.
Physiopathologic alterations in hemorrhage and hemorrhagic shock.

Evans et al. have reported a protein, which occurs in the first 20 minutes of serious hemorrhage in the rats, depolarizing several cells in a number of species [45]. Boulanger et al. have confirmed this finding in dogs with serious hemorrhage [46]. Jones et al. noted that this substance reduced both the contractility and velocity in the isolated and perfused rat hearts, reporting that this depolarizing protein was potentially effective in the development of cardiogenic shock [47]. This led to the conclusion that this hypothetical protein should be the similar underlying cause for three types of circulatory shock.

The experiments testing this hypothesis and looking for the significant consequences of cell depolarization isolated adenosine as the stimulating factor [48]. It was demonstrated that adenosine enhanced the ATPase activity and provided survival for hours during the experimental hemorrhagic shock in rats. Following these results, the stimulation of the Na/K ATPase pump showed the significance of inhibition in shock states. The inhibition of the pump should have a critical effect on mortality [49] (**Figure 1**).

3. Diagnosis

The early recognition of hemorrhagic shock and stopping hemorrhage is lifesaving as it takes only 2 hours from its start until death [50]. In order to limit the severity level and duration of shock and to replace mounted oxygen debt, a prompt control of the origin of hemorrhage and the restoration of the intravascular volume and oxygen transfer capacity is essential [51].

Traumatic injuries are the fourth and are the first reason for deaths under the age of 45 in the United States. About 80% of traumatic injuries are blunt and the majority of the deaths progress as secondary following the hypovolemic shock. Intraperitoneal bleeding occurs in 12% of blunt traumas, and it is essential to be promptly detected. The optimal test should be rapid, accurate, and noninvasive. Diagnostic peritoneal lavage (DPL) was historically conducted in the diagnosis of hemoperitoneum. While DPL is extremely sensitive (96–99%) and specific (98%), it is an invasive procedure with a complication rate more than 1%. However, it is quite confusing to assess hemodynamically unstable patients for whom it is late and who are brought out of the emergency service [52].

In an emergency situation, ultrasonography can provide guiding insights into a patient's condition or injury pattern and is considered to be a highest priority technological tool that deserves evaluation. The ultrasound protocols used comprised focused assessment with sonography for trauma (FAST), prehospital lung ultrasound (PLUS), and focused echocardiography in emergency life support (FEEL). By combining the standard examination according to the FAST protocol (detection of internal bleeding) with pleural and lung ultrasound (PLUS) and echocardiography (FEEL), important life-threatening conditions, such as pneumothorax and cardiac tamponade, can be ruled out [53].

In irreversible shock, sodium accumulates within the cell due to the inhibition of Na/K ATPase pump. The direction of exchange of sodium and calcium is reversed, and calcium starts accumulating within the cells. Increasing levels of intracellular calcium causes proteolytic enzyme activation leading to degradation of the organelles of cells and at end cell death [54]. This definitely irreversible condition was first observed by Holden et al. under the electron microscope [55].

3.1 Assessment of hemorrhagic shock

The recently introduced physiological or therapeutic classification of hemorrhagic shock is based on basic physiological principles. It takes the fluid-blood replacement resistant hypotension and natural hemostatic mechanisms of the body into account as well as considering the role of the I-R and SIR triggered by ischemia [56].

In critical shock conditions, the circulating blood volume is insufficient, and brain and heart internal circulations are merely holding as a result of the systemic vasoconstriction from chemoreceptor and central nervous system receptor stimulation. Although the endogenous vasomotor/vasoconstrictor compensatory mechanisms are impaired in severe shock, blood volume sufficient to maintain the perfusion exists. In moderate shock, the compensatory mechanism is ongoing, while a mild shock state means only a little blood loss [56].

The total blood volume in relation to body weight is determined to be 70 ml/kg in adults, 80 ml/kg in infants, and between 80 and 90 ml/kg in newborns. Transfusion blood or erythrocyte suspension of 10 U or more in volume is defined as a massive blood transfusion, receiving more attention how to determine the required amount. Cancio et al. pointed out the need for identifying logistic requirements during combat to prevent mortality [57].

To measure the efficacy of fluid replacement, it was attempted to measure the diameter of the vena cava by ultrasound before and after the fluid resuscitation. A failure of an increase in the diameter suggested an inadequate treatment [58]. Ferrada et al. examined the inferior vena cava in echocardiography in order to quantify the volume status in severely injured patients. They used this technique to determine pharmacological interventions and monitor the fluid treatment [59].

3.2 Signs and symptoms

It is difficult to identify the signs and symptoms of hemorrhagic shock, especially if hemorrhage is originated from occult source. The presence of hypotension is an insensitive marker due to compensatory mechanisms until the blood volume loss reaches up to 30% of the total blood volume. Early posttrauma hypotension is associated with multiple organ failure (MOF) and development of infectious complications [60]. Nonspecific clinical symptoms including anxiety, tachypnea, and weakened peripheral pulses and mottled, pale, and cold extremities can be more indicative for diagnosis of shock. In regard to classification for severity of shock, for a 70-kg male patient in Class I shock, the blood volume loss is less than 750 ml, which accounts for 15% of the total blood volume, and the only clinical symptom may be a mild form of anxiety. Class II hemorrhage involves blood volume loss to 1500 ml, accounting for 30% of total blood volume. Patients look moderately anxious with a narrow pulse around 120 beats per minute. The respiratory rate is increased and reached over 20 breaths per minute. In Class III hemorrhage, blood volume loss is up to 2000 cc, accounting for 40% of total blood volume. The patient has tachycardia with a heart rate up to 140 beats/min, while the blood pressure is reduced. The patient is observed to be severely anxious, and the loss of consciousness may occur. Class IV patients are lethargic with severe hypotension and tachycardia. The respiration rate is over 35/min. Promising technologies, such as portable incident darkfield microscopy allowing for a simultaneous assessment of the compensatory reserve index and the microvascular bed, may help clinicians to promptly diagnose the patients in shock [2, 61, 62].

Potential bleeding source, such as hematemesis or hematochezia, significant vaginal bleeding, or bleeding from an aneurysm of the abdominal aorta should be identified. Bleeding from the extremities can easily be observed after trauma; however, the intensity of bleeding may not be severe in shock states. The body regions including the proximal thigh and retroperitoneal region can accumulate large amounts of blood, and this volume loss can easily be missed unless it is examined during the initial assessments. The intracavitary spaces in the body like the chest, abdomen, and the pelvis should immediately be examined after trauma by radiologic imaging [2]. An immediate examination of these cavities with chest and pelvic radiograms and focused assessment with sonography for trauma (FAST) can help diagnose the potential sites of bleeding [63]. Ultrasound is also used in the diagnostic evaluation of ectopic pregnancies, abdominal aortic aneurysm ruptures, and uterine hemorrhages, which may remain hidden as bleeding foci. Echocardiography is used for assessing cardiac filling and contractility [64] (**Table 1**).

3.3 Laboratory measures

Blood gas analysis and the markers of hypoperfusion may help quantify the base deficit and the lactate levels. The ratio of heart rate to systolic arterial pressure termed as shock index and better predicts massive transfusion compared with traditional vital signs in trauma patients. In a retrospective study including 302 primary postpartum hemorrhage patients, Sohn et al. confirmed that an increased initial shock index is associated with the need for massive transfusion, and also lactate is a better predictor for blood requirements in trauma patients. Also, it is a robust predictor of requirement for massive transfusion in hemodynamically stable shock patients [65].

In a study, Lee et al. lactate has a prognostic role in patients with nonvariceal upper gastrointestinal bleeding higher lactate clearance rate (%/hr) within 24 hours after admission was associated with lower 30-day rebleeding rate. Higher initial, maximal, and average lactate levels within 24 hour after admission were associated with higher 30-day mortality rate and a more frequent admission over 7 days [66].

Hemoglobin and international normalized ratio (INR) values are used to determine the need for a massive blood transfusion in patients with severe hemorrhage [67]. Thrombocyte count and fibrinogen levels should be examined and treated to return to normal levels. Electrolyte levels, especially the levels of calcium and potassium, should be monitored at frequent intervals because fluctuations may occur during resuscitation with blood or blood products [33, 68]. Finally, any presence of coagulopathies should be diagnosed and resuscitation with blood products should be monitored by evaluating the clot-formation kinetics by means of viscoelastic testing such as thromboelastography or rotational thromboelastometry [69]. All these tests allow for determining the severity of shock, the extent to which the blood bank resources will be used, and will identify the type of coagulopathy.

3.4 Radiology

A computed tomography scan, which is commonly used for diagnostic means, should be immediately performed in critical patients for whom the origin of the

Critical HS	Shock with heart and brain involvement or > 40% TBV loss (impending CV collapse) → Stand-by surgery for source control
Severe HS	Shock with hypotension not responding to blood/fluid load-test (unstably unstable) → Rapid surgery for source control
Moderate/ Mild HS	Moderate shock is hypotensive shock responding with normotension and reverse tachycardia trend to blood/ fluid overload (unstably stable); mild shock is normotensive tachycardic from start → Investigate, Ponder surgery, Interventional radiology/ Non-operative intervention

*Hypotension may occur at ≥ 20% and is always present at ≥ 30% TBV loss; **by response is meant reverse tachycardia trend and normalization of pressure; HS: Haemorrhagic shock; TBV: Total blood volume; CV: Cardiovascular

Table 1.
Summary of hemorrhage/hemorrhagic shock and treatment modalities.

bleeding cannot be identified once the clinical picture is stable. CT remains the gold standard for diagnosing intra-abdominal injuries detecting as little as 100 cc of intraperitoneal fluid [52]. CT prompt approaches with intraoperative exploration, angiography, embolization, or gastrointestinal endoscopy may help in achieving better diagnostic and treatment outcomes [2].

Ultrasound has severe benefits on evolution and treatment of trauma patients. Bedside examination, easy way and cheap, never needs contrast and radiation source, reproducibility are advantages of it. In Europe, during the 1970s, the use of ultrasound to detect intraperitoneal fluid was first described. FAST is an ultrasound protocol for assessing hemoperitoneum and hemopericardium. Sensitivity of this protocol is 85–96% and specificity is over 98%. In the subset of hypotensive trauma patients, the sensitivity of the FAST exam approaches 100%. Experienced physicians perform the FAST exam less than 5 minutes, and its use decreases time to surgical intervention, patient length of stay, and rates of CT and DPL. Recently, many institutions have introduced the Extended FAST (eFAST) protocol into their trauma algorithms. The eFAST examines each hemithorax for the presence of hemothoraces and pneumothoraces [52].

4. Resuscitation

4.1 Prehospital care

Time is everything. Causa prima: optimization should be performed in cardiogenic shock, and treatment should be aimed at the underlying cause in hemorrhagic and septic shock. Survival of the patients with time-sensitive disorders like myocardial infarction or stroke can be made possible with prehospital arrangements, which should be performed in the patients with severe hemorrhage as well [70]. Minimizing the bleeding and limiting fluid resuscitation with large peripheral vascular access and immediate transfer to a center for ultimate treatment are limited options for prehospital care. Recent findings have demonstrated that when the patient can immediately be transported to the healthcare center for treatment, applying tourniquets to the proximal extremities to the origin of bleeding is lifesaving without leading to dysfunction or amputation of the extremities [71, 72]. Recent guidelines accept application of tourniquets in patients in whom direct compression cannot be performed during the first-aid procedures or during the prehospital interventions [73, 74]. In large injuries or injuries in joints such as groin and axilla, where tourniquets cannot be applied, a group of newly introduced homeostatic dressings have been demonstrated to be of benefit [75]. Canon demonstrated that, in a patient with a penetrating injury in the torso, delaying the intravenous fluid treatment starting from the urban treatment center until admission to the hospital for final treatment contributes to survival probably by preventing the development of dilutional coagulopathy [76].

Bickell et al. compared the outcomes of immediate and delayed fluid therapies in hypotensive patients with penetrating injuries and found out that survival rates at 62 and 70% were higher and serious complication rates from 30 to 23% were lower in delayed fluid treatment. In contrast to the predictions, the delayed fluid treatment was not disadvantageous but timesaving. The principal motivation of the treatment is to ensure a fast recovery in the patient with an acute injury favoring the transport of the patient compared to primary stabilization [77]. A number of experimental studies on animals' standard resuscitation associated with decreased oxygen delivery, increased rates of hemorrhage, reperfusion injuries, organ failures, and coagulopathies [16].

Duton et al. challenged the findings reported by Bickel et al. and suggested to limit the fluid therapy maintain systolic blood pressure around 70 mmHg using an intermediate approach rather than 100 mmHg as it is in the conventional standard methods. The results did not demonstrate any significant benefit in mortality [78].

In regard to damage control resuscitation (DCR), Holcomb suggested an exchange of plasma with limited amounts of volume and crystalloids and proposed an early use of plasma with limited support for systolic blood pressure [79]. Plasma helps prevent coagulopathy due to acidosis and hypothermia. In the daily clinical practice, the patients treated with conventional methods were compared with the patients to whom DCR was applied, resulting in findings favoring DCR. Increasing the blood volume may prevent the development of both acidosis and hypothermia. Plasma contains coagulation factors activated by temperature and brings the hydrogen ion concentrations to normal levels [80].

There is not any proof on that fluids are superior over each other in patients with trauma in the literature. Due to the fact that colloidal fluids quickly increase oncotic pressure, they are much faster than the plasma expansion colloidal fluids. Although crystalloids are cheap, benefits of colloid applications on survival could not be proved in the studies [81]. In a review of clinical studies dating back to 2002 with safety data documented in ICU patients who received hydroxyethyl starch (HES), gelatin, dextran, or albumin, Groeneveld et al. showed that impaired coagulation, clinical bleeding, and acute kidney injury were frequently reported after HES infusion [82].

Although blood to plasma ratios have not been definitely established yet, their increase from 1:8 to 1:1.4 provided a decrease in the mortality rates from 64 to 9% in injured patients with approximately the same severity [83]. Kashuk et al. reported that blood-plasma ratios of 1:2 improved the mortality rates and that fluid replacements with lactated ringer solution resulted in increased international normalized ratios [84]. A multi-center study reported that the daily clinical use of plasma-red blood cell ratios at 1:1 or more in civilians reduced the 24-hour mortality rates by half [85].

In the treatment of hemorrhagic shock, Velasco et al. brought resuscitation with hypertonic saline solution (HTS) to the forefront. Their studies were conducted both on animals and on the patients in hemorrhagic or septic shock using either HTS alone or HTS and 6% dextrane combination [86]. Vassar et al. reported the efficacy of the latter combination in injured patients in their country [87]. The purpose of this combination lied on the fact that HTS moved the intracellular fluid to the extracellular space, while dextrane kept a significant amount of that fluid in the vascular bed. The relative efficacy of 7.5% NaCl did not cause a significant change in the survival rates regardless of its use either alone or in combination with dextrane; however, it has been demonstrated that this mode of treatment increased the costs [88]. The Resuscitation Outcomes Consortium found out that neither HTS nor hypertonic dextrane solution provided benefits compared to the fluid resuscitation with normal saline solution during the prehospitalization period in a mixed population of patients with either penetrating or blunt injuries [89]. Similarly, albumin did not provide any benefits over crystalloid solutions [90]. A recent retrospective analysis of a cohort, where trauma patients in the war were compared, demonstrated that a prehospital transfusion of an erythrocyte suspension or plasma or a combination of both, all provided significant benefits on survival. However, a number of studies being conducted currently have reported that they do not provide benefits in the daily practice [91]. Current practice shows that the radial pulse should be maintained in the patients with serious hemorrhage in the prehospital interventions, and crystalloid solutions should be used in relatively smaller quantities to keep the patients conscious [92].

4.2 Treatment

A successful resuscitation requires to stop the hemorrhage at all sources and to replace the intravascular volume immediately. These allow for preventing the mounting oxygen debt and replacing it [51]. In the trauma patients, a combination of damage-control surgery and damage-control resuscitation helps to achieve these objectives. In several hemorrhage cases except trauma, the patients similarly benefit from controlling the bleeding upon identifying the hemorrhage source and from resuscitation with blood and blood products [93–95].

The arrival of a patient with hemorrhage at the hospital first requires restoration of the intravascular volume with fluid replacement and hemorrhage control. The strategies in replacing the intravascular volume include the conventional fluid resuscitation with plasma, platelet, red blood cells, or whole blood. Massive blood transfusion can be performed with universal blood products including packed red cells, plasma, platelets, and cryoprecipitate in predetermined volumes accompanied with the administration of several pharmaceutical agents like calcium and tranexamic acid at the patient bedside. These treatment protocols provide benefits for patients with acute hemorrhage in regard to survival [95]. Multiple scoring systems guide the therapeutic teams in identifying the need for massive blood transfusion. Any delays in actualizing the treatment protocols increase the mortality rates [96].

A panel moderated by Sheldon et al. announced a warning stating that blood is the most dangerous drug we have ever used [97]. Potentially, the best alternative to replace the blood is the crystalloid solutions without colloid; its use should be followed by type-specific blood according to the specific need of a patient. The required multiple component therapy is provided by transfusing a single unit of whole blood. Increasing the hematocrit levels over 30% provides no benefits in injuries [98]. In a review evaluating the use of whole blood and blood expanders during the Vietnam war, Sheldon et al. suggested the use of type-specific fresh whole blood preferably [99]. Although the experts in the area agree that blood is the best fluid replacement therapy in hemorrhagic patients, blood transfusion is not free of risks. Therefore, the use of "blood substitutes" or administration of a blood component therapy or acellular oxygen carriers should be considered [98]. Gervin and Fischer have reported type-specific noncross-matched blood as a safer alternative option to the use of cross-matched blood [100].

Red blood cell, plasma, and platelet ratios provide clinical values; however, the ratios have not been definitely established yet. A systemic review and two prospective studies reported that plasma, platelet, and red blood cell ratios around 1:1:1 were safe and decreased the mortality rates in trauma-associated hemorrhages. The general use is to administer six units of plasma and one unit of platelets processed by apheresis for each six units of red blood cells, which constitute an equivalent to six units of pooled thrombocytes [95, 101, 102]. A platelet to red blood cell ratio of over 1:2 has been demonstrated to reduce the mortality in the first 48 hours; however, plasma use at these ratios has not provided any benefits [103]. Barry et al. a total of 17 studies were included in this meta-analysis and including total of 10,610 patients. High fresh frozen plasma (FFP) to packed red blood cell ratios result low posthemorrhage mortality; however, the need for further optimization is highlighted as evidenced by reported increase in post-damage control resuscitation (DCR) sepsis, MOF, and hospital lengths of stay among survivors [104].

All of these blood products contain citrate as an anticoagulant, which is metabolized rapidly by a healthy human liver. However, the use of high volumes of blood products may reach toxic doses in the patients in hemorrhagic shock and may lead to the development of life-threatening hypoglycemia and progressive coagulopathy

[68, 105]. Empirically, 1 gram of calcium chloride infusion can be administered following four units of blood product infusion, and the electrolyte levels should be monitored at frequent intervals.

Resuscitation with isotonic crystalloids has been in use for decades since the historical treatments for hemorrhage. However, isotonic crystalloids provide no intrinsic benefits other than increasing the intravascular volume temporarily. Complication rates are increased after high-volume infusions of isotonic crystalloids. The potential complications may include respiratory failure, compartment syndromes in the abdomen or in the extremities, and coagulopathy. In acute hemorrhagic trauma patients, it is recommended to administer crystalloid infusions in the first 6 hours of admission to the hospital, but the volume of infusion should not exceed 3 l [106]. Blood products are not included in this limit. No benefits of prehospital resuscitation with colloid, dextran, and hypertonic saline infusions have been demonstrated as discussed previously.

Pruit et al. found out that fluid resuscitation with normal saline was sufficient to replace both the blood loss and the sequestrated extravascular fluid in males with a moderate level of hemorrhage [107]. Lactated ringer's solution has found to be superior probably because it does not contain acetate or magnesium, and its chlorine content is low [108]. Recent studies stress that infusion of normal saline may lead to hyperchloremic acidosis. In addition, caution is advised against uncontrolled use of crystalloids [109, 110]. The experiences during the times of war showed that administration of blood in combination with protein-free fluids did not cause edema and did not lower the serum albumin levels in severely injured persons [111].

Procoagulant hemostatic such as activated recombinant factor VII, tranexamic acid, prothrombin complex concentrate, and fibrinogen concentrate can be included in the treatment in patients with hemorrhage [112]. The use of procoagulant hemostatic is off-label in patients receiving warfarin and in patients with hemophilia except for the use of prothrombin complex concentrate in the former group of patients and the use of activated recombinant factor VII and tranexamic acid in the latter, respectively. Vasopressin, included in the treatment of patients in hemorrhagic shock, reduces the need for administering blood products and fluids [113].

Prolonged hemostasis in pelvic fractures or in patients with a ruptured aneurysm of aorta or with gastrointestinal bleeding causes an increased need for blood transfusion, elevates the risk levels for mortality, or it may cause both of them simultaneously [114–116]. The duration of emergency department stay should be less than 10 minutes to make a diagnosis and start the initial treatment for trauma patients with hemorrhage in the body in order to keep the mortality risk at a relatively lower level [116]. Patients bleeding out of their extremities, who were applied tourniquets, should be immediately operated to perform a vascular exploration. In a patient bleeding into more than one space in the body, vascular exploration should be performed in the space where most of the bleeding occurs in order to reduce mortality [117].

Regardless of the origin of bleeding, the patients with abdominal or pelvic hemorrhage may benefit from the endovascular occlusion of the aorta as a temporary measure. This approach is called as resuscitative endovascular balloon occlusion of aorta (REBOA). In severe bleeding, this approach reduces the perfusion pressure distal to the origin of bleeding, increases the afterload, and the remaining blood volume is redirected especially to the brain and heart. REBOA reduces intraoperative mortality in patients with a ruptured aneurysm of the abdominal aorta [118]. The method can also be used in gastrointestinal bleeding or in peripartum hemorrhages [119].

Aoki et al. reported that the use of vasopressor agents increases mortality in the traumatic hemorrhagic shock in the retrospective cohort study [120].

5. Conclusion

The definite treatment of hemorrhage is to stop the bleeding in its source as soon as possible. However, almost all of these hemorrhages occur at locations away from the hospitals. The time from the start of the bleeding until the time of intervention and the ultimate treatment is critical in the management of hemorrhages occurring due to an illness or due to trauma. Then, the primary approach should aim to shorten this period. Critical time is considerably exceeded when the time required for fluid resuscitation is added to the time elapsed at the scene where hemorrhage occurred. Crystalloid solutions are always at our disposal, and they are cheap and available fluids for intravenous use. Physiological saline administration in high volumes is a cause for increased mortality. No kinds of crystalloid fluids are superior to the other. What can be their alternatives? Type-specific blood and blood products have limitations in their supply, storage, and transport to the event scene. If the supply of these products and their storage can be achieved especially in the absence of cold chain facilities, they can provide solutions to the existing issues; however, the near future is not promising at all in this respect. There is continuing research on the use of 0-type whole blood and the use of freeze-dried plasma in the management of patients with trauma-associated hemorrhage [121, 122].

Systems, preventing the blood loss mechanically, such as REBOA can be developed. Generally, the first people to arrive at the scene are paramedics and young doctors. The required time and feasibility of applying these systems to a patient with weakened or no peripheral pulses in the adverse conditions of the scene during the induced sense of panic should be reviewed and estimated in detail.

We may suggest that hemorrhage and hemorrhagic shock has been an issue since the initial existence of humanity. Initiated by a toxin hypothesis, the understanding in physiopathology of shock has already been advanced; however, our achievements in terms of creating solutions to the existing problems are still limited. Technology progresses at a faster pace in terms of creating a trauma, causing injuries, and killing people compared to its advances in maintaining survival.

Conflict of interest

There is no conflict of interest

Author details

Fevzi Sarper Türker
Elazığ Town Hospital, Cardiovascular Surgery Clinic, University of Health Sciences, Elazığ, Turkey

*Address all correspondence to: sarperturker@gmail.com

References

[1] Kauvar DS, Lefering R, Wade CE. Impact of hemorrhage on trauma outcome: An overview of epidemiology, clinical presentations, and therapeutic considerations. Journal of Trauma and Acute Care Surgery. 2006;**60**(6 Suppl): S3-S11

[2] Cannon JW. Hemorrhagic shock. The New England Journal of Medicine. 2018;**378**:370-379. DOI: 10.1056/NEJMra1705649

[3] Lozano R, Naghavi M, Foreman K, et al. Global and regional mortality from 235 causes of death for 20 age groups in 1990 and 2010: A systematic analysis for the Global Burden of Disease Study 2010. Lancet. 2012;**380**:2095-2128

[4] Halmin M, Chiesa F, Vasan SK, et al. Epidemiology of massive transfusion: A binational study from Sweden and Denmark. Critical Care Medicine. 2016;**44**:468-477

[5] Mitra B, Gabbe BJ, Kaukonen K-M, Olaussen A, Cooper DJ, Cameron PA. Longterm outcomes of patients receiving a massive transfusion after trauma. Shock. 2014;**42**:307-312

[6] Celsus AC. (trans. W.G. Spencer). De Medicina, vol. 3, books 7-8. London, UK: Loeb Classical Library; 1938

[7] LeDran HF. A Treatise, or Reflections, Drawn from Practice on Gunshot Wounds. John Clarke: London, UK; 1743

[8] Cannon WB. Traumatic Shock. New York, NY: D Appleton & Co.; 1923

[9] Dale HH. Conditions conducive to the production of shock by histamine. Journal of Experimental Pathology. 1920;**1**:103

[10] Artz CP, Fitts CT. Replacement therapy in shock. Journal of Trauma. 1962;**2**:358-369

[11] Shires GT. Pathophysiology and fluid replacement in hypovolemic shock. Annals of Clinical Research. 1977;**8**:144-150

[12] Kinney JM, Wells RE. Problems of ventilation after injury and shock. Journal of Trauma. 1962;**2**:370-385

[13] Lansing AM, Stevenson JAF, McLachlin AD. The use of vasopressor agents in the treatment of shock. Journal of Trauma. 1962;**2**:386-398

[14] Nickerson M, Gourzis JT. Blockade of sympathetic vasoconstriction in the treatment of shock. Journal of Trauma. 1962;**2**:399-411

[15] Nickson C. Trauma mortality and the golden hour. Critical Care Compendium. 3 Apr 2015

[16] Gann DS, Drucker WR. Hemorrhagic shock. Journal of Trauma and Acute Care Surgery. 2013;**75**(5):888-895. DOI: 10.1097/TA.0b013e3182a686ed

[17] Chaudry IH. Cellular mechanisms in shock and ischemia and their correction. The American Journal of Physiology. 1983;**245**:R117-R134

[18] Bernard C. Leçons sur le diabète et la glycogenèse animale. 1st ed. Paris, France: Baillière; 1877

[19] Cuthbertson DP. Observations on the disturbance of metabolism by injury to the limbs. The Quarterly Journal of Medicine. 1932;**1**:233

[20] Stoner HB, Threlfall CJ. The Biochemical Response to Injury. Oxford, England: Blackwell; 1960

[21] Stoner HB. Energy metabolism after injury. Journal of Clinical Pathology. 1970;**23**(Suppl 4):47-55

[22] Engle F. The significance of metabolic changes during shock. Annals of the New York Academy of Sciences; Sep 1952. https://doi.org/10.1111/j.1749-6632.1952.tb26554.x

[23] Pearce FJ, Drucker WR. Glucose infusion arrests the decompensatory phase of hemorrhagic shock. Journal of Trauma. 1987;**27**:1213-1220

[24] Gann DS, Foster AH. Endocrine and metabolic response to injury. In: Schwartz SI, editor. Principles of Surgery. New York, NY: McGraw-Hill; 1993. pp. 1-59

[25] Zhang Q, Raoof M, Chen Y, et al. Circulating mitochondrial DAMPs cause inflammatory responses to injury. Nature. 2010;**464**:104-107

[26] Tisherman SA, Alam HB, Rhee PM, et al. Development of the emergency preservation and resuscitation for cardiac arrest from trauma clinical trial. Journal of Trauma and Acute Care Surgery. 2017;**83**:803-809

[27] White NJ, Ward KR, Pati S, Strandenes G, Cap AP. Hemorrhagic blood failure: Oxygen debt, coagulopathy, and endothelial damage. Journal of Trauma and Acute Care Surgery. 2017;**82**(Suppl 1):S41-S49

[28] Hoffman M, Cichon LJH. Practical coagulation for the blood banker. Transfusion. 2013;**53**:1594-1602

[29] Chang R, Cardenas JC, Wade CE, Holcomb JB. Advances in the understanding of trauma-induced coagulopathy. Blood. 2016;**128**:1043-1049

[30] Moore HB, Moore EE, Liras IN, et al. Acute fibrinolysis shutdown after injury occurs frequently and increases mortality: A multicenter evaluation of 2,540 severely injured patients. Journal of the American College of Surgeons. 2016;**222**:347-355

[31] Brown LM, Call MS, Margaret Knudson M, et al. A normal platelet count may not be enough: The impact of admission platelet count on mortality and transfusion in severely injured trauma patients. The Journal of Trauma. 2011;**71**(Suppl 3):S337-S342

[32] Wohlauer MV, Moore EE, Thomas S, et al. Early platelet dysfunction: An unrecognized role in the acute coagulopathy of trauma. Journal of the American College of Surgeons. 2012;**214**:739-746

[33] Sihler KC, Napolitano LM. Complications of massive transfusion. Chest. 2010;**137**:209-220

[34] Cosgriff N, Moore EE, Sauaia A, KennyMoynihan M, Burch JM, Galloway B. Predicting life-threatening coagulopathy in the massively transfused trauma patient: Hypothermia and acidoses revisited. The Journal of Trauma. 1997;**42**:857-861

[35] Tompkins RG. Genomics of injury: The Glue Grant experience. Journal of Trauma and Acute Care Surgery. 2015;**78**:671-686

[36] Baue AE, Tragus ET, Parkins WM. A comparison of isotonic and hypertonic solutions and blood on blood flow and oxygen consumption in the initial treatment of hemorrhagic shock. Journal of Trauma. 1967;**7**:743-756

[37] Drucker WR, Holden WD, Kingsbury B, Hofmann N, Graham L. Metabolic aspects of hemorrhagic shock. II: Metabolic studies on the need for erythrocytes in the treatment of hypovolemia due to hemorrhage. Journal of Trauma. 1962;**2**:567-584

[38] Haller JA, Ward MJ, Cahill JL. Metabolic alterations in shock: The effect of controlled reduction of blood flow on oxidative metabolism and catecholamine response. Journal of Trauma. 1967;**7**:727-742

[39] Gann DS, Pirkle JC. Role of cortisol in the restitution of blood volume after

hemorrhage. The American Journal of Surgery. 1975;**130**:565-569

[40] Pirkle JC, Gann DS. Expansion of the interstitial fluid is required for full restitution of blood volume after hemorrhage. Journal of Trauma. 1976;**16**:937-947

[41] Byrnes GJ, Pirkle JC, Gann DS. Cardiovascular stabilization after hemorrhage depends upon volume restitution and extracellular osmolality. Journal of Trauma. 1978;**18**:623-1975

[42] Gann DS, Carlson DE, Byrnes GJ, Pirkle JC Jr, Allen-Rowlands CF. Impaired restitution of blood volume after large hemorrhage. Journal of Trauma. 1981;**21**:598-603

[43] Shires GT. Shock and Related Problems, Clinical Surgery International. Edinburgh, Scotland: Churchill Livingston; 1984

[44] Shires GT 3rd, Peitzman AB, Illner H, Shires GT. Changes in red blood cell transmembrane potential, electrolytes, and energy content in septic shock. Journal of Trauma. 1983;**23**:769-774

[45] Evans JA, Darlington DN, Gann DS. A circulating factor(s) mediates cell depolarization in hemorrhagic shock. Annals of Surgery. 1991;**21**:549-557

[46] Boulanger BR, Evans JA, Lilly MP, Shurtleff DM, Williams JC, Gann DS. A circulating protein that depolarizes cells increases after hemorrhage in dogs. Journal of Trauma. 1993;**34**:591-598

[47] Jones RO, Carlson DE, Gann DS. A circulating shock protein that depolarizes cells in vitro depresses myocardial contractility and rate in isolated rat hearts. The Journal of Trauma. 1994;**37**:752-758

[48] Darlington DN, Gann DS. Adenosine stimulates Na/K ATPase, and prolongs survival in hemorrhagic shock. The Journal of Trauma. 2005;**58**:1-6

[49] Eastridge BJ, Darlington DN, Evans JA, Gann DS. A circulating shock protein depolarizes cells in hemorrhage and sepsis. Annals of Surgery. 1994;**219**:298-305

[50] Tisherman SA, Schmicker RH, Brasel KJ, et al. Detailed description of all deaths in both the shock and traumatic brain injury hypertonic saline trials of the Resuscitation Outcomes Consortium. Annals of Surgery 2015;**261**:586-590. 28. National Academies of Sciences, Engi

[51] Barbee RW, Reynolds PS, Ward KR. Assessing shock resuscitation strategies by oxygen debt repayment. Shock. 2010;**33**:113-122

[52] Bloom BA, Gibbons RC. Focused Assessment with Sonography for Trauma (FAST). StatPearls [Internet]. Treasure Island (FL): StatPearls Publishing; 2018

[53] Scharonow M, Weilbach C. Prehospital point-of-care emergency ultrasound: A cohort study. Scandinavian Journal of Trauma, Resuscitation and Emergency Medicine. 2018 Jun 18;**26**(1):49. DOI: 10.1186/s13049-018-0519-9

[54] Trump BF, Berezesky IK. The mechanisms of calcium-mediated cell injury and cell death. New Horizons. 1996;**4**:139-150

[55] Holden WD, DePalma RG, Drucker WR. Ultrastructural changes in hemorrhagic shock. Electron microscopic study of liver, kidney and striated muscle cells in rats. Annals of Surgery. 1965;**162**:517-536

[56] Bonanno FG. Hemorrhagic shock: The "physiology approach". Journal of Emergencies, Trauma, and Shock. 2012;**5**(4):285-295. DOI: 10.4103/0974-2700.102357

[57] Cancio LC, Wade CE, West SA. Predictions of mortality and of the need

for massive transfusion in casualties at combat support hospitals in Iraq. The Journal of Trauma. 2008;**64**:S51-S56

[58] Yanagawa Y, Sakamoto T, Okada Y. Hypovolemic shock evaluated by sonographic measurement of the inferior vena cava during resuscitation in trauma patients. The Journal of Trauma. 2007;**63**:1245-1248

[59] Ferrada P, Murthi S, Anand RJ, Bochicchio GV, Scalea T. Transthoracic rapid echocardiographic examination real-time evaluation of fluid status in critically ill trauma patients. The Journal of Trauma. 2011;**70**:56-64

[60] Franklin GA, Boaz PW, Spain DA, Lukan JK, Carrillo EH, Richardson JD. Prehospital hypotension as a valid indicator of trauma team activation. The Journal of Trauma. 2000;**48**:1034-1037

[61] Nadler R, Convertino VA, Gendler S, et al. The value of noninvasive measurement of the compensatory reserve index in monitoring and triage of patients experiencing minimal blood loss. Shock. 2014;**42**:93-98

[62] Hutchings S, Naumann DN, Harris T, Wendon J, Midwinter MJ. Observational study of the effects of traumatic injury, haemorrhagic shock and resuscitation on the microcirculation: A protocol for the MICROSHOCK study. BMJ Open. 2016;**6**:e010893

[63] Rozycki GS, Ballard RB, Feliciano DV, Schmidt JA, Pennington SD. Surgeon performed ultrasound for the assessment of truncal injuries: Lessons learned from 1540 patients. Annals of Surgery. 1998;**228**:557-567

[64] Shokoohi H, Boniface KS, Pourmand A, et al. Bedside ultrasound reduces diagnostic uncertainty and guides resuscitation in patients with undifferentiated hypotension. Critical Care Medicine. 2015;**43**:2562-2569

[65] Sohn CH, Kim YJ, Seo DW, Won HS, Shim JY, Lim KS, et al. Blood lactate concentration and shock index associated with massive transfusion in emergency department patients with primary postpartum haemorrhage. British Journal of Anaesthesia. 2018 Aug;**121**(2):378-383. DOI: 10.1016/j.bja.2018.04.039 Epub 2018 Jun 8

[66] Lee SH, Min YW, Bae J, Lee H, Min BH, Lee JH, et al. Lactate parameters predict clinical outcomes in patients with nonvariceal upper gastrointestinal bleeding. Journal of Korean Medical Science. 2017 Nov;**32**(11):1820-1827. DOI: 10.3346/jkms.2017.32.11.1820

[67] Callcut RA, Cotton BA, Muskat P, et al. Defining when to initiate massive transfusion: A validation study of individual massive transfusion triggers in PROMMTT patients. Journal of Trauma and Acute Care Surgery. 2013;**74**:59-65

[68] MacKay EJ, Stubna MD, Holena DN, et al. Abnormal calcium levels during trauma resuscitation are associated with increased mortality, increased blood product use, and greater hospital resource consumption: A pilot investigation. Anesthesia and Analgesia. 2017;**125**:895-901

[69] Gonzalez E, Moore EE, Moore HB, et al. Goal-directed hemostatic resuscitation of trauma-induced coagulopathy: A pragmatic randomized clinical trial comparing a viscoelastic assay to conventional coagulation assays. Annals of Surgery. 2016;**263**:1051-1059

[70] National Academies of Sciences, Engineering, and Medicine. A National Trauma Care System: Integrating Military and Civilian Trauma Systems to Achieve Zero Preventable Deaths after Injury. Washington, DC: National Academies Press; 2016

[71] Schroll R, Smith A, McSwain NE Jr, et al. A multi-institutional analysis of prehospital tourniquet use. Journal

of Trauma and Acute Care Surgery. 2015;**79**:10-14

[72] Kragh JF Jr, Walters TJ, Baer DG, et al. Survival with emergency tourniquet use to stop bleeding in major limb trauma. Annals of Surgery. 2009;**249**:1-7

[73] Singletary EM, Charlton NP, Epstein JL, et al. Part 15: First aid: 2015 American Heart Association and American Red Cross guidelines update for first aid. Circulation. 2015;**132**(Suppl 2): S574-S589

[74] Bulger EM, Snyder D, Schoelles K, et al. An evidence-based prehospital guideline for external hemorrhage control: American College of Surgeons Committee on Trauma. Prehospital Emergency Care. 2014;**18**:163-173

[75] Achneck HE, Sileshi B, Jamiolkowski RM, Albala DM, Shapiro ML, Lawson JH. A comprehensive review of topical hemostatic agents: Efficacy and recommendations for use. Annals of Surgery. 2010;**251**:217-228

[76] Bickell WH, Wall MJ Jr, Pepe PE, et al. Immediate versus delayed fluid resuscitation for hypotensive patients with penetrating torso injuries. The New England Journal of Medicine. 1994;**331**:1105-1109

[77] Bickell WH, Wall MJ Jr, Pepe PE, Martin RR, Ginger VF, Allen MK, et al. Immediate versus delayed fluid resuscitation for hypotensive patients with penetrating torso injuries. The New England Journal of Medicine. 1994;**331**:1105

[78] Dutton RP, Mackenzie CF, Scalea TM. Hypotensive resuscitation during active hemorrhage: Impact on in-hospital mortality. The Journal of Trauma. 2002;**52**:1141-1146

[79] Holcomb JB. Damage control resuscitation directly addressing the early coagulopathy of tissues. The Journal of Trauma. 2007;**62**:307-310

[80] Duchesne JC, Kimonis K, Marr AB, Rennie KV, Wahl G, Wells JE, et al. Damage control resuscitation in combination with damage control laparotomy: A survival advantage. The Journal of Trauma. 2010;**69**:46-52

[81] Bougle A, Harrois A, Duranteau J. Resuscitative strategies in traumatic hemorrhagic shock. Annals of Intensive Care. 2013;**3**:1

[82] Groeneveld AB, Navickis RJ, Wilkes MM. Update on the comparative safety of colloids: A systematic review of clinical studies. Annals of Surgery. 2011;**253**:470-448

[83] Borgman MA, Spinella PC, Perkins JG, Grathwohl KW, Repine T, Beekley AC, et al. The ratio of blood products transfused affects mortality in patients receiving massive transfusions at a combat support hospital. The Journal of Trauma. 2007;**64**(4):805-815

[84] Kashuk JL, Moore EE, Johnson JL, Haenel J, Wilson M, Moore JB, et al. Postinjury life threatening coagulopathy: Is 1:1 fresh frozen plasma:packed red blood cells the answer? The Journal of Trauma. 2008;**65**:261-270

[85] Wafaisade A, Maegele M, Lefering R, Braun M, Peiniger S, Neugebauer E, et al. High plasma to red blood cell ratios are associated with lower mortality rates in patients receiving multiple transfusion ($4 \leq$ red blood cell units < 10) during acute trauma resuscitation. The Journal of Trauma. 2011;**70**:81-89

[86] Velasco IT, Pontieri V, Rocha è Silva M Jr, Lopes OU. Hyperosmotic NaCl and severe hemorrhagic shock. The American Journal of Physiology. 1980;**239**:H664-H673

[87] Vassar MJ, Perry CA, Holcroft JW. Prehospital resuscitation of hypotensive

trauma patients with 7.5% NaCl versus 7.5% NaCl with added dextran: A controlled trial. The Journal of Trauma. 1993;**34**(5):622-632

[88] Freshman SP, Battistella FD, Matteucci M, Wisner DH. Hypertonic saline (7.5%) versus mannitol: A comparison for therapy of acute head injuries. The Journal of Trauma. 1993;**35**:344-348

[89] Bulger EM, May S, Kerby JD, et al. Out-of-hospital hypertonic resuscitation after traumatic hypovolemic shock: A randomized, placebo controlled trial. Annals of Surgery. 2011;**253**:431-441

[90] Roberts I, Blackhall K, Alderson P, Bunn F, Schierhout G. Human albumin solution for resuscitation and volume expansion in critically ill patients. Cochrane Database of Systematic Reviews. 2011;**11**:CD001208

[91] Shackelford SA, Del Junco DJ, PowellDunford N, et al. Association of prehospital blood product transfusion during medical evacuation of combat casualties in Afghanistan with acute and 30-day survival. JAMA. 2017;**318**:1581-1591

[92] Cotton BA, Jerome R, Collier BR, et al. Guidelines for prehospital fluid resuscitation in the injured patient. The Journal of Trauma. 2009;**67**:389-402

[93] Chovanes J, Cannon JW, Nunez TC. The evolution of damage control surgery. The Surgical Clinics of North America. 2012;**92**:859-875

[94] Duchesne JC, McSwain NE Jr, Cotton BA, et al. Damage control resuscitation: The new face of damage control. The Journal of Trauma. 2010;**69**:976-990

[95] Cannon JW, Khan MA, Raja AS, et al. Damage control resuscitation in patients with severe traumatic hemorrhage: A practice management guideline from the Eastern Association for the Surgery of Trauma. Journal of Trauma and Acute Care Surgery. 2017;**82**:605-617

[96] Meyer DE, Vincent LE, Fox EE, et al. Every minute counts: Time to delivery of initial massive transfusion cooler and its impact on mortality. Journal of Trauma and Acute Care Surgery. 2017;**83**:19-24

[97] Sheldon GF, Watkins GM, Glover JL, Greenburg AG, Friedman BA. Panel: "present use of blood and blood products". The Journal of Trauma. 1981;**21**:1005-1012

[98] Fortune JB, Feustel PJ, Saifi J, Stratton HH, Newell JC, Shah DM. Influence of hematocrit on cardiopulmonary function after acute hemorrhage. The Journal of Trauma. 1987;**27**:243-249

[99] Sheldon GF, Lim RC, Blaisdell FW. The use of fresh blood in the treatment of critically injured patients. The Journal of Trauma. 1975 Aug;**15**:670-677

[100] Gervin AS, Fischer R. Resuscitation of trauma patients with typespecific uncrossmatched blood. The Journal of Trauma. 1984;**24**(4):327-331

[101] Holcomb JB, del Junco DJ, Fox EE, et al. The prospective, observational, multicenter, major trauma transfusion (PROMMTT) study: Comparative effectiveness of a timevarying treatment with competing risks. JAMA Surgery. 2013;**148**:127-136

[102] Holcomb JB, Tilley BC, Baraniuk S, et al. Transfusion of plasma, platelets, and red blood cells in a 1:1:1 vs a 1:1:2 ratio and mortality in patients with severe trauma: The PROPPR randomized clinical trial. JAMA. 2015;**313**:471-482

[103] Etchill EW, Myers SP, McDaniel LM, et al. Should all massively

transfused patients be treated equally? An analysis of massive transfusion ratios in the nontrauma setting. Critical Care Medicine. 2017;**45**:1311-1316

[104] Barry N, Mubang RN, Wojda TR, Evans DC, Sharpe RP, et al. An exploratory hypothesis-generating meta-analytic study of damage control resuscitation acute hemorrhagic shock: Examining the behavior of patient morbidity and mortality in the context of plasma to packed red blood cell ratios. International journal of Academic Medicine. 2016;**2**(2):159

[105] Spahn DR, Bouillon B, Cerny V, et al. Management of bleeding and coagulopathy following major trauma: An updated European guideline. Critical Care. 2013;**17**:R76

[106] Shafi S, Collinsworth AW, Richter KM, et al. Bundles of care for resuscitation from hemorrhagic shock and severe brain injury in trauma patients—Translating knowledge into practice. Journal of Trauma and Acute Care Surgery. 2016;**81**:780-794

[107] Pruitt BA, Moncrief JA, Mason AD. Efficacy of buffered saline as the sole replacement fluid following acute measured hemorrhage in man. The Journal of Trauma. 1967;**7**:767-782

[108] Traverso LW, Lee WP, Langford MJ. Fluid resuscitation after an otherwise fatal hemorrhage: I. Crystalloid solutions. The Journal of Trauma. 1986;**26**:168-175

[109] Healey MA, Davis RE, Lui FC. Lactated Ringer's is superior to normal saline in a model of massive hemorrhage and resuscitation. The Journal of Trauma. 1998;**45**:899

[110] Balogh Z, McKinley BA, Holcomb JB. Both primary and secondary abdominal compartment syndrome can be predicted early and are harbingers of multiple organ failure. The Journal of Trauma. 2003;**54**:848-859

[111] Cloutier CT, Lowery BD, Carey LC. The effect of hemodilutional resuscitation on serum protein levels in humans in hemorrhagic shock. The Journal of Trauma. 1961;**9**:517-521

[112] Schöchl H, Schlimp CJ. Trauma bleeding management: The concept of goaldirected primary care. Anesthesia and Analgesia. 2014;**119**:1064-1073

[113] Cohn SM, McCarthy J, Stewart RM, Jonas RB, Dent DL, Michalek JE. Impact of low-dose vasopressin on trauma outcome: Prospective randomized study. World Journal of Surgery. 2011;**35**:430-439

[114] Salhab M, Farmer J, Osman I. Impact of delay on survival in patients with ruptured abdominal aortic aneurysm. Vascular. 2006;**14**:38-42

[115] Laine L, Laursen SB, Dalton HR, Ngu JH, Schultz M, Stanley AJ. Relationship of time to presentation after onset of upper GI bleeding with patient characteristics and outcomes: A prospective study. Gastrointestinal Endoscopy. 2017;**86**:1028-1037

[116] Meizoso JP, Ray JJ, Karcutskie CA IV, et al. Effect of time to operation on mortality for hypotensive patients with gunshot wounds to the torso: The golden 10 minutes. Journal of Trauma and Acute Care Surgery. 2016;**81**:685-691

[117] Hirshberg A, Wall MJ Jr, Allen MK, Mattox KL. Double jeopardy: Thoracoabdominal injuries requiring surgical intervention in both chest and abdomen. The Journal of Trauma. 1995;**39**:225-229

[118] Morrison JJ, Galgon RE, Jansen JO, Cannon JW, Rasmussen TE, Eliason JL. A systematic review of the use of resuscitative endovascular balloon occlusion of the aorta in the management of hemorrhagic shock. Journal of Trauma and Acute Care Surgery. 2016;**80**:324-334

[119] Raux M, Marzelle J, Kobeiter H, et al. Endovascular balloon occlusion is associated with reduced intraoperative mortality of unstable patients with ruptured abdominal aortic aneurysm but fails to improve other outcomes. Journal of Vascular Surgery. 2015;**61**:304-308

[120] Aoki M, Abe T, Saitoh D, Hagiwara S, Oshima K. Use of vasopressor increases the risk of mortality in traumatic hemorrhagic shock: A nationwide cohort study in Japan. Critical Care Medicine. 2018. DOI: 10.1097/CCM.0000000000003428

[121] Yazer MH, Jackson B, Sperry JL, Alarcon L, Triulzi DJ, Murdock AD. Initial safety and feasibility of cold-stored uncrossmatched whole blood transfusion in civilian trauma patients. Journal of Trauma and Acute Care Surgery. 2016;**81**:21-26

[122] Pusateri AE, Given MB, Schreiber MA, et al. Dried plasma: State of the science and recent developments. Transfusion. 2016;**56**(Suppl 2):S128-S139

Chapter 5

Sepsis and Septic Shock

Alaap Mehta, Ali Khalid and Mamta Swaroop

Abstract

Sepsis and septic shock are life-threatening conditions that remain an enormous burden of morbidity and mortality to millions of patients globally and cause organ dysfunction, leading to death in as many as one in four patients, often even more. Early management and appropriate treatment are essential to improve outcomes and reduce morbidity and mortality. In 2016, the Third International Consensus Definition for Sepsis and Septic Shock (Sepsis-3) defined sepsis *as life-threatening organ dysfunction resulting from dysregulated host responses to infection*, and defined septic shock as *a subset of sepsis in which underlying circulatory, cellular, and metabolic abnormalities are profound enough to substantially increase the risk of mortality*. That same year the group also implemented the application of the sequential organ failure assessment (SOFA) score over the systemic inflammatory response syndrome (SIRS) score. Sepsis in pregnancy remains a leading cause of maternal morbidity and mortality worldwide, with no current standard definition for severe sepsis for the pregnant or peripartum woman. The prevalence of pediatric septic shock is on the rise and brings with it the consequences of long-term morbidity and also death. Since the advent of programs for early recognition and treatment, mortality has decreased. Even so, globally, many children succumb to septic shock despite evidence-based care and years of research.

Keywords: sepsis, septic shock, pediatrics, obstetrics, SIRS, SOFA, qSOFA

1. Introduction

Sepsis and septic shock are life-threatening conditions that remain an enormous burden of morbidity and mortality to millions of patients globally and cause organ dysfunction, leading to death in as many as one in four patients, often even more [1]. Early management and appropriate treatment are essential to improve outcomes and reduce morbidity and mortality.

Sepsis is a multifaceted disorder, developing from a dysregulated response by the host to an infectious nidus, and is associated with acute organ dysfunction and a high risk of mortality.

The incidence of sepsis is high, and remains one of the leading causes of death worldwide [2]. The reported incidence is increasing, which is likely a reflection on the older population with more comorbidities. Even though incidence is not known, estimates indicate that sepsis is a leading cause of morbidity and mortality globally. Even though sepsis is a deadly disease, data now shows the after effects of sepsis to be quite traumatic; often showing long term physical, physiological and cognitive disabilities [3].

Over the past 30 years, with the help of an extensive amount of research and better-quality clinical processes, the treatment and recognition of sepsis has happened at a faster pace [2]. At the World Health Assembly in 2017, the World Health Organization (WHO) made sepsis a global health priority and passed a resolution to improve the prevention, diagnosis and management of sepsis [4].

In this chapter, we will examine the current definitions of sepsis and septic shock. We will explore the current guidelines in the diagnosis of sepsis. As we delve into the diagnosis, we will discuss the pathophysiology, clinical presentation, risk factors, etiologies, and finally, management strategies and treatments of the adult, pregnant and pediatric populations.

2. Sepsis and septic shock in adults

2.1 Definitions of sepsis and septic shock

The first definition of sepsis, published in 1992, was based on the presence of a suspected or proven infection with two or more criteria of the systemic inflammatory response syndrome (SIRS) [5]. Sepsis was defined, as the presence of two or more positive SIRS criteria with a confirmed or suspected infection as the underlying cause. If signs of organ dysfunction were seen, the diagnosis was changed to severe sepsis. Septic shock was defined by the presence of acute circulatory failure and arterial hypotension along with features of sepsis. Until recently, the definitions of sepsis, septic shock and organ dysfunction remained the same for more than 20 years (**Figure 1**). Due to the inaccuracies of the past definition and the SIRS criteria, new guidelines were published by the surviving sepsis campaign (SSC) in 2016, a multidisciplinary task force started by the Society of Critical Care Medicine in the United States and the European Society of Intensive Care Medicine [6, 7]. Since there is no gold standard test for sepsis, the task force decided to come up with definitions and clinical criteria that were clear, useful, and valid [3]. Instead of using the SIRS criteria to determine if a patient is in going into sepsis, the new guidelines suggest using the sequential organ failure assessment (SOFA) score and a quick SOFA score for more emergent cases, a topic that will be discussed in length in the next section.

In 2016, the Third International Consensus Definition for Sepsis and Septic Shock (Sepsis-3) defined sepsis as *a life-threatening organ dysfunction resulting from dysregulated host responses to infection*, and defined septic shock as *a subset of sepsis in which underlying circulatory, cellular, and metabolic abnormalities are profound enough to substantially increase the risk of mortality* (**Table 1**) [2]. Septic shock is also *defined as persisting hypotension that requires vasopressors to achieve a mean arterial pressure* ≥65 mmHg *despite adequate fluid resuscitation and a lactic acid level* >2 mmol/L [7]. These new definitions focused on organ dysfunction rather than inflammation.

2.2 SIRS versus SOFA

The same task force that changed the definition also implemented the use of the sequential organ failure assessment (SOFA) score over the SIRS criteria. Even though SOFA is not considered the gold standard for diagnosis, its use is recommended over SIRS.

SIRS was based on an inflammatory response to an infectious inoculation (**Figure 2**). Throughout its utilization, the surviving sepsis guidelines, specifically the SIRS criteria, were widely criticized. Many thought the definition was not helpful largely because the definition place a large emphasis on inflammation,

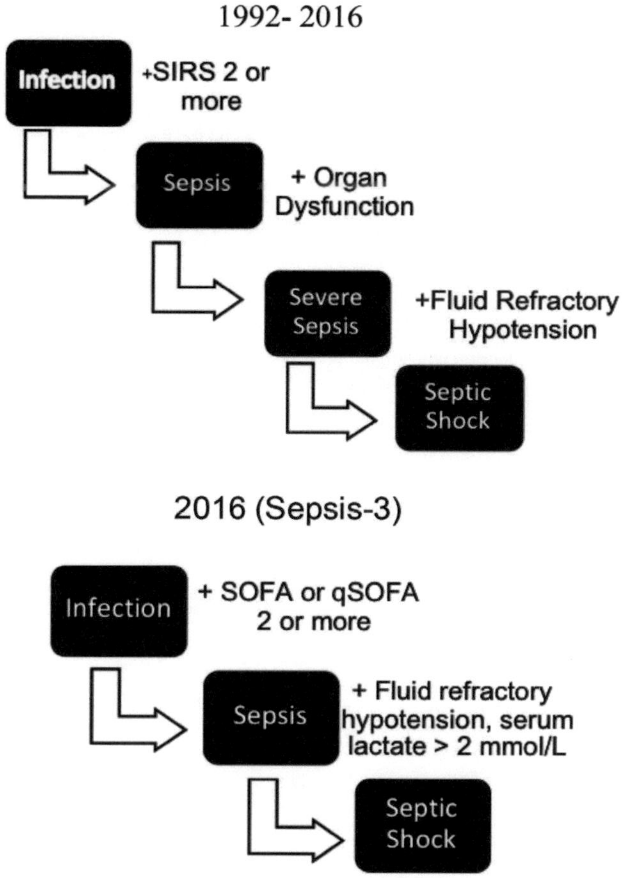

Figure 1.
Sepsis and septic shock definitions over the years [9]. Abbreviations: SIRS, systemic inflammatory response syndrome; SOFA, sequential organ failure assessment; and qSOFA, quick sequential organ failure assessment.

causing many patients without bacterial or viral infections to receive empiric antibiotic therapy and over-resuscitation [10]. The SIRS criteria were also thought to be remarkably sensitive, not taking into account any outside factors, multi-drug resistance and the ability to attain source control [3]. Based on the old definition of sepsis using the SIRS criteria, patients may have been incorrectly identified as being septic. One study showed a positive SIRS score in 87% of all ICU admissions, yet 14.3% of those with 2 or more SIRS criteria did not have infection [5, 7]. Moreover, in another study, 12.1% of patients had SIRS-negative sepsis, which is approximately a miss of 1 in 8 patients diagnosed with sepsis [11].

Due to these inaccuracies in the SIRS criteria, the new Sepsis-3 definitions recommend using the SOFA score; however, it is not commonly used or known outside of the critical care world [7]. The SOFA score is an aggregate score, from 0 to 4, for each organ system, including respiratory, coagulation, liver, cardiovascular, renal and central nervous systems [12]. An acute increase in the total score of 2 or more reflects an overall mortality risk in patients suspected of infection [7]. Calculating the SOFA score at the bedside or in a noncritical care unit and in patients who do not have full laboratory testing, is challenging. Since the SOFA score is based on biochemical criteria, the task force developed the clinical qSOFA screening tool which is based on respiratory rate, systolic blood pressure and altered mental state (**Figure 2**) [13]. If 2 of the 3 clinical variables

Sepsis-3 new terms and definitions
• Sepsis is defined as life threatening organ dysfunction caused by dysregulated host responses to infection.
• Organ dysfunction can be identified as an acute change if you have ≥2 points on the SOFA score in relation to an infection • Baseline SOFA score can be assumed to be zero in patients with no preexisting organ dysfunction and a score of ≥2 reflects an overall mortality risk of approximately 10% in a general hospital population with suspected infection.
• Layman terms—sepsis is a life-threatening condition that arises when the body's response to an infection injures its own tissues and organs.
• Patients with suspected infection who are likely to have a prolonged ICU stay or to die in the hospital can be identified at the bedside with qSOFA (altered mental status, respiratory rate >22, systolic blood pressure <100 mmHg).
• Septic shock is a subset of sepsis in which underlying circulatory and cellular/metabolic abnormalities are severe enough to increase mortality.
• Patients with septic shock have preexisting sepsis with persisting hypotension requiring vasopressors to maintain MAP ≥ 65 mmHg and having a serum lactate level >2 mmol/L despite adequate volume resuscitation.
Abbreviations: MAP, mean arterial pressure; qSOFA, quick SOFA; SOFA, sequential [8] organ failure assessment; and ICU, intensive care unit.

Table 1.
Sepsis-3 terms and definitions [3, 6].

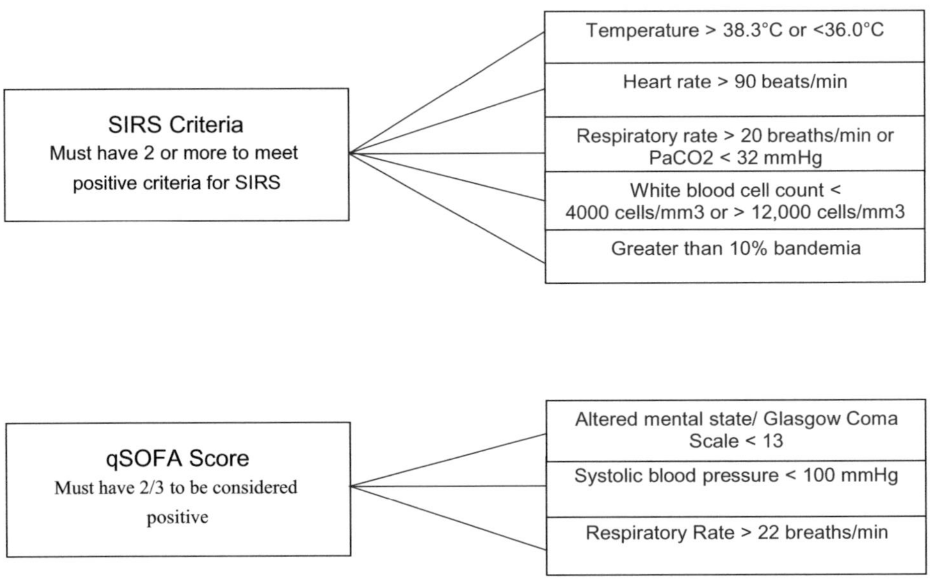

Figure 2.
Comparison of SIRS versus qSOFA [7, 13, 15]. Abbreviations: SIRS, systemic inflammatory response syndrome; SOFA, sequential organ failure assessment; and qSOFA, quick SOFA.

are positive, the predictive validity is similar to the entire SOFA score when used outside the ICU setting [14].

2.3 Pathophysiology

Sepsis is a clinical syndrome with an array of disease courses of which is not completely understood. It is characterized by a varied response to infection, started by recognition of pathogen associated molecular patterns (PAMPs) from invasive microorganisms [16]. PAMPs are conservative antigens that are recognized by four classes of receptors: Toll-like receptors, C-type lectin receptors, retinoic acid inducible gene 1-like receptors and nucleotide-binding oligomerization domain-like receptors [17]. Cell lysis and spillover of intracellular molecules into the extracellular space is seen due to the resulting inflammatory response to the pathogen. The net result is an increased capillary permeability and vasodilation leading to hypotension that results in tissue hypo-perfusion [16].

In sepsis, a hypercoagulable state is achieved due to the changes in the clotting factors. There is an increase of tissue factor which causes a decrease of antithrombin, subsequently causing an increase in plasma thrombin. At the same time there is decreased production of protein C and an increase in plasminogen activator inhibitor type 1 which all inhibits fibrinolysis. Increased coagulation and hypotension in sepsis can lead to multi organ failure, the most severe and life threatening consequence of sepsis [18]. During severe sepsis, and altered coagulation is almost always seen leading to disseminated intravascular coagulation (DIC). The mechanisms of how cell injury and sepsis-induced organ dysfunction occur are not fully understood and continue to be an ongoing investigation [2].

2.4 Etiology

Sepsis can be caused by any type of infecting organism and can originate from communities, hospitals or other health care facilities [2]. The most common culprit is pneumonia, which accounts for about half of all cases, followed closely by intra-abdominal infections and urinary tract infections [19]. The most common gram positive bacteria seen are *Staphylococcus aureus* and *Streptococcus pneumoniae*, whereas *Escherichia coli*, Klebsiella species, and *Pseudomonas aeruginosa* are the most common gram-negative bacteria seen [20].

2.5 Risk factors

Most risk factors for sepsis mainly rely on the patient's predisposition to infection. The main groups of patients are but not limited to; young or old age, patients with immunosuppressive diseases (e.g., AIDS) or ones taking immunosuppressive medications, cancer patients, alcoholics, patients with indwelling catheters, or other patients that have altered skin integrity all predispose them to infection [2, 21]. Age, sex, race, or ethnic groups have an influence on the incidence of severe sepsis. It is seen that sepsis mainly occurs in infants and elderly people, in males and African Americans rather than females Caucasians respectively [19, 22].

2.6 Clinical presentation

In sepsis, a person's response to an infection presents as signs of infection together with acute organ dysfunction, which can lead to multiple organ failure, acidosis, and death [21]. The clinical manifestations of sepsis varies, depending on the where the infection happens, the type of organism, the pattern of acute organ dysfunction, the health status of the patient, and what happens prior to initiation of treatment. Acute organ dysfunction is most commonly seen in the respiratory and cardiovascular systems. Respiratory compromise is classically manifested as acute respiratory distress syndrome (ARDS), which is defined as hypoxemia with bilateral infiltrates of noncardiac origin. Cardiovascular compromise is manifested primarily as hypotension or an elevated serum lactate level [18]. Patients often present to the emergency department with general malaise, fever, tachycardia, tachypnea, or altered mental status. Health professionals should look at lactate levels, white blood cell counts (leukocytosis or leukopenia), increases in plasma C-reactive protein or procalcitonin concentrations to help determine if a patient is becoming septic [2].

2.7 Clinical significance of lactate production

Lactate production in sepsis is multifactorial and incompletely understood. Most patients with sepsis and elevated lactate have a hyperdynamic circulation with adequate oxygen delivery. The source of lactate production is from the rapid rate of glycolysis and increased anaerobic production that does not always take place in the muscle, so other tissues/cells are possible major contributors. Its greatest utility is as a guide to therapeutic response, an indicator of severity, and a prognostic tool for mortality [7].

2.8 Management/treatment

The management and treatment of sepsis and septic shock should be dealt with as a medical emergency. Screening patients for signs and symptoms of sepsis and septic shock helps to identify and intervene when needed [21]. Proper treatment should focus on when to intervene and being able to find the source of the infection. An important part of the initial management of sepsis is to make sure there is an aggressive assessment to identify unknown sources of infection using appropriate laboratory testing and diagnostic imaging [2]. In addition, early initiation of appropriate antimicrobial therapy after blood cultures have been taken, restoring tissue perfusion by administering the proper amount of fluids, and advanced interventions guided by assessment of the adequacy of resuscitation and resolution of organ dysfunction should be part of the initial sepsis management [21, 23].

The surviving sepsis campaign (SSC) issued guidelines for the management of sepsis and septic shock. It is divided into two sections: an initial management section and a management section. The initial management section indicates what to do within the first 6 h after the patient presents with signs and symptoms that imply sepsis, and the management section indicates what to do when the patient is transferred to the ICU. The main points of the initial management section is to make sure that cardiorespiratory resuscitation takes place and to make sure that the immediate threats of infection have been controlled. Intravenous fluids and vasopressors are used to resuscitate the patient and oxygen therapy and mechanical ventilation are used if needed [18]. For patients with hemodynamic instability, as defined by either hypotension (systolic blood pressure <90 mmHg, MAP <70 mmHg, or a decrease in systolic blood pressure of >40 mmHg from baseline) or elevated lactate concentration (≥4 mmol/L), the SSC recommends rapid administration of 30 mL/kg crystalloid fluids started within the first hour [21, 24].

To determine the type of empirical antibiotic therapy needed, many factors are considered before choosing the initial therapy; the suspected site of infection, the setting where the infection developed, medical history, and local microbial-susceptibility patterns. There is an increased chance of death if the improper therapy is chosen of if there is a delay in treatment, so intravenous broad spectrum antibiotics should be started immediately to cover all pathogens until sensitivity of the blood culture comes back [25]. The 2017 SSC recommendations state that IV antimicrobials should be started immediately, the initial choice should be broad spectrum coverage and the antibiotic spectrum should be narrowed when pathogens have been isolated and sensitivities have been established. A decrease in antibiotic usage should be considered when the patient's condition improves [26].

Septic shock is a consequence of sepsis and one of the criteria to determine if the patient is in septic shock is if the patient is hypotensive and requires vasopressor therapy even if adequate fluids have been administered [27]. In patients with septic shock, vasopressor therapy is often needed to help maintain perfusion pressure [2]. The first-line vasopressor recommended in septic shock is norepinephrine, based on multiple randomized controlled studies and meta-analysis comparing dopamine and norepinephrine. Use of norepinephrine was found to be superior with regard to mortality and adverse cardiac events [28]. Epinephrine has potent inotropic and vasoconstrictive effects, but is less commonly used as a first-line agent in septic shock, which is typically associated with a hyperdynamic circulation [7]. Vasopressin reduces the dose of catecholamine vasopressors, but does not appear to affect patient mortality [2]. It is often used as a replacement dose after initiation of norepinephrine [29].

3. Sepsis and septic shock in obstetrics

3.1 Introduction

Sepsis during pregnancy remains a leading cause of maternal morbidity and mortality worldwide [30]. In the USA, infection accounted for 14% and sepsis 4.3% of all maternal deaths between 2006 and 2010. In the UK between 2006 and 2012, genital tract sepsis accounted for 7% of all maternal deaths [8]. Even with advances in hygiene and antibiotic use, sepsis still accounts for 15% of maternal deaths a year worldwide. Due to inadequate resources and improper hygiene, it is mainly seen in low-income countries that maternal death is 3 times higher compared to high-income countries [31]. The failure to recognize sepsis and institute prompt treatment underlies most cases of maternal sepsis with poor outcomes. Pregnant women are at higher risk of developing infection due to the physiological changes that take place along with possible trauma and surgical interventions. These infections can go unnoticed until there is substantial clinical deterioration. The initial alteration of hemodynamics may be falsely attributed to labor pain or blood loss subsequent to delivery. Normal laboratory values in pregnant patients are different compared to the non-pregnant population. The definitions and criteria used to determine if a patient is in sepsis has not been fully investigated in pregnancy. There are currently efforts taking place to help implement early warning systems and revise the definition of sepsis to help diagnose sepsis earlier in a pregnant patient. It has been shown that early recognition, diagnosis and management of maternal sepsis lead to better maternal and fetal outcomes [9]. Overall, diagnosing sepsis in a pregnant woman can be very difficult due to differing normal values. In this section we will go over causes, clinical presentation, diagnosis and treatment for sepsis and septic shock during pregnancy.

3.2 Definition of sepsis during pregnancy

Compared to the non-pregnant population, there is currently no standard definition for severe sepsis for pregnant and peripartum women [32]. There are multiple physiological changes that occur in an obstetric patient during the antepartum and postpartum periods, which can make it difficult to identify if the patient is going into sepsis using the qSOFA scoring system.

3.3 Identification and scoring systems in pregnancy

Sepsis is something can occur at any time during one's pregnancy and can even happen during the postpartum period, something that everyone should be aware of [33].

During pregnancy, sepsis generally still follows the same rules versus a non-pregnant person, but it can be difficult to determine if a pregnant woman is in sepsis due to the changes in the baseline normal lab values seen; a non-pregnant patient's normal lab values are different compared to a pregnant patient's normal lab values. The physiological changes of pregnancy overlap with hemodynamic changes associated with the initial presentation of sepsis [9]. Before 2016, the SIRS criteria were the main source to diagnose a pregnant patient. The pitfalls with the SIRS criteria were that physiologic maternal lab values would almost result in a diagnosis of SIRS. During pregnancy, the maternal heart rate is often >100, usually due to intravascular volume changes, PCO_2 is normally at 32–34 mmHg, and WBC commonly increases to 14,000 or even as high as 30,000, usually secondary to adrenocorticoid-mediated leukocytosis. After the Society of Critical Care Medicine redefined its criteria via the Sepsis-3 model, a qSOFA score was used instead of SIRS. As mentioned before, this score included three important points: altered mental status, hypotension (systolic <100 mmHg) and tachypnea (respiratory rate > 22). In terms of the qSOFA and SOFA score, there continues to be a struggle to reach a clear cut definition for pregnant patients. Due to their normal lab values, it makes it difficult to diagnose a pregnant patient with sepsis using the current definitions. For example, many patients have systolic blood pressures that are <100 mmHg and they are in no distress or their respiratory rate will increase with movement due to the extra effort it takes because of the large uterus, mainly during the third trimester [15]. With that being said, the diagnosis of sepsis during pregnancy is currently being made based on clinical suspicion, with a greater emphasis on signs of organ dysfunction rather than infection when determining the timing of intervention [33].

In the last decade, there has been development of early warning scoring systems to help identify septic patients at risk for poor outcomes. Unfortunately, many of these systems have not shown much use in the maternal population, such as the Modified Early Warning System (MEWS). These systems do not take into account the physiological changes that occur during pregnancy, something that overlaps with clinical criteria for diagnosing sepsis in the general population. Even though there is a high recommendation to develop maternal warning systems, there has been clear evidence that shows a lack of outcome benefit and validation studies have shown high sensitivity but low specificity. There needs to be further work done to improve the ability of the early warning systems to improve their ability to predict those with signs of early sepsis and at risk of deterioration. A major factor, that is, delaying the development is deciding which vital signs to use and what values are a sign of normality in the obstetric population [9].

Due to the inconsistencies in defining maternal sepsis, there are delays in diagnosis and treatment, something that can prove to be deadly to the pregnant population [15].

3.4 Immunological changes during pregnancy

During pregnancy, the maternal immune system will go through changes that will help protect the fetus from the maternal inflammatory response. There is downregulation of cell-mediated immunity, with decreased T-cell activity secondary to a decrease in numbers or reduction in the CD4/CD8 ratio, with an intact or upregulated humoral response to balance this change. Because of these changes, there is an increased chance to develop certain infections, such as Listeria, and more severe manifestations of some viral and fungal infections [34].

3.5 Risk factors of sepsis during pregnancy

Several risk factors have been identified during pregnancy, leading to the development of guidelines to help prevent sepsis in this patient population [9]. There are many reasons that sepsis can occur during pregnancy and postpartum. The pregnant woman can develop the same type of infections as in the non-pregnant population, but since there is a decrease in cell-mediated immune response, the infection can cause a more severe response. It is now routine to screen and treat asymptomatic bacteriuria and sexually transmitted diseases in early pregnancy and to administer antibiotic prophylaxis for cesarean deliveries [9, 35].

A woman can develop an infection at many sites during the course of her pregnancy. One common area is the genitalia, where urinary tract infections are very common due to the high levels of progesterone [32]. An untreated or improperly treated urinary tract infection can lead to pyelonephritis, a common severe infection that occurs during pregnancy. It usually affects the right kidney, because of compression of the pregnant uterus, with offending organisms similar to non-pregnant patients, *E. coli* being the major pathogen [32].

Chorioamnionitis is another cause of serious obstetric infection and is associated with increased risk of premature delivery and neonatal sepsis. The infection usually starts from the cervicovaginal area, and migrates to the amnion, decidua, and amniotic fluid. The infection is typically polymicrobial; commonly consisting of genital Mycoplasma, *Streptococcus agalactiae* and *Escherichia coli*. Risk factors for infection include prolonged labor, membrane rupture, digital vaginal examinations, young age, and alcohol use [32].

Pneumonia, which is associated with a high rate of morbidity and mortality compared to the non-pregnant population, may be caused by a bacterial, viral or fungal organism. The most common pneumonia pathogens seen in pregnancy are Varicella and Influenza A and B. Acute respiratory distress syndrome (ARDS) is a possible outcome due to respiratory infections in pregnancy [31].

Other risk factors include obesity, caesarean section, prolonged rupture of membranes, mastitis, poor nutrition, chronic hypertension, anemia, lack of prenatal care, immunosuppression, and diabetes mellitus [36]. All of these risk factors can cause sepsis and eventually lead to septic shock in the pregnant population.

3.6 Causative organisms of sepsis during pregnancy

The major contributor to sepsis during pregnancy is group A streptococcus (GAS). It spreads directly through contact with open skin sores, perineal contamination or by mucus or droplet contamination. Group B streptococcus can cause urosepsis, endometritis, mastitis, wound infections and meningitis [37]. In urinary tract infections during pregnancy, *Escherichia coli* is the most common pathogen, and if left untreated, it can lead to sepsis. *S. aureus*, *E. coli*, and anaerobes are common causes of bacteremia after cesarean section. *Listeria monocytogenes* is more classically associated with fetal loss [31]. HIV, AIDS, *Pneumocystis carinii* pneumonia, tuberculosis, and malaria are significant causes for maternal sepsis in low and middle income countries [38].

3.7 Management and treatment of sepsis during pregnancy

Even though the obstetric population were not specifically considered when the Surviving Sepsis Program were making the guidelines for treatment, those guidelines can still be used as a basis for treatment of sepsis and septic shock [21]. Early recognition of sepsis is associated with improved mortality and outcome. In a young, healthy pregnant patient, it may be difficult to identify sepsis and a delay in treatment may occur. With that being said a few warning signs to be considered that may alert severe sepsis include fever or hypothermia, tachycardia, tachypnea, diarrhea, vaginal discharge, leukopenia or leukocytosis, elevated lactate, metabolic acidosis, thrombocytopenia, or other manifestations of coagulopathy [39].

Pregnant women who develop sepsis are usually infected with multiple organisms. The initial choice of antibiotic should have broad spectrum coverage and base it off of guidelines and patterns of resistance [40]. The initial treatment should include coverage against Group A Streptococcus and *Escherichia coli* because they are the most common contributors to sepsis in pregnancy and responsible for a significant proportion of deaths [9].

In a septic pregnant patient, one big challenge is being able to manage fluids. The SSC guidelines recommend crystalloid at an initial 30 mL/kg bolus. This recommendation can be too aggressive in the obstetric population, but there is evidence that shows balanced crystalloid solutions are associated with a lower mortality in sepsis as compared to normal saline [41, 42].

Vasopressors can be used in sepsis mediated hypotension and septic shock. If hypotension does occur, the surviving sepsis campaign (SCC) recommends norepinephrine as the first line agent. These SCC guidelines are based on evidence from non-pregnant patients and there is little data on the effect that vasopressors have on placental blood flow in a pregnant woman [9].

4. Sepsis and septic shock in pediatrics

4.1 Introduction

The prevalence of pediatric septic shock, causing death and long term mobility, has increased over the years, and prior to implementation of early recognition programs and treatment, mortality remained unchanged [43, 44]. Even with millions of dollars being spent and years of research being done, many children still suffer from septic shock [45]. Morbidity in children following severe sepsis is now similar to that in critically ill adults [46]. Due to the high rates of morbidity, mortality and costs associated with pediatric sepsis, there is an increased burden on healthcare communities [47]. As reported by Watson et al., pediatric sepsis patients had an average hospital stay of 31 days and about 2 billion dollars are spent a year for their care [48]. The mainstays of pediatric sepsis treatment, according to the international guidelines, is prompt administration of antibiotics, rapid resuscitation and supportive care of organ dysfunction [1].

Adults and children differ in physiology, predisposing diseases, and sites of infection which necessitates differing diagnostic criteria and management strategies [49]. Among children who develop sepsis worldwide, 49% have a comorbid condition that leaves them vulnerable to infection. The most common comorbidities in children who develop sepsis are age specific; infants have chronic lung disease or congenital heart disease, while children ages one through nine have underlying neuromuscular disease and adolescents have pre-existing cancer [50].

4.2 Diagnosis

The definition of adult sepsis has undergone continuing revision to keep pace with the high volume of published research; however, it is only recently that attention has been given to the pediatric patient and the many caveats that separate the pediatric patient from the adult. Prior to 2005, there was not a standard definition for pediatric sepsis which resulted in a lack of uniformity among sepsis studies [49]. In 2005, the Pediatric Sepsis Consensus Congress (PSCC) met to standardize the definition of sepsis. Defining sepsis in the pediatric patient is made more difficult due to age specific vital signs, and their tremendous physiologic reserve which often masks the seriousness of their condition. The PSCC divided age into six distinct categories in order to take into account age specific vital signs as well as age specific

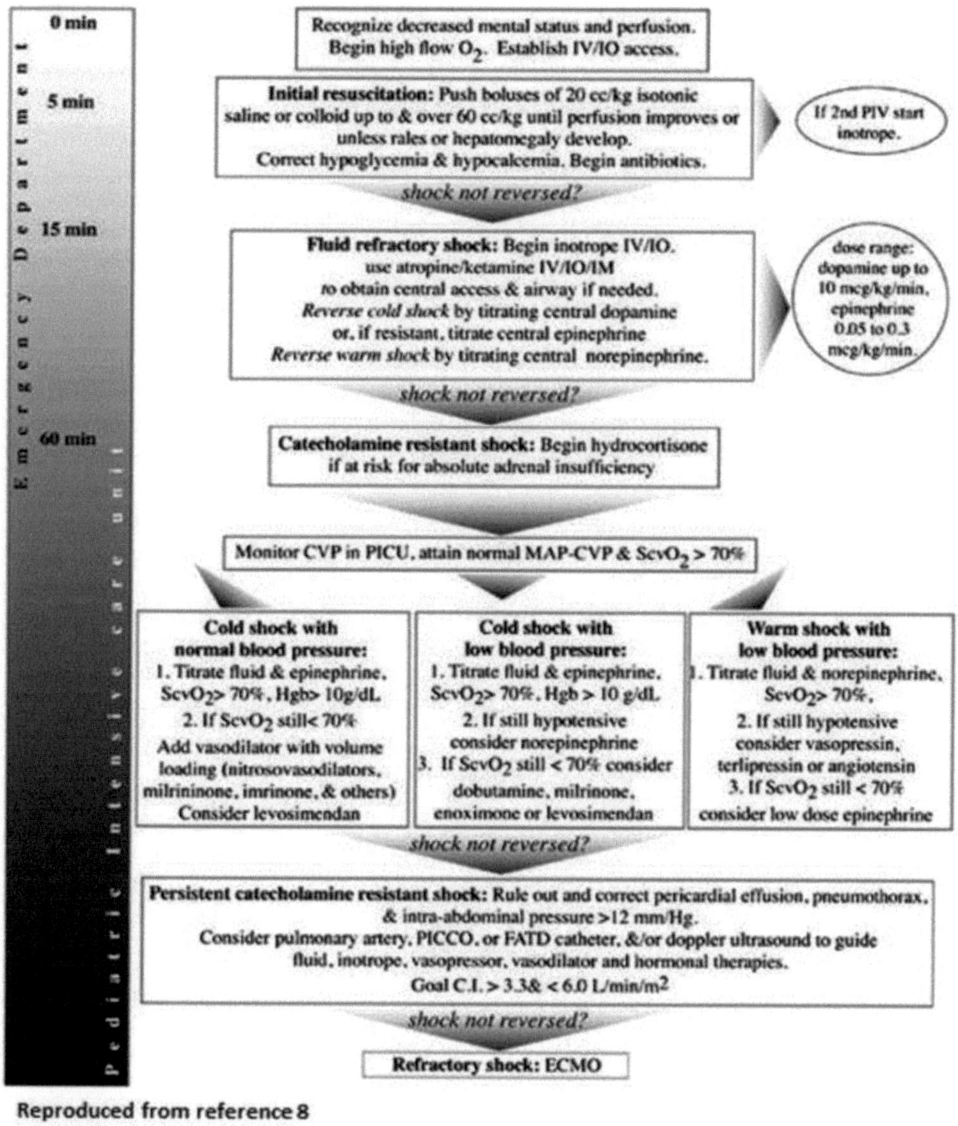

Figure 3.
Survive sepsis campaign pediatric treatment protocol [21].

risk factors for invasive infections which in turn affect antibiotic coverage guidelines [51]. Pediatric severe sepsis is defined as two or more systemic inflammatory response syndrome criteria, confirmed or suspected invasive infection, and cardiovascular dysfunction, acute respiratory distress syndrome, or two or more organ dysfunctions. Determination of altered physiology is specific to age dependent vital signs [49, 52]. At present, there is no single biomarker that has proven specific or sensitive enough to diagnose sepsis or prognosticate outcome in selected cohorts. Similar to studies of sepsis in adults, there is active research examining both clinical and research measurements applicable to a pediatric population [49].

4.3 Management

The current guidelines for treatment are summarized in the pediatric section of the surviving sepsis campaign (**Figure 3**) [49]. Early and aggressive source control should be a top priority; this includes drainage, debridement, and surgical intervention. Empiric antibiotic therapy should be administered within 1 hour of clinical suspicion and can be administered IV, IM or PO; antibiotics should not be delayed for blood cultures but every attempt should be made to obtain blood cultures prior to the first dose of antibiotics. Fluid resuscitation should be aggressive and administered as boluses of 20 mL/kg crystalloid given over 5–10 min via intravenous or intraosseous access. Early and aggressive fluid resuscitation has been shown to decrease mortality [21].

5. Conclusion

Sepsis and Septic Shock continue to be a growing concern in the world. Even though there is no current gold standard to diagnose sepsis and septic shock, the new guidelines allow the healthcare professional to determine if the patient could possibly go into sepsis and septic shock. The new guidelines help identify sepsis at an early stage in the adult population, but still show concerns in the pregnant and pediatric population. Due to the different normal lab values in a pregnant patient, SOFA cannot be accurately used to diagnose a patient. Defining sepsis in the pediatric patient is made more difficult due to age specific vital signs, and their tremendous physiologic reserve which often masks the seriousness of their condition. Sepsis and septic shock can be very deadly and the health care professional should be aware of the determining factors in the non-pregnant, pregnant and pediatric populations.

Acknowledgements

Funding for this manuscript was provided by The Everest Foundation.

Author details

Alaap Mehta*, Ali Khalid and Mamta Swaroop
Northwestern University, Chicago, Illinois, USA

*Address all correspondence to: alaapm@gmail.com

References

[1] Rhodes A et al. Surviving sepsis campaign: international guidelines for management of sepsis and septic shock: 2016. Intensive Care Medicine. 2017;**43**(3):304-377

[2] Cecconi M et al. Sepsis and septic shock. Lancet. 2018;**392**(10141):75-87

[3] Singer M et al. The third international consensus definitions for sepsis and septic shock (Sepsis-3). JAMA. 2016;**315**(8):801-810

[4] Reinhart K et al. Recognizing sepsis as a global health priority—A WHO resolution. The New England Journal of Medicine. 2017;**377**(5):414-417

[5] Vincent JL et al. Sepsis in European intensive care units: Results of the SOAP study. Critical Care Medicine. 2006;**34**(2):344-353

[6] J AC, Pinheiro I, Menezes Falcao L. Rethinking the concept of sepsis and septic shock. European Journal of Internal Medicine. 2018;**54**:1-5

[7] Gotur DB. Sepsis in a panorama: What the cardiovascular physician should know. Methodist DeBakey Cardiovascular Journal. 2018;**14**(2):89-100

[8] Abir G et al. Clinical and microbiological features of maternal sepsis: A retrospective study. International Journal of Obstetric Anesthesia. 2017;**29**:26-33

[9] Burlinson CEG et al. Sepsis in pregnancy and the puerperium. International Journal of Obstetric Anesthesia. 2018;**36**:96-107

[10] Shankar-Hari M et al. Judging quality of current septic shock definitions and criteria. Critical Care. 2015;**19**:445

[11] Kaukonen KM, Bailey M, Bellomo R. Systemic inflammatory response syndrome criteria for severe sepsis. The New England Journal of Medicine. 2015;**373**(9):881

[12] Vincent JL et al. The SOFA (sepsis-related organ failure assessment) score to describe organ dysfunction/failure. On behalf of the working group on sepsis-related problems of the European Society of Intensive Care Medicine. Intensive Care Medicine. 1996;**22**(7):707-710

[13] van der Woude SW et al. Classifying sepsis patients in the emergency department using SIRS, qSOFA or MEWS. The Netherlands Journal of Medicine. 2018;**76**(4):158-166

[14] Seymour CW et al. Assessment of clinical criteria for sepsis: For the third international consensus definitions for sepsis and septic shock (Sepsis-3). JAMA. 2016;**315**(8):762-774

[15] Vaught AJ. Maternal sepsis. Seminars in Perinatology. 2018;**42**(1):9-12

[16] Larsen FF, Petersen JA. Novel biomarkers for sepsis: A narrative review. European Journal of Internal Medicine. 2017;**45**:46-50

[17] Takeuchi O, Akira S. Pattern recognition receptors and inflammation. Cell. 2010;**140**(6):805-820

[18] Angus DC, van der Poll T. Severe sepsis and septic shock. The New England Journal of Medicine. 2013;**369**(21):2063

[19] Angus DC et al. Epidemiology of severe sepsis in the United States: Analysis of incidence, outcome, and associated costs of care. Critical Care Medicine. 2001;**29**(7):1303-1310

[20] Opal SM et al. Systemic host responses in severe sepsis analyzed by causative microorganism and treatment effects of drotrecogin alfa (activated). Clinical Infectious Diseases. 2003;**37**(1):50-58

[21] Dellinger RP et al. Surviving sepsis campaign: International guidelines for management of severe sepsis and septic shock: 2012. Critical Care Medicine. 2013;**41**(2):580-637

[22] Mayr FB et al. Infection rate and acute organ dysfunction risk as explanations for racial differences in severe sepsis. JAMA. 2010;**303**(24):2495-2503

[23] Hollenberg SM et al. Practice parameters for hemodynamic support of sepsis in adult patients: 2004 update. Critical Care Medicine. 2004;**32**(9):1928-1948

[24] Rivers E et al. Early goal-directed therapy in the treatment of severe sepsis and septic shock. The New England Journal of Medicine. 2001;**345**(19):1368-1377

[25] Paul M et al. Systematic review and meta-analysis of the efficacy of appropriate empiric antibiotic therapy for sepsis. Antimicrobial Agents and Chemotherapy. 2010;**54**(11):4851-4863

[26] Rhodes A et al. Surviving sepsis campaign: international guidelines for management of sepsis and septic shock: 2016. Critical Care Medicine. 2017;**45**(3):486-552

[27] Shankar-Hari M et al. Developing a new definition and assessing new clinical criteria for septic shock: For the third international consensus definitions for sepsis and septic shock (Sepsis-3). JAMA. 2016;**315**(8):775-787

[28] De Backer D et al. Comparison of dopamine and norepinephrine in the treatment of shock. The New England Journal of Medicine. 2010;**362**(9):779-789

[29] Sacha GL, Bauer SR, Lat I. Vasoactive agent use in septic shock: Beyond first-line recommendations. Pharmacotherapy. 2019;**39**(3):369-381

[30] Say L et al. Global causes of maternal death: A WHO systematic analysis. The Lancet Global Health. 2014;**2**(6):e323-e333

[31] Bamfo JE. Managing the risks of sepsis in pregnancy. Best Practice & Research. Clinical Obstetrics & Gynaecology. 2013;**27**(4):583-595

[32] Chebbo A et al. Maternal sepsis and septic shock. Critical Care Clinics. 2016;**32**(1):119-135

[33] Kendle AM, Louis J. Recognition and treatment of sepsis in pregnancy. Journal of Midwifery & Women's Health. 2018;**63**(3):347-351

[34] Lapinsky SE. Obstetric infections. Critical Care Clinics. 2013;**29**(3):509-520

[35] Smaill FM, Grivell RM. Antibiotic prophylaxis versus no prophylaxis for preventing infection after cesarean section. Cochrane Database of Systematic Reviews. 2014;**10**:CD007482

[36] Parfitt SE et al. Sepsis in obstetrics: Clinical features and early warning tools. MCN: American Journal of Maternal Child Nursing. 2017;**42**(4):199-205

[37] Muller AE et al. Morbidity related to maternal group B streptococcal infections. Acta Obstetricia et Gynecologica Scandinavica. 2006;**85**(9):1027-1037

[38] McIntyre J. Mothers infected with HIV. British Medical Bulletin. 2003;**67**:127-135

[39] Sriskandan S. Severe peripartum sepsis. The Journal of the Royal College of Physicians of Edinburgh. 2011;**41**(4):339-346

[40] Barton JR, Sibai BM. Severe sepsis and septic shock in pregnancy. Obstetrics and Gynecology. 2012;**120**(3):689-706

[41] Angus DC et al. A systematic review and meta-analysis of early goal-directed therapy for septic shock: The ARISE, ProCESS and ProMISe investigators. Intensive Care Medicine. 2015;**41**(9):1549-1560

[42] Raghunathan K et al. Association between the choice of IV crystalloid and in-hospital mortality among critically ill adults with sepsis. Critical Care Medicine. 2014;**42**(7):1585-1591

[43] Acker SN et al. Head injury and unclear mechanism of injury: Initial hematocrit less than 30 is predictive of abusive head trauma in young children. Journal of Pediatric Surgery. 2014;**49**(2):338-340

[44] Ames SG et al. Infectious etiologies and patient outcomes in pediatric septic shock. Journal of the Pediatric Infectious Diseases Society. 2017;**6**(1):80-86

[45] Alder MN, Opoka AM, Wong HR. The glucocorticoid receptor and cortisol levels in pediatric septic shock. Critical Care. 2018;**22**(1):244

[46] Syngal P, Giuliano JS Jr. Health-related quality of life after pediatric severe sepsis. Healthcare (Basel). 2018;**6**(3):1-7

[47] Marshall JC. Understanding the global burden of pediatric sepsis. American Journal of Respiratory and Critical Care Medicine. 2015;**191**(10):1096-1098

[48] Watson RS et al. The epidemiology of severe sepsis in children in the United States. American Journal of Respiratory and Critical Care Medicine. 2003;**167**(5):695-701

[49] Mathias B, Mira JC, Larson SD. Pediatric sepsis. Current Opinion in Pediatrics. 2016;**28**(3):380-387

[50] Watson RS, Carcillo JA. Scope and epidemiology of pediatric sepsis. Pediatric Critical Care Medicine. 2005;**6**(3 Suppl):S3-S5

[51] Goldstein B et al. International pediatric sepsis consensus conference: Definitions for sepsis and organ dysfunction in pediatrics. Pediatric Critical Care Medicine. 2005;**6**(1):2-8

[52] Ruth A et al. Pediatric severe sepsis: Current trends and outcomes from the pediatric health information systems database. Pediatric Critical Care Medicine. 2014;**15**(9):828-838

Chapter 6

Anaphylactic Shock

Stephen DeTurk, Shravan Reddy, Anna Ng Pellegrino and John Wilson

Abstract

Anaphylaxis is a life threatening hypersensitivity reaction that can cause shock. Epidemiology studies show anaphylaxis and anaphylactic shock is relatively rare, but its incidence is increasing. A review of the pathophysiology of anaphylaxis can provide insight into clinical decisions. Diagnosing anaphylaxis can be difficult as symptoms and history are not always obvious. Diagnostic guidelines provide an objective tool to assess for anaphylaxis. Early intervention during anaphylaxis may prevent development of shock. Management is focused on circulation support with epinephrine and IV fluids, and airway maintenance. Following an acute anaphylactic reaction, patients should be provided with a referral for follow up and educated on avoidance of triggers and use of epinephrine autoinjectors.

Keywords: anaphylaxis, anaphylactic shock, distributive shock, management

1. Introduction

In this chapter, we will learn the differences between anaphylaxis and anaphylactic shock. Epidemiology of anaphylactic shock will be reviewed. We will also discuss the biochemical markers and mediators most noted to triggering an anaphylactic reaction. Lastly, we will provide a review on clinical manifestations and management of an anaphylactic reaction in a nonclinical setting and in a clinical setting.

Throughout this chapter anaphylaxis will be defined according to the World Allergy Organization (WAO) definition '*a severe, life-threatening generalized or systemic hypersensitivity reaction*' [1]. This includes Gell-Combs Type I hypersensitivity, as well anaphylactoid reactions that are immunologically and nonimmunological mediated.

There are few studies on anaphylactic shock, and most recommendations for anaphylactic shock management come from major allergy organizations: WAO, AAAA/ACAAI, and EAACI. The recommendations of these groups for management of anaphylactic shock are presented in this chapter. Recent changes in anaphylaxis definitions require a review of the immunologic and nonimmunologic biochemical pathways of anaphylaxis.

1.1 Definitions

1.1.1 Anaphylactoid reactions

Reactions that occur via mechanisms other than IgE mediated mast cell degranulation have been referred to as *Anaphylactoid reactions*. However, the WAO, AAAA/ACAAI, and EAACI have recommended stoppage of the term [2]. Throughout this chapter reactions that would be included in this term will be referred to as anaphylaxis.

1.1.2 Anaphylaxis

Anaphylaxis is typically taught as Gell-Combs classification type 1 hypersensitivity, that is IgE mediated. However, the World Allergy Organization (WAO) proposed a new expanded definition of anaphylaxis '*a severe, life-threatening generalized or systemic hypersensitivity reaction*' [3]. This new definition of anaphylaxis now includes reactions previously categorized as 'anaphylactoid reactions'.

1.1.3 Anaphylactic shock

End manifestation of anaphylaxis, occurs when there is inadequate tissue perfusion causing end organ damage.

2. Epidemiology

Studies have estimated that the incidence of anaphylaxis is between 0.05 and 2.0% of the population [4], although the actual incidence is not clear. Issues previously identified with epidemiologic studies include variations in definitions, under reporting of anaphylaxis, and unclear use of incidence and prevalence of disease [5].

Although the actual incidence is not clear, there have been multiple studies showing that the incidence of anaphylaxis in the United States has increased in recent years [6–9], although the case fatality rate has decreased [8]. Similar findings are reported in other countries, with UK reporting increasing rates of anaphylaxis [10–12], but no increase in the incidence of fatal anaphylaxis [10]. In Australia the incidence of anaphylaxis [13–15] and fatal anaphylaxis has increased as well [16]. One study on the incidence of anaphylaxis with circulatory symptoms found a rate of approximately 8–9 cases per 100,000 persons per year [17]. Severe anaphylaxis, including respiratory or circulatory symptoms, occurs more frequently at a rate of about 1–3 per 10,000 people [18].

Factors that may affect the incidence of anaphylaxis include geography, seasonal variations, age, and gender [19]. Demographic factors associated with higher incidence include living in northern areas of US [7, 20].

3. Pathophysiology

Anaphylaxis is caused by massive release of biochemical mediators from mast cell and basophils. Mast cells activation occurs mainly via antigen crosslinking of IgE bound to FcεRI receptors on cell membranes. However, other membrane receptors can activate mast cells as well or potentiate IgE activation [21]. The multiple activation pathways allow for immunologic (e.g. IgE mediated) and/or nonimmunologic activation (e.g. drug directly interacting with receptors) (**Figure 1**: mechanisms of mast cell degranulation). Some antigens may mediate effects via several mechanisms simultaneously (e.g. vespid venom, NSAIDs, opiates). In non-IgE mediated anaphylaxis, symptoms can occur on first exposure to an antigen as prior exposure and sensitization is not required.

Reproduced from Spoerl et al. [22] in agreement with publishing under terms of the Creative Commons Attribution (CC BY) license.

3.1 Triggers and cell activation

In IgE mediated anaphylaxis, an immunogen cross links membrane bound IgE in previously sensitized mast cell. Immunogens are typically large foreign proteins

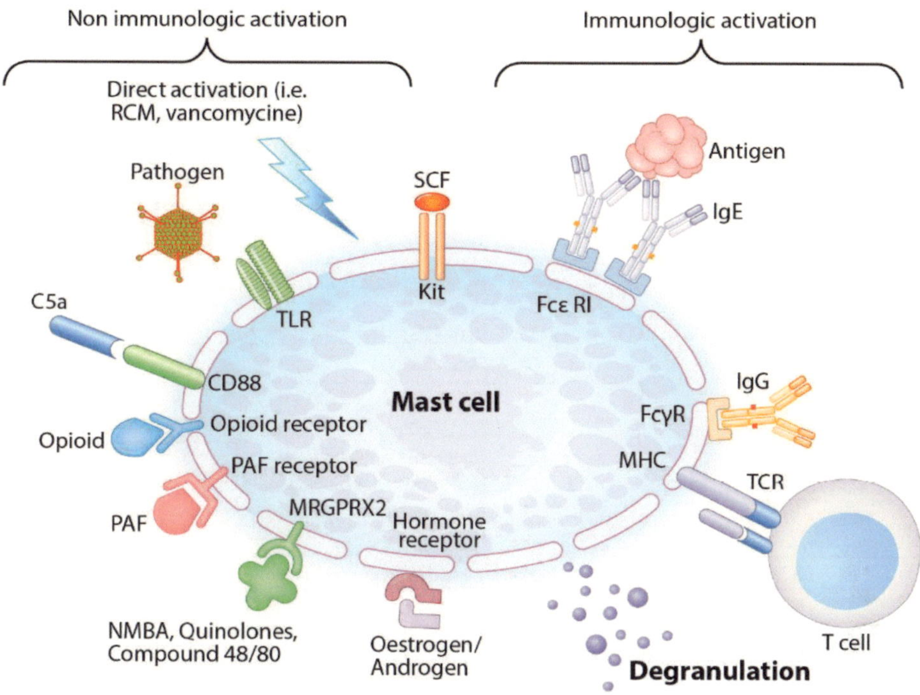

Figure 1.
Mechanisms of mast cell degranulation. Abbreviations: RCM, radiocontrast media; TLR. Toll-like receptor; SCF, stem cell factor; FcεRI, high affinity IgE receptor; FcγR, IgG receptor; TCR, T-cell receptor; NMBA, neuromuscular blocking agent; PAF, platelet activating factor; MHC, major histocompatibility complex.

with multiple epitope binding sites (e.g. proteins in insect venom and certain foods) [23]. Antigens that are too small to cross link IgE (e.g. penicillin) must first bind to larger carrier molecules in order to elicit an immune response. Common triggers of IgE-mediated anaphylaxis include various food, venom and medications are summarized in **Table 1**: IgE-dependent triggers and discussed in more detail below.

3.1.1 Food

The most common foods causing anaphylaxis varies by region, in North America the most common food allergies includes milk, egg, peanuts, tree nuts, fish, shellfish, wheat, soy, and sesame [24]. Allergenic proteins have been identified for these common causes as well as in rice, barley, buckwheat, mustard, celery, potato, carrots, and apples [25].

Most cases of anaphylaxis due to food occurs in children or those with known food allergies, and fatal cases are rare [7, 8, 10]. When fatal, the cause of death is more often due to respiratory arrest, although shock can occur as well. Arrest occurs later compared to medication or venom, typically occurring 25–35 min after exposure [26].

3.1.2 Venom

Stinging insects belonging to the order Hymenoptera produce venoms that can cause anaphylaxis. The important insects from this order include bees, vespids (wasps, yellow jackets, hornets) and stinging ants [27]. Vespid venom additionally activates complement in an IgE independent mechanism, which may potentiate anaphylaxis [28]. In addition to hymenoptera venom, bites from rattlesnakes [29],

Foods	Milk Eggs Peanuts Tree nuts Fish Shellfish Soy Wheat Sesame
Bites/venoms	Hymenoptera venom (bee, vespids*, ants) Tick Rattlesnake Hamster
Medications	Antibiotics NSAIDs* Chemotherapy Neuromuscular blocker* Radiocontrast* Opioids*

**Non-IgE mediated mechanisms identified as alternative or additional mechanism.*

Table 1.
IgE-dependent triggers [9, 24, 27, 29–32].

hamsters [30], and ticks [31] have been implicated as causes of anaphylaxis. Fatal cases due stings are more often due to shock than respiratory distress, arrest typically occurs 10–15 min after exposure [26].

3.1.3 Medications

The most common medications causing anaphylaxis are beta-lactam antibiotics, NSAIDs, neuromuscular blocking agents, and chemotherapy [9, 32] . However, nearly any medication has the potential to cause anaphylaxis, some drugs that have been implicated includes intravenous iron [33], gelatin found in a vaccines [34], dextran [35], and human serum albumin [36]. In addition to IgE mediated mechanisms, other mechanisms of inducing anaphylaxis have been identified for multiple drugs [37]. This includes complement or contact activation (e.g. radiocontrast media, pegylated compounds, liposomal drugs [38], and heparin contaminated with oversulfated chondroitin sulfate (OSCS) [39]) and direct mast cell activation (e.g. opiates and neuromuscular blockers [37]). There have been multiple reports of anaphylaxis occurring to biologic agents, where the patient had IgG but no detectable IgE antibody to the therapy [40]. In medication induced anaphylaxis, shock is more common in severe cases than respiratory distress [26, 41]. Arrest occurs can occur rapidly after exposure, most cases in less than 5 min [26].

3.2 Biochemical mediators and clinical pharmacology

Once activated, mast cells and basophils release a cascade of mediators which cause physiologic changes, activate other immunology pathways, and attract other immune cells. Preformed mediators are released immediately upon activation including histamine, tryptase, heparin, and chymase. Over several minutes additional mediators are generated including platelet activating factor, leukotrienes, and prostaglandins (**Table 2**). Various cytokines and chemokines are generated over several hours further propagate the inflammatory response [37, 42].

Immediate release	Histamine	Vasodilation, edema, bronchoconstriction, mucus secretion, change myocardial contractility
	Tryptase	Vasodilation, edema, bronchoconstriction
	Chymase	Vasodilation, edema, mucus secretion
	Heparin	Initiates formation of bradykinin causing edema
	TNFa	Bronchoconstriction
Rapid generation (min)	PAF	Vasodilation, edema, bronchoconstriction, platelet activation, decrease myocardial contractility
	LTs C4, D4	Potent vasoactive and spasmogenic agents
	Prostaglandin D2	Bronchospasm and increase mucus secretion

Table 2.
Physiologic effects of mediators [42, 49].

Histamine has long been considered the principal mediator of anaphylaxis, and concentrations of histamine correlate with symptom severity [42]. Histamine acts on receptors to cause vasodilation and increased permeability [43, 44], bronchoconstriction, and increase mucus secretion. In the heart H2 receptors have positive chronotropic and ionotropic effects and causes coronary vasodilation, while the H1 receptor causes coronary vasoconstriction [45].

Platelet activating factor (PAF) has been increasingly recognized as important in the pathophysiology of anaphylaxis. In PAF receptor knockout mice, symptoms of anaphylaxis are reduced [46]. In humans PAF levels in the serum directly correlates with the severity of anaphylaxis symptoms [47]. In addition to activating platelets, PAF causes vasodilation, increased vascular permeability, decreased myocardial contractility, bronchoconstriction, and initiates allergic response through stimulation of other mediators [48, 49].

4. Signs and Symptoms

Anaphylaxis causes a generalized systemic reaction affecting multiple organ systems, symptoms involving the skin occur in 80–90% of cases, respiratory tract in 70%, GI in 45%, CV in 45%, and CNS involvement in 15% [50, 51]. The cardiovascular and respiratory systems are the principal shock organs in fatal anaphylaxis. Death occurs in most often due to shock or acute respiratory distress, but DIC and epinephrine overdose have also been cited as cause of death [26, 52–55]. Most fatal cases of anaphylaxis due to medication or venoms are a result of shock, in food related anaphylaxis respiratory involvement is the main cause of death although shock is still possible [26, 56].

Anaphylaxis develops rapidly with symptoms developing in minutes. Biphasic reactions, where symptoms resolve and then reappear later occurs around 20% of the time [57]. A systematic review of biphasic reactions found the medium time between resolution of initial symptoms and onset of delayed symptoms to be 11 h, with a range of 0.2–72 h [58].

4.1 Cardiovascular changes

Cardiovascular manifestations of anaphylaxis develop due to direct and indirect effects of mediators on the vasculature and heart. Increased vascular permeability causes rapid fluid extravasation, with up to 35% of plasma volume shift occurring in a matter of minutes [59, 60]. Vascular smooth muscle relaxation causes vasodilation and a rapid decrease in SVR [61, 62]. Rapid drop in measured CVP suggests that venodilation plays a major as well. The combined effects as extravasation and venodilation cause significant reduction in preload. This can be severe enough to cause Empty ventricle syndrome, has been documented in autopsies of patients who died from anaphylaxis [63].

Arrhythmias and myocardial infarction can also be seen in anaphylaxis. Arrhythmias may develop due to the combined direct effect of mediators, and hemodynamic changes previously described. Myocardial infarctions seen in anaphylaxis may be due to decreased venous return and direct effects of mediators on coronary arteries causing vasospasm or disruption of atherosclerotic plaques [64, 65].

Compensatory response to these changes includes rise in heart rate, ejection fraction, and cardiac index [61, 62]. Although Tachycardia is typical in anaphylaxis, although bradycardia may be seen as well. Bradycardia occurs due to a compensatory *Bezold-Jarisch* reflex, and has been found to have lower mortality rates when compared to cases of anaphylactic shock with tachycardia [66, 67]. Atropine therefore should not be administered, as it would counteract this protective effect and may increase mortality [68].

4.2 Respiratory changes

The entire respiratory tract can be affected in anaphylaxis, involving the upper airway and/or lower airway [69]. Upper airway symptoms develop due to fluid extravasation causing mucosal edema [70]. Some symptoms of upper airway involvement include angioedema, stridor, dysphagia, and rhinorrhea [50, 71]. Lower airway obstruction occurs due to mucosal edema, bronchospasm, and mucous plugging [70]. Oxygen saturation may decrease secondary to respiratory effects of anaphylaxis limiting airflow. When there is diffuse lower respiratory tract involvement, decreased oxygen saturation can persist despite endotracheal intubation [72]. When PaO2 is adequate, tissue oxygenation can still be compromised causing anaerobic metabolism. In one study on rats, tissue oxygenation of muscle decreased faster in anaphylaxis compared to nicardipine induced hypotension. The anaphylactic group also showed a greater increase in lactate and lactate-pyruvate ratio indicating depletion of intracellular energy storage [73].

4.3 Mucocutaneous, gastrointestinal, and neurologic changes

Mucocutaneous symptoms (e.g. flushing, pruritus, angioedema, and urticaria) are common in anaphylaxis, however in cases of shock cutaneous symptoms are often absent. Vasodilation and increased vasculature permeability leads to flushing and angioedema [74]. In addition to vascular changes, urticaria develops due inflammatory cell infiltration and neuropeptide release from sensory nerves [75]. Gastrointestinal symptoms include nausea, vomiting, diarrhea, and abdominal pain [76]. These symptoms are likely due to intestinal smooth muscle contraction and alterations in water and electrolyte absorption [77, 78]. Neurologic changes are mostly secondary to hypotension and decreased perfusion and may manifest as dizziness, confusion, syncope/presyncope, or headache [50]. More serious effects including seizure and stroke may also be seen but are rare [74, 79].

5. Diagnosing

It is often difficult to recognize anaphylaxis, and many cases go undiagnosed [80, 81]. Early intervention in acute anaphylaxis reduces risk of severe reaction and need for hospitalization [82]. In order to aid in diagnosis of anaphylaxis, diagnostic criteria have been developed (**Table 3**). In the clinic or emergency department, it may be unclear if the patient had been exposed to an allergen. In the ICU or operating room, rapid development of symptoms after administering medication makes recognizing anaphylaxis easier. Following the acute phase of anaphylaxis, serum tryptase and histamine should be measured to aid immunologist in confirming the diagnosis of anaphylaxis during follow-up care [83, 84]. Plasma tryptase remains elevated for 6 h following the onset of symptoms, but histamine levels remain elevated for just 1 h [85, 86]. Urinary histamine metabolites remain elevated for a longer period and may therefore be more useful than plasma histamine for confirming anaphylaxis [86].

5.1 Diagnostic criteria

Anaphylaxis is likely when one of the following criteria is fulfilled:
1. Acute onset of an illness (minutes to several hours) with involvement of the skin and/or mucosal tissue and at least one:
a. Respiratory compromise
b. Reduced blood pressure or symptoms of end-organ damage
2. Two or more of the following that occur rapidly after exposure to a likely allergen for that patient
a. Involvement of the skin-mucosal tissue
b. Respiratory compromise
c. Reduced blood pressure or associated symptoms
d. Persistent gastrointestinal symptoms
3. Reduced blood pressure after exposure to known allergen for that patient (minutes to several hours)
a. Adults: systolic blood pressure of less than 90 mm Hg or greater than 30% decrease from that person's baseline
b. Infants and children: low systolic blood pressure (age-specific) or greater than 30% decrease in systolic blood pressure

Table 3.
Clinical criteria for diagnosing anaphylaxis, modified from [3, 87].

5.2 Differential diagnosis

There are several conditions which may mimic certain characteristics of anaphylaxis. Acute anxiety can present as dyspnea and near syncope with hyperventilation. Hypoglycemia can precipitate an altered sensorium and syncope. Vasovagal episodes can involve nausea with vomiting, hypotension, pallor, bradycardia, diaphoresis and syncope. Additional considerations include severe reactive airway disease, vocal cord dysfunction and non-allergy mediated angioedema. Vasovagal episodes can involve nausea with vomiting, hypotension, pallor, bradycardia, diaphoresis and syncope [50, 88].

6. Management

There is a general lack of evidence basis for the treatment of anaphylaxis [89], but multiple expert guidelines highlight the chief treatment as epinephrine, oxygen, and fluids [86, 90, 91].

6.1 Principal treatment

Epinephrine is the first line treatment of anaphylaxis, and delayed administration increases the likelihood of poor outcomes [54, 55, 92]. Despite this, use of epinephrine in anaphylaxis is infrequent and often delayed [80]. There are no contraindications for use of epinephrine in anaphylaxis, and it should still be administered in patients with history of heart disease [93].

Epinephrine exerts its effects via alpha and beta adrenergic receptors in a dose-dependent response where beta receptors effects are dominant at low doses, but alpha receptors effects are seen at higher doses. The α1 receptors cause vasoconstriction increasing peripheral vascular resistance and blood pressure and improving coronary and cerebral perfusion. The β1 receptors exert positive chronotropic and inotropic effects which improves cardiac output and increases blood pressure. In the respiratory system, β2 receptors stimulation results in bronchodilation, and relief and respiratory symptoms. β receptors also inhibit release of mediators from mast cells and basophils, via increased cAMP production [94].

In most situations intramuscular administration is preferred, but IV epinephrine can be used in the ICU. IM epinephrine should be given in 0.2–0.5 mg doses (1:1000 dilution), and repeated every 5 min depending on the resolution of symptoms [86]. Studies showed that peak epinephrine concentrations were higher when epinephrine was given IM into the thigh, compared to IM administration in the arm or subcutaneous administration [95]. Multiple doses of epinephrine may be required to reverse symptoms [96]. Care should be taken to closely monitor pulse and blood pressure when epinephrine is administered intravenously as there is greater risk of severe adverse effects compared to intramuscular administration including arrhythmias and myocardial infarctions [97].

Following epinephrine administration, patients should continue to be assessed for worsening signs of anaphylaxis. Patients should be placed on pulse oximeter and given high flow oxygen as needed. Patients in anaphylactic shock should be placed in supine or Trendelenburg position to increase blood return to the heart. Patients who are sitting upright can have a significant decrease in preload leading to empty ventricle syndrome and PEA [98].

Due to the intravascular depletion, fluid is often necessary to maintain pressure. Crystalloids or colloids may be used, although physicians should be aware of the anaphylactic potential of some colloid solutions. Normal saline (0.9% saline) should be chosen over other crystalloids as it remains in the intravascular space longer than dextrose solutions [86, 99]. Caution should taken while giving fluids to patients with heart failure to prevent fluid overload.

6.2 Adjunct treatments

Antihistamines are often given as adjunct therapy in anaphylaxis, however there is no evidence to support or advise against their use in anaphylaxis [100]. Steroids may be used to prevent biphasic anaphylaxis [86], although there is no evidence to support the use of steroids in acute treatment of anaphylaxis [101, 102].

Nebulized albuterol or other beta-2 agonists may be useful to treat respiratory distress due to bronchoconstriction. While there is no clinical trial on use of these medications in anaphylaxis, their effectiveness in treating other allergic diseases offers some basis for their use [90].

6.3 Additional consideration

Beta blockers may complicate the treatment of anaphylaxis, as some of the beneficial effects of epinephrine will be diminished [103]. In patients on beta-blockers who do not respond to epinephrine and fluids, other vasopressors should be considered. Glucagon has been reported to be a successful treatment in several case reports of patients on beta blockers who experienced anaphylactic shock [104].

Glucagon mechanism of action is via direct activation of adenylate cyclase, bypassing the blocked adrenergic receptors.

Vasopressin or phenylephrine can be used to increase systemic vascular resistance without further increasing heart rate. Dopamine or norepinephrine can be added in cases of relative bradycardia [105]. Mechanical support with ECMO has been reported to be successful at treating refractory anaphylaxis with profound myocardial dysfunction [106].

Methylene blue has been reported to be an effective treatment in cases of severe anaphylaxis not responding to epinephrine [88], as well as cases of anaphylaxis without hypotension. Methylene blue inhibits NO mediated vasodilation via competitive inhibition of guanylate cyclase decreasing cyclic GMP production and subsequent vasodilation [107]. This mechanism acts independent of adrenergic receptors, and may be effective in patients with refractory anaphylactic shock [108].

6.4 Follow up

Before discharging a patient that experienced anaphylaxis, they should be referred to an immunologist for a thorough evaluation. Labs to assess for anaphylaxis (i.e. tryptase, histamine) should be drawn to assist allergist in making a diagnosis. Patients should also receive a prescription for an epinephrine autoinjector, along with education on how to use it [87].

7. Conclusions

Anaphylaxis is a rapidly acting life-threatening hypersensitivity reaction. Diagnosis of anaphylaxis can be difficult, and early recognition and treatment is essential to prevent development of shock. Shock is more common in cases due to medication compared to food, although shock can occur. The primary treatment in anaphylactic shock is epinephrine, fluids, and oxygen. Additional medications including antihistamines, steroids, and inhaled beta-agonist should be used as needed. In patients who do not respond to epinephrine, other vasopressors or mechanical support can be used.

Abbreviations

AAAAI	American Academy of Allergy, Asthma and Immunology
ACAAI	American College of Allergy, Asthma and Immunology
EAACI	European Academy of Allergy and Clinical Immunology
WAO	World Allergy Organization
Ig	immunoglobulin
Antigen	molecule capable of interacting with Ig, includes immunogens and haptens
Immunogen	molecule that can interact with Ig and cause an immune response
Hapten	molecule that can interact with Ig, but cannot cause immune response on its own

Author details

Stephen DeTurk[1*], Shravan Reddy[2], Anna Ng Pellegrino[3] and John Wilson[4]

1 Research Department, St. Luke's University Health Network, USA

2 Warren Family Medicine Residency, St. Luke's University Health Network, USA

3 Department of Anesthesia, St. Luke's University Health Network, USA

4 Department of Emergency Medicine, St. Luke's University Health Network, USA

*Address all correspondence to: stephen.deturk1@sluhn.org

References

[1] Johansson SGO, Bieber T, Dahl R, Friedmann PS, Lanier BQ, Lockey RF, et al. Revised nomenclature for allergy for global use: Report of the Nomenclature Review Committee of the World Allergy Organization, October 2003. The Journal of Allergy and Clinical Immunology. 2004;**113**(5):832-836

[2] Simons FER, Ardusso LRF, Bilo MB, Cardona V, Ebisawa M, El-Gamal YM, et al. International consensus on (ICON) anaphylaxis. World Allergy Organization Journal. 2014;7:9

[3] Sampson HA, Munoz-Furlong A, Bock A, Schmitt M, Bass R, Chowdhury BA, et al. Symposium on the definition and management of anaphylaxis: Summary report. The Journal of Allergy and Clinical Immunology. 2005;**115**(3):584-591

[4] Lieberman P, Camargo CA, Bohlke K, Jick H, Miller RL, Sheikh A, et al. Epidemiology of anaphylaxis: Findings of the American College of Allergy, Asthma and Immunology epidemiology of Anaphylaxis Working Group. Annals of Allergy, Asthma & Immunology. 2006;**97**(5):596-602

[5] Tanno LK, Bierrenbach AL, Simons FER, Cardona V, Thong BYH, Molinari N, et al. Critical view of anaphylaxis epidemiology: Open questions and new perspectives. Allergy, Asthma & Clinical Immunology. 2018;**14**:11

[6] Lin RY, Anderson AS, Shah SN, Nurruzzaman F. Increasing anaphylaxis hospitalizations in the first 2 decades of life: New York State, 1990-2006. Annals of Allergy, Asthma & Immunology. 2008;**101**(4):387-393

[7] Jerschow E, Lin RY, Scaperotti MM, McGinn AP. Fatal anaphylaxis in the United States, 1999-2010: Temporal patterns and demographic associations. Journal of Allergy and Clinical Immunology. 2014;**134**(6):1318

[8] Ma L, Danoff TM, Borish L. Case fatality and population mortality associated with anaphylaxis in the United States. The Journal of Allergy and Clinical Immunology. 2014;**133**(4):1075-1083

[9] Graudins LV, Trubiano JA, Zubrinich CM, Elliott AS, Aung AK. Medication-related anaphylaxis treated in hospital: Agents implicated, patient outcomes, and management lessons. Pharmacoepidemiology and Drug Safety. 2018;**27**(9):1029-1033

[10] Turner PJ, Gowland MH, Sharma V, Ierodiakonou D, Harper N, Garcez T, et al. Increase in anaphylaxis-related hospitalizations but no increase in fatalities: An analysis of United Kingdom national anaphylaxis data, 1992-2012. Journal of Allergy and Clinical Immunology. 2015;**135**(4):956

[11] Gupta R, Sheikh A, Strachan D, Anderson HR. Increasing hospital admissions for systemic allergic disorders in England: Analysis of national admissions' data. British Medical Journal. 2003;**327**(7424):1142-1143

[12] Sheikh A, Alves B. Hospital admissions for acute anaphylaxis: Time trend study. British Medical Journal. 2000;**320**(7247):1441

[13] Poulos LM, Waters AM, Correll PK, Loblay RH, Marks GB. Trends in hospitalizations for anaphylaxis, angioedema, and urticaria in Australia, 1993-1994 to 2004-2005. The Journal of Allergy and Clinical Immunology. 2007;**120**(4):878-884

[14] Liew WK, Williamson E, Tang MLK. Anaphylaxis fatalities and admissions in Australia. The Journal of Allergy and Clinical Immunology. 2009;**123**(2):434-442

[15] Mullins RJ, Dear KBG, Tang MLK. Time trends in Australian hospital anaphylaxis admissions in 1998-1999 to 2011-2012. The Journal of Allergy and Clinical Immunology. 2015;**136**(2):367-375

[16] Mullins RJ, Wainstein BK, Barnes EH, Liew WK, Campbell DE. Increases in anaphylaxis fatalities in Australia from 1997 to 2013. Clinical and Experimental Allergy. 2016;**46**(8):1099-1110

[17] Helbling A, Hurni T, Mueller UR, Pichler WJ. Incidence of anaphylaxis with circulatory symptoms: A study over a 3-year period comprising 940 000 inhabitants of the Swiss Canton Bern. Clinical and Experimental Allergy. 2004;**34**(2):285-290

[18] Moneret-Vautrin DA, Morisset M, Flabbee J, Beaudouin E, Kanny G. Epidemiology of life-threatening and lethal anaphylaxis: A review. Allergy. 2005;**60**(4):443-451

[19] Yu JE, Lin RY. The epidemiology of anaphylaxis. Clinical Reviews in Allergy and Immunology. 2018;**54**(3):366-374

[20] Sheehan WJ, Graham D, Ma L, Baxi S, Phipatanakul W. Higher incidence of pediatric anaphylaxis in northern areas of the United States. The Journal of Allergy and Clinical Immunology. 2009;**124**(4):850-852

[21] Gilfillan AM, Tkaczyk C. Integrated signalling pathways for mast-cell activation. Nature Reviews. Immunology. 2006;**6**(3):218-230

[22] Spoerl D, Nigolian H, Czarnetzki C, Harr T. Reclassifying anaphylaxis to neuromuscular blocking agents based on the presumed patho-mechanism: IgE-mediated, pharmacological adverse reaction or "innate hypersensitivity"? International Journal of Molecular Sciences. 2017;**18**(6):1223

[23] Huby RDJ, Dearman RJ, Kimber I. Why are some proteins allergens? Toxicological Sciences. 2000;**55**(2):235-246

[24] Sicherer SH, Sampson HA. Food allergy. The Journal of Allergy and Clinical Immunology. 2010;**125**(2):S116-SS25

[25] Sampson HA. Food allergy. Part 1: Immunopathogenesis and clinical disorders. The Journal of Allergy and Clinical Immunology. 1999;**103**(5):717-728

[26] Pumphrey RS, editor. Fatal anaphylaxis in the UK, 1992-2001. In: Novartis Found Symp. Vol. 1999. Chichester; New York: John Wiley; 2004

[27] Reisman RE. Insect stings. The New England Journal of Medicine. 1994;**331**(8):523-527

[28] Vanderlinden PWG, Hack CE, Kerckhaert JAM, Struyvenberg A, Vanderzwan JC. Preliminary-report—Complement activation in wasp-sting anaphylaxis. Lancet. 1990;**336**(8720):904-906

[29] Hogan DE, Dire DJ. Anaphylactic shock secondary to rattlesnake bite. Annals of Emergency Medicine. 1990;**19**(7):814-816

[30] Lim DL, Chan RME, Wen H, Van Bever HPS, Chua KY. Anaphylaxis after hamster bites—Identification of a novel allergen. Clinical and Experimental Allergy. 2004;**34**(7):1122-1123

[31] Mateos-Hernandez L, Villar M, Moral A, Rodriguez CG, Arias TA, de la Osa V, et al. Tick-host conflict: Immunoglobulin E antibodies

to tick proteins in patients with anaphylaxis to tick bite. Oncotarget. 2017;**8**(13):20630-20644

[32] Park HK, Kang MG, Yang MS, Jung JW, Cho SH, Kang HR. Epidemiology of drug-induced anaphylaxis in a tertiary hospital in Korea. Allergology International. 2017;**66**(4):557-562

[33] Bailie GR, Clark JA, Lane CE, Lane PL. Hypersensitivity reactions and deaths associated with intravenous iron preparations. Nephrology Dialysis Transplantation. 2005;**20**(7):1443-1449

[34] Pool V, Braun MM, Kelso JM, Mootrey G, Chen RT, Yunginger JW, et al. Prevalence of anti-gelatin IgE antibodies in people with anaphylaxis after measles-mumps-rubella vaccine in the United States. Pediatrics. 2002;**110**(6):9

[35] Zinderman CE, Landow L, Wise RP. Anaphylactoid reactions to dextran 40 and 70: Reports to the United States Food and Drug Administration, 1969 to 2004. Journal of Vascular Surgery. 2006;**43**(5):1004-1009

[36] Stafford CT, Lobel SA, Fruge BC, Moffitt JE, Hoff RG, Fadel HE. Anaphylaxis to human-serum albumin. Annals of Allergy. 1988;**61**(2):85-88

[37] Kemp SF, Lockey RF. Anaphylaxis: A review of causes and mechanisms. The Journal of Allergy and Clinical Immunology. 2002;**110**(3):341-348

[38] Szebeni J. Complement activation-related pseudoallergy: A stress reaction in blood triggered by nanomedicines and biologicals. Molecular Immunology. 2014;**61**(2):163-173

[39] Kishimoto TK, Viswanathan K, Ganguly T, Elankumaran S, Smith S, Pelzer K, et al. Contaminated heparin associated with adverse clinical events and activation of the contact system. The New England Journal of Medicine. 2008;**358**(23):2457-2467

[40] Finkelman FD, Khodoun MV, Strait R. Human IgE-independent systemic anaphylaxis. The Journal of Allergy and Clinical Immunology. 2016;**137**(6):1674-1680

[41] Renaudin JM, Beaudouin E, Ponvert C, Demoly P, Moneret-Vautrin DA. Severe drug-induced anaphylaxis: Analysis of 333 cases recorded by the Allergy Vigilance Network from 2002 to 2010. Allergy. 2013;**68**(7):929-937

[42] Stone SF, Brown SGA. Mediators released during human anaphylaxis. Current Allergy and Asthma Reports. 2012;**12**(1):33-41

[43] Dale HH, Richards A. The vasodilator action of histamine and of some other substances. The Journal of Physiology. 1918;**52**(2-3):110-165

[44] Majno G, Palade G. Studies on inflammation: I. The effect of histamine and serotonin on vascular permeability: An electron microscopic study. The Journal of Cell Biology. 1961;**11**(3):571-605

[45] Bristow MR, Ginsburg R, Harrison DC. Histamine and the human-heart—The other receptor system. The American Journal of Cardiology. 1982;**49**(1):249-251

[46] Ishii S, Kuwaki T, Nagase T, Maki K, Tashiro F, Sunaga S, et al. Impaired anaphylactic responses with intact sensitivity to endotoxin in mice lacking a platelet-activating factor receptor. The Journal of Experimental Medicine. 1998;**187**(11):1779-1788

[47] Vadas P, Gold M, Perelman B, Liss GM, Lack G, Blyth T, et al. Platelet-activating factor, PAF acetylhydrolase, and severe anaphylaxis. The New England Journal of Medicine. 2008;**358**(1):28-35

[48] Cuss F, Dixon CS, Barnes P. Effects of inhaled platelet activating factor on pulmonary function and bronchial responsiveness in man. The Lancet. 1986;**328**(8500):189-192

[49] Montrucchio G, Alloatti G, Camussi G. Role of platelet-activating factor in cardiovascular pathophysiology. Physiological Reviews. 2000;**80**(4):1669-1699

[50] Simons FER. Anaphylaxis. The Journal of Allergy and Clinical Immunology. 2010;**125**(2):S161-SS81

[51] Brown SGA. Clinical features and severity grading of anaphylaxis. The Journal of Allergy and Clinical Immunology. 2004;**114**(2):371-376

[52] Pumphrey RSH. Lessons for management of anaphylaxis from a study of fatal reactions. Clinical and Experimental Allergy. 2000;**30**(8):1144-1150

[53] Pumphrey RSH, Gowland MH. Further fatal allergic reactions to food in the United Kingdom, 1999-2006. The Journal of Allergy and Clinical Immunology. 2007;**119**(4):1018-1019

[54] Bock SA, Munoz-Furlong A, Sampson HA. Further fatalities caused by anaphylactic reactions to food, 2001-2006. The Journal of Allergy and Clinical Immunology. 2007;**119**(4):1016-1018

[55] Bock SA, Munoz-Furlong A, Sampson HA. Fatalities due to anaphylactic reactions to foods. The Journal of Allergy and Clinical Immunology. 2001;**107**(1):191-193

[56] Pumphrey RSH, Roberts ISD. Postmortem findings after fatal anaphylactic reactions. Journal of Clinical Pathology. 2000;**53**(4):273-276

[57] Tole JW, Lieberman P. Biphasic anaphylaxis: Review of incidence, clinical predictors, and observation recommendations. Immunology and Allergy Clinics of North America. 2007;**27**(2):309

[58] Lee S, Bellolio MF, Hess EP, Erwin P, Murad MH, Campbell RL. Time of onset and predictors of biphasic anaphylactic reactions: A systematic review and meta-analysis. The Journal of Allergy and Clinical Immunology: In Practice. 2015;**3**(3):408

[59] Fisher M. Blood-volume replacement in acute anaphylactic cardiovascular collapse related to anesthesia. British Journal of Anaesthesia. 1977;**49**(10):1023-1026

[60] Fisher MM. Clinical observations on the pathophysiology and treatment of anaphylactic cardiovascular collapse. Anaesthesia and Intensive Care. 1986;**14**(1):17-21

[61] Nicolas F, Villers D, Blanloeil Y. Hemodynamic pattern in anaphylactic shock with cardiac-arrest. Critical Care Medicine. 1984;**12**(2):144-145

[62] Beaupre PN, Roizen MF, Cahalan MK, Alpert RA, Cassorla L, Schiller NB. Hemodynamic and two-dimensional trans-esophageal echocardiographic analysis of an anaphylactic reaction in a human. Anesthesiology. 1984;**60**(5):482-484

[63] Brown SGA. The pathophysiology of shock in anaphylaxis. Immunology and Allergy Clinics of North America. 2007;**27**(2):165

[64] Brown AFT. Anaphylactic shock—Mechanisms and treatment. Journal of Accident & Emergency Medicine. 1995;**12**(2):89-100

[65] Kounis NG. Kounis syndrome (allergic angina and allergic myocardial infarction): A natural paradigm? International Journal of Cardiology. 2006;**110**(1):7-14

[66] Campagna JA, Carter C. Clinical relevance of the Bezold-Jarisch reflex. Anesthesiology. 2003;**98**(5):1250-1260

[67] Demetriades D, Chan LS, Bhasin P, Berne TV, Ramicone E, Huicochea F, et al. Relative bradycardia in patients with traumatic hypotension. The Journal of Trauma. 1998;**45**(3):534-539

[68] Dewachter P, Mouton-Faivre C, Emala CW. Anaphylaxis and anesthesia: Controversies and new insights. Anesthesiology. 2009;**111**(5):1141-1150

[69] Kemp SF, Lockey RF. In: Castells MC, editor. Pathophysiology and Organ Damage in Anaphylaxis. Totowa: Humana Press Inc; 2011. 33-46 p

[70] Brown SG. Anaphylaxis: Clinical concepts and research priorities. Emergency Medicine Australasia. 2006;**18**(2):155-169

[71] Lieberman P, Kemp SF, Oppenheimer J, Lang DM, Bernstein IL, Nicklas RA, et al. The diagnosis and management of anaphylaxis: An updated practice parameter. The Journal of Allergy and Clinical Immunology. 2005;**115**(3):S483-S523

[72] Smith PL, Kageysobotka A, Bleecker ER, Traystman R, Kaplan AP, Gralnick H, et al. Physiologic manifestations of human anaphylaxis. The Journal of Clinical Investigation. 1980;**66**(5):1072-1080

[73] Dewachter P, Jouan-Hureaux V, Franck P, Menu P, de Talance N, Zannad F, et al. Anaphylactic shock—A form of distributive shock without inhibition of oxygen consumption. Anesthesiology. 2005;**103**(1):40-49

[74] Lieberman P. Anaphylaxis. Medical Clinics of North America. 2006;**90**(1):77

[75] Tharp M. Chronic urticaria: Pathophysiology and treatment approaches. The Journal of Allergy and Clinical Immunology. 1996;**98** (6 Pt 3):S325

[76] Vighi G, Marcucci F, Sensi L, Di Cara G, Frati F. Allergy and the gastrointestinal system. Clinical and Experimental Immunology. 2008;**153**(s1):3-6

[77] Scott R, Diamant S, Gall D. Motility effects of intestinal anaphylaxis in the rat. American Journal of Physiology-Gastrointestinal and Liver Physiology. 1988;**255**(4):G505-GG11

[78] Perdue M, Chung M, Gall D. Effect of intestinal anaphylaxis on gut function in the rat. Gastroenterology. 1984;**86**(3):391

[79] Jain J, Banait S, Srivastava AK, Lodhe R. Stroke intracerebral multiple infarcts: Rare neurological presentation of honey bee bite. Annals of Indian Academy of Neurology. 2012;**15**(2):163-166

[80] Sclar DA, Lieberman PL. Anaphylaxis: Underdiagnosed, underreported, and undertreated. The American Journal of Medicine. 2014;**127**(1):S1-S5

[81] Aun MV, Kalil J, Giavina-Bianchi P. Adults and children with anaphylaxis in the emergency room: Why it is not recognized? Current Opinion in Allergy and Clinical Immunology. 2018;**18**(5):377-381

[82] Fleming JT, Clark S, Camargo CA, Rudders SA. Early treatment of food-induced anaphylaxis with epinephrine is associated with a lower risk of hospitalization. Journal of Allergy and Clinical Immunology-in Practice. 2015;**3**(1):57-62

[83] Laroche D, Gomis P, Gallimidi E, Malinovsky JM, Mertes PM. Diagnostic value of histamine and tryptase concentrations in severe anaphylaxis

with shock or cardiac arrest during anesthesia. Anesthesiology. 2014;**121**(2):272-279

[84] Schwartz LB. Diagnostic value of tryptase in anaphylaxis and mastocytosis. Immunology and Allergy Clinics of North America. 2006;**26**(3):451

[85] Laroche D, Vergnaud MC, Sillard B, Soufarapis H, Bricard H. Biochemical markers of anaphylactoid reactions to drugs—Comparison of plasma histamine and tryptase. Anesthesiology. 1991;**75**(6):945-949

[86] Lieberman P, Nicklas RA, Oppenheimer J, Kemp SF, Lang DM, Bernstein DI, et al. The diagnosis and management of anaphylaxis practice parameter: 2010 update. The Journal of Allergy and Clinical Immunology. 2010;**126**(3):477-480

[87] Sampson HA, Munoz-Furlong A, Campbell RL, Adkinson NF Jr, Bock SA, Branum A, et al. Second symposium on the definition and management of anaphylaxis: Summary report—Second National Institute of Allergy and Infectious Disease/Food Allergy and Anaphylaxis Network symposium. The Journal of Allergy and Clinical Immunology. 2006;**117**(2):391-397

[88] Lee JK, Vadas P. Anaphylaxis: Mechanisms and management. Clinical and Experimental Allergy. 2011;**41**(7):923-938

[89] Simons FER. Pharmacologic treatment of anaphylaxis: Can the evidence base be strengthened? Current Opinion in Allergy and Clinical Immunology. 2010;**10**(4):384-393

[90] Simons FER, Ardusso LRF, Bilo MB, El-Gamal YM, Ledford DK, Ring J, et al. World Allergy Organization anaphylaxis guidelines: Summary. The Journal of Allergy and Clinical Immunology. 2011;**127**(3):587-593

[91] Muraro A, Roberts G, Worm M, Bilo MB, Brockow K, Rivas MF, et al. Anaphylaxis: Guidelines from the European Academy of Allergy and Clinical Immunology. Allergy. 2014;**69**(8):1026-1045

[92] Sampson HA, Mendelson L, Rosen JP. Fatal and near-fatal anaphylactic reactions to food in children and adolescents. The New England Journal of Medicine. 1992;**327**(6):380-384

[93] Kemp SF, Lockey RF, Simons FER. World allergy org ad hoc C. epinephrine: The drug of choice for anaphylaxis. A statement of the World Allergy Organization. 2008;**63**(8):1061-1070

[94] Brown AFT. Therapeutic controversies in the management of acute anaphylaxis. Journal of Accident & Emergency Medicine. 1998;**15**(2):89-95

[95] Estelle F, Simons R, Gu XC, Simons KJ. Epinephrine absorption in adults: Intramuscular versus subcutaneous injection. The Journal of Allergy and Clinical Immunology. 2001;**108**(5):871-873

[96] Korenblat P, Lundie MJ, Dankner RE, Day JH. A retrospective study of epinephrine administration for anaphylaxis: How many doses are needed? Allergy and Asthma Proceedings. 1999;**20**(6):383-386

[97] McLean-Tooke A, Goulding M, Bundell C, White J, Hollingsworth P. Postmortem serum tryptase levels in anaphylactic and non-anaphylactic deaths. Journal of Clinical Pathology. 2014;**67**(2):134-138

[98] Pumphrey RSH. Fatal posture in anaphylactic shock. The Journal of Allergy and Clinical Immunology. 2003;**112**(2):451-452

[99] Simons FER, Ardusso LRF, Bilo MB, El-Gamal YM, Ledford DK, Ring J, et al. World allergy organization guidelines for the assessment and Management of Anaphylaxis. The Journal of Allergy and Clinical Immunology. 2011;**127**(3):22

[100] Sheikh A, Ten Broek V, Brown SG, Simons FE. H1-antihistamines for the treatment of anaphylaxis: Cochrane systematic review. Allergy. 2007;**62**(8):830-837

[101] Choo KJL, Simons FER, Sheikh A. Glucocorticoids for the treatment of anaphylaxis. Cochrane Database of Systematic Reviews. 2012;**4**:CD007596

[102] Choo KJL, Simons E, Sheikh A. Glucocorticoids for the treatment of anaphylaxis: Cochrane systematic review. Allergy. 2010;**65**(10):1205-1211

[103] Toogood JH. Beta-blocker therapy and the risk of anaphylaxis. Canadian Medical Association Journal. 1987;**136**(9):929-933

[104] Thomas M, Crawford I. Glucagon infusion in refractory anaphylactic shock in patients on beta-blockers. Emergency Medicine Journal. 2005;**22**(4):272-273

[105] LoVerde D, Iweala OI, Eginli A, Krishnaswamy G. Anaphylaxis. Chest. 2018;**153**(2):528-543

[106] Raper RF, Fisher MM. Profound reversible myocardial depression after anaphylaxis. Lancet. 1988;**1**(8582):386-388

[107] Bauer CS, Vadas P, Kelly KJ. Methylene blue for the treatment of refractory anaphylaxis without hypotension. The American Journal of Emergency Medicine. 2013;**31**(1):3

[108] Lo JCY, Darracq MA, Clark RF. A review of methylene blue treatment for cardiovascular collapse. The Journal of Emergency Medicine. 2014;**46**(5):670-679

Chapter 7

Neurogenic Shock

Anna Volski and Daniel J. Ackerman

Abstract

Neurogenic shock is a state characterized by hypotension, bradycardia, and other evidence of autonomic dysfunction. The most common cause is acute spinal cord injury (SCI), which will be the subject of our focus. Because the typical autonomic reflexes may be either abolished or dysregulated, appropriate treatment requires an understanding of the neuroanatomic substrate for the change. In this chapter, we will explore the root cause for neurogenic shock, differentiating it from spinal shock, and discuss those patients at risk and generally accepted treatment paradigms. The timeframe for manifestation of neurogenic shock is variable and it can quickly progress to cause secondary injury or death, so appropriate monitoring requires a high level of suspicion and diligence.

Keywords: neurogenic, shock, hypotension, bradycardia, hypothermia, autonomic, sympathetic, vasomotor, dysreflexia, spinal cord

1. Introduction

Imagine that you are in the trauma bay receiving a patient with a suspected high spinal cord injury due to a motor vehicle crash. Emergency medical responders sign out to you that the blood pressure has been fine on the way in, 110/60 mmHg with a heart rate in the 60s. As you complete your primary survey and get the patient on to your monitors you find the pressure has plummeted to 80/50 but rather than tachycardia the patient's heart rate is only 45. The rhythm is sinus bradycardia, the hemoglobin on your initial lab is 14.4 g/dl and there is no clear source of blood loss.

All too often neurogenic shock is an under-recognized but deadly cause of hypotension, bradycardia, and other complications related to spinal cord injury. In this chapter, we examine the definition, diagnosis, and treatment taking special care to differentiate it from spinal shock. We also briefly discuss autonomic dysreflexia and the role that neurogenic shock and autonomic dysreflexia can play in the rehabilitation setting.

2. Methods

Searches were conducted using the PubMed database for "neurogenic shock." The Lewis Katz School of Medicine online textbook library was also referenced using the same search terms, as were hard copies of reference textbooks 10 and 11.

IntechOpen

3. Background

3.1 History

The contemporary understanding of "neurogenic shock" was born with Alfred Blalock's "classification of peripheral circulatory failure," which he described in articles between 1927 and 1942. His "pure" types of shock included cardiogenic, hematogenic (better known as hypovolemic), neurogenic, and vasogenic (anaphylactic and septic) [1]. In descriptions of the neurogenic type, Blalock wrote: "the primary alteration is vasodilatation dependent on diminished constrictor tone as a result of influences acting through the nervous system," a description that has persisted [2]. At the time, Blalock associated neurogenic shock with spinal cord injury, spinal anesthesia, and vasovagal syncope [2]. Though our definition of neurogenic shock has evolved since Blalock's time, his classification system remains, and so do the challenges of defining, identifying, and managing neurogenic shock.

3.2 Neurogenic shock vs. spinal shock

Neurogenic shock is considered distributive in nature and refers to the loss of vasomotor tone and the instability that subsequently follows due to an imbalance in the autonomic nervous system (ANS) [3, 4]. Loss of sympathetic tone leads to unopposed parasympathetic control, manifested by refractory hypotension and bradycardia [3]. Other aspects of neurogenic shock include temperature dysregulation, autonomic dysreflexia, and orthostatic hypotension [5]. Aside from bradycardia and hypotension, many patients develop autonomic dysreflexia defined as a profound autonomic response to what would typically be a mild stimulus such as bladder or bowel distension [6]. The presence of a focal neurological deficit is not required for diagnosis, and although this is most often encountered in the setting of an acute SCI, theoretically any damage resulting in the loss of cerebral control of the autonomic nervous system may place a patient at risk for neurogenic shock. Neurogenic and spinal shocks are distinct consequences of spinal cord injury and the terms should not be used interchangeably.

Neurogenic shock most often occurs after an acute injury above T6, with a possible incidence of 29% in the cervical SCI population and 19% in the thoracic SCI population [4]. The onset may be variable in relation to the timing of the injury, but in SCI patients it most commonly manifests within 2 h of the trauma [7]. In most patients it is transient and may last for 1–6 weeks after injury [5, 8].

Conversely, spinal shock is the transient loss of reflexes and sensorimotor function that manifests acutely after injury to the spinal cord. It is a symptom of underlying spinal cord injury and the term "shock" in this situation does not refer to cardiovascular instability. Spinal shock is characterized by flaccid paralysis, anesthesia, and areflexia or hyporeflexia [3, 7]. Note that often enough the two may be present in the same patient but their natural course and treatment are distinct; furthermore there are often other potential causes for shock in the trauma patient (e.g. hypovolemic secondary to acute blood loss) clouding the diagnosis. It has been proposed that there are four phases of complete spinal shock resolution: hyporeflexia or areflexia (0–24 h), initial return of reflexes (1–3), early hyperreflexia (day 4 – 1 month) and spasticity (1–12 months) [7]. The total duration of spinal shock depends on the definition of its resolution. Resolution has been defined as the appearance of any reflex, the appearance of the bulbocavernosus reflex, return of reflex detrusor functions, or the return of deep tendon reflexes [7, 9]. Depending on which definition you use, spinal shock can last anywhere from days to months.

	Spinal shock	Neurogenic shock
Definition	Transient loss of reflexes and sensorimotor function below level of injury	Loss of sympathetic tone with unopposed parasympathetic control, leading to cardiovascular instability
Blood pressure	Hypotension	Hypotension
Heart rate	Bradycardia	Bradycardia
Associated autonomic symptoms	Difficulty breathing, bowel and bladder dysfunction, priapism	Autonomic dysreflexia, orthostatic hypotension, temperature dysregulation
Motor	Flaccid paralysis	Varies with injury
Reflexes	Areflexia or hyporeflexia in early stage, hyperreflexia in later stage of resolution	Varies with injury
Duration	Days to months	Most often 1–6 weeks
Treatment	Stabilization and treatment of underlying injury	Fluids and vasopressors with appropriate temperature monitoring

Table 1.
Comparison between spinal shock and neurogenic shock [3–5, 7–9].

Spinal shock and neurogenic shock may occur at the same time in a patient, complicating management, but they are not synonymous (see **Table 1**). Perhaps the most significant distinction is the difference in their management. The mainstay of treatment of neurogenic shock is fluids and vasopressors. As a transient symptom of spinal cord injury, spinal shock is expected to resolve on its own, in a predictable manner. Once spinal shock resolves, the underlying injury may be more accurately assessed.

4. Anatomic and epidemiologic considerations

The autonomic nervous system constitutes the involuntary control of many crucial systems of the body. Described as a system of visceral sensory inputs and motor responses, it maintains homeostasis and responds to both internal and external stimuli by manipulating the balance between its main divisions, the sympathetic and parasympathetic systems [10]. Although much of the autonomic system includes spinal reflex arcs with visceral motor neurons originating in ganglia lying peripheral to the spinal cord, there is overarching control exerted by multiple systems in the brain (**Figure 1**) [5]. It is the loss of this input from above that produces the dysfunction of the system, leading to shock [3]. The ANS maintains control of vital functions in the heart, vasculature, lungs, liver, digestive and para-digestive organs, glands, and reproductive organs. Although there are many involved neuropeptides, norepinephrine is the most common effector molecule in the sympathetic division and exerts it influence on both alpha and beta receptors, as well as the adrenal gland [10].

Estimating the true incidence of neurogenic shock is difficult for multiple reasons. The overall definition is reasonably broad, and a patient may experience multiple subtypes of shock at the same time. Furthermore, there may not be a simple direct imaging correlate that is easily elucidated (for example, one can see a significant anterior or lateral cord injury and correlate the physical symptoms to the level of the lesion, but isolating the level of injury in the intermediolateral

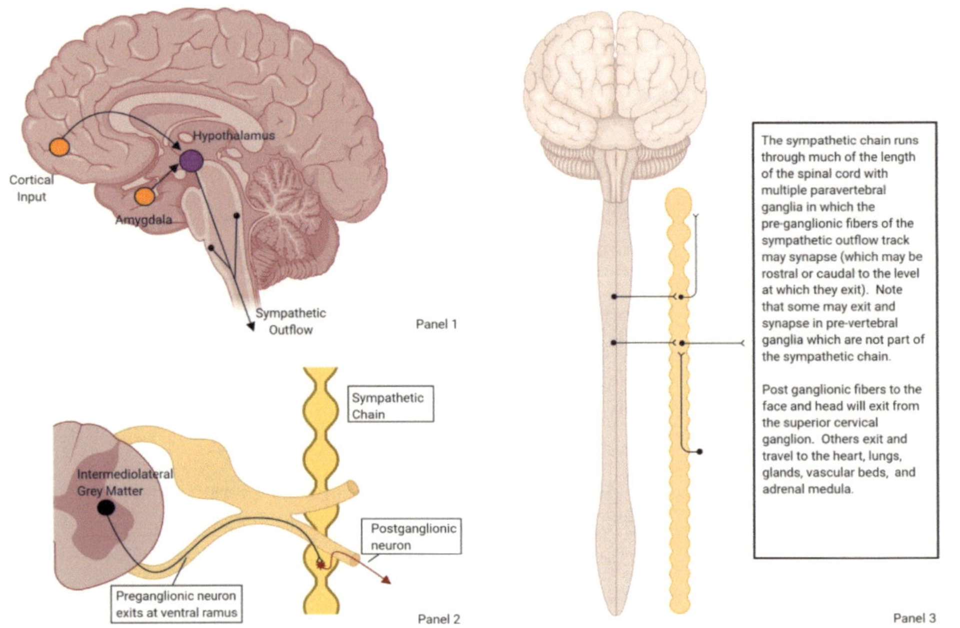

Figure 1.
Overview of sympathetic outflow. Panel 1 (top left): CNS control of the sympathetic nervous system originates in multiple brainstem areas and nuclei as well as the hypothalamus, which also receives input from the cortex and amygdala. The combined input creates a sympathetic outflow tract which descends the spinal cord to the intermediolateral gray matter. Panel 2 (bottom left): At multiple levels from T1 through the rostral lumbar spine the preganglionic neurons will exit through the ventral rami and then jump to the sympathetic chain where they may ascend, descend, or synapse at that level before exiting again as part of the spinal nerves. Panel 3 (right): Zoomed out view of the sympathetic chain with multiple Para-vertebral ganglia in which the preganglionic neurons may synapse. The exiting post ganglionic noradrenergic neurons provide direct sympathetic input to the heart, lungs, glands, vascular beds, and adrenal medulla. Note that some sympathetic neurons may exit and not synapse in the sympathetic chain but travel to pre-ganglionic neurons to synapse (such as the celiac and mesenteric ganglia) [10, 11]. Created with Biorender.com.

gray matter and ruling out other causes of shock is more challenging). Studies of incidence after SCI have been widely variable, ranging from 14 to 44% depending on the criteria used [4]. Extrapolating from a range of papers, criteria have ranged from systolic blood pressures (SBP) <70 mmHg up to <100 mmHg, and heart rates (HR) <50 beats per minute (BPM) up to ≤90 BPM in various combinations [12]. Examples include SBP <90 mmHG or HR <50 BPM as a cutoff, more recently others have used SBP <100 mmHG and HR <80 BPM, and still others simultaneous SBP <90 mmHg and HR <80 BPM with some variability in terms of whether or not lab values accounting for hypovolemia were examined as a confounder [4]. In one cohort of patients with isolated spinal cord injury (the majority of which were related to blunt trauma), defining neurogenic shock as SBP <100 mmHg, HR <80 BPM or both, out of 490 cases the incidence of hypotension was 25.8% and of classic neurogenic shock (hypotension and bradycardia) was only 19.3% [13]. What is suggested but not thoroughly quantified in the literature is that the incidence is highest in cervical spine injury and somewhat less for upper thoracic injury (above T6) while SCI lower than T6 would be considered rarely associated with neurogenic shock [3]. There is also not a single consensus in regard to penetrating vs. blunt trauma as to which is more likely to lead to neurogenic shock. Considering that SCI accounts for only about 5% of major trauma cases, a lack of experience may play a role in limiting identification and definitive management even at centers of reasonably high volume [13].

5. Initial evaluation and stabilization

5.1 Identification of patients

Case Presentation: 70 y/o male presents by air to a level I trauma center following a bike accident wherein he was thrown down a hill. It is unclear if he was wearing a helmet. He was initially resuscitated by bystanders as he was in cardiac arrest, and then intubated in the field prior to arrival (GCS 3-T). At the time of arrival he is found to have bradycardia with HR 53 BPM and initial BP was 112/74 with mildly low body temp 96.3 F (35.7 C). He became more bradycardia and did not respond to atropine requiring another brief round of cardiopulmonary resuscitation. Although the initial hemoglobin on his arterial blood gas (ABG) was 13.3 g/dl, he was also transfused four units of packed red blood cells (PRBC's). Computed Tomography (CT) of the head and cervical spine showed an occipital condyle fracture as well as a type III (low) dens fracture with 6 mm distraction and a c2 spinous process fracture (**Figure 2**). Pressor support with norepinephrine was initiated and preparations were made for trans-venous pacing in the event of refractory bradycardia. Magnetic resonance imaging (MRI) the following day confirmed a likely distraction injury with cord edema and hemorrhage (**Figure 3**). Interestingly, his hemoglobin by hospital day 1 had increased to 17.5 g/dl suggesting that his perceived response to transfusion may have been related to volume resuscitation and pressers rather than the PRBC's. He continued to have issues with bradycardia but did not require trans-venous pacing. Considering his severe high cervical spine injury with resultant tetraparesis and complications he was transitioned to comfort directed care on hospital day 3.

Case Discussion: The case above illustrates the complexities in early identification of neurogenic shock as a distinct entity. Because the signs of neurogenic shock are somewhat variable in terms of timeframe from injury to onset, and in light of differences between individual patients and systems in regard to fluid resuscitation in the field, a high index of suspicion is necessary from the time of initial evaluation through the early hours and days of intensive care. Any patient presenting with a spinal cord injury should be considered to be at risk with those having higher level

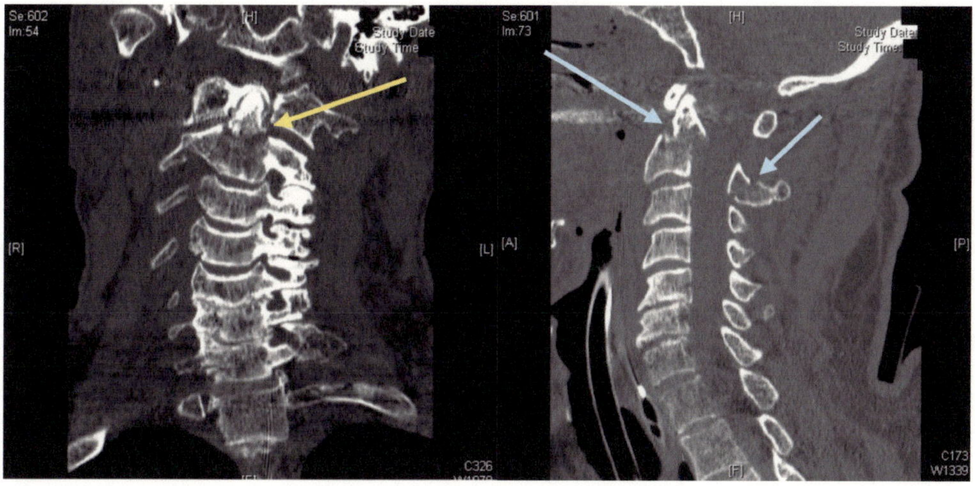

Figure 2.
Coronal (left pane) and sagittal (right pane) CT scan views of the cervical spine showing a type III odontoid fracture (yellow arrow), C1/C2 fracture distraction (long blue arrow) and C2 spinous process fracture (short blue arrow). Created with Biorender.com.

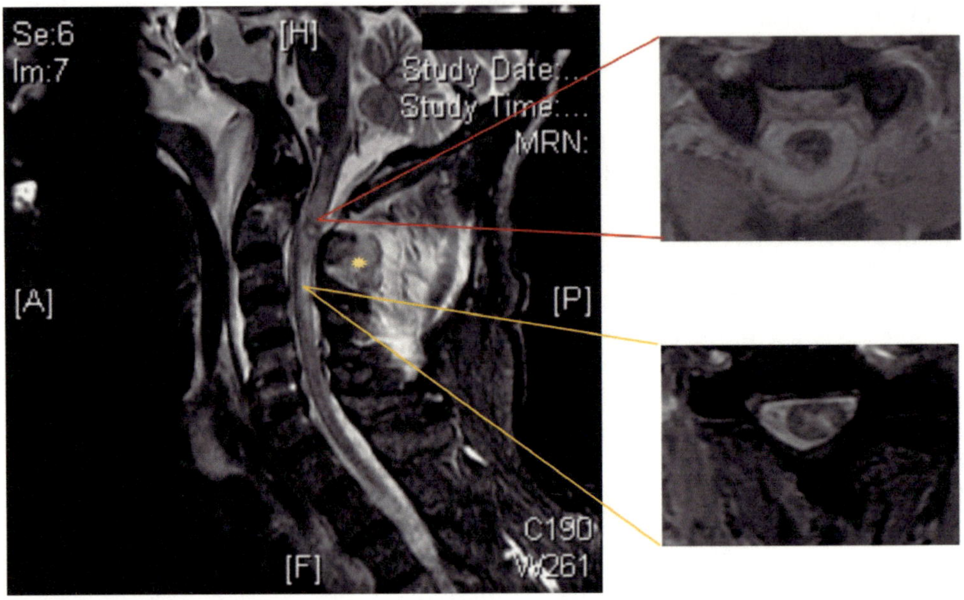

Figure 3.
Sagittal STIR c-spine MRI (left pane) with noted intra-axial edema and hemorrhage at the base of the odontoid (red triangle and top axial slice), more inferior cord edema (yellow triangle and bottom axial slice), and significant posterior compartment paravertebral edema (yellow star). Created with Biorender.com.

injuries at higher risk (**Figure 1**). The authors suggest that the American Spinal Injury Association Autonomic Standards Assessment Form [14] is a reasonable place to start and takes into account blood pressure, heart rate, sweating, temperature regulation, the bronchopulmonary system, and the lower urinary tract and bowel. Even with this tool, however, no specific definition of bradycardia/hypotension is forthcoming; thus it will need to be set by individuals and institutions. As there is no single accepted treatment cutoff for the bradycardia and hypotension, it may be important for systems to consider their patient population in relation to prior studies and establish parameters for automatic physician notification during hemodynamic monitoring with reasonable case reviews to establish the best local standard.

It is agreed, however, that the profound systemic hypotension that characterizes neurogenic shock may lead to hypoperfusion of the spinal cord with subsequent ischemia and secondary injury [15]. To improve outcomes, prompt and aggressive treatment of hypotension should be undertaken in a monitored intensive care unit, with adequate cardiopulmonary and ventilatory support [8]. Medical treatment consists of sufficient fluid administration as well as vasopressor therapy for sustaining blood pressure and maintaining perfusion [4]. That being said, it should be noted that the data regarding pressor use in SCI may be conflicting in this regard, as a distinction needs to be made between pressor use in an attempt to stabilize or improve the motor and sensory loss related to SCI, and that to preclude hypotension and bradycardia related to neurogenic shock from causing complications such as systemic hypoperfusion and cardiac arrest among others. According to one author, up to 100% of patients suffering from neurogenic shock may also have bradycardia, with 71% reported as having severe bradycardia (HR < 46 BPM) and 16% progressing to cardiac arrest [16].

5.2 Patient management

Fluid resuscitation is the first line therapy for hypotension in the setting of neurogenic shock [17]. Maintenance of blood volume influences both blood pressure and blood flow around the site of injury [8]. If there is an inadequate response to fluid resuscitation, agents with α_1 and β_1 adrenergic receptor activity should ideally be used to increase sympathetic activation [15]. What is otherwise considered routine care such as suctioning, as well as abdominal changes such as elevated bladder and bowel pressures, are known to produce wide swings in heart rate and blood pressure that may be refractory to treatment [18]. These changes should be anticipated and prevented as much as possible.

Blood pressure can be further augmented through the administration of intravenous vasopressor agents. These include norepinephrine, epinephrine, dopamine, phenylephrine, as well as concurrent atropine in patients with significant bradycardia [15]. There are some prior reports of transitioning individuals that need extended treatment with a non-intravenous agent to propantheline, aminophylline, theophylline, and ephedrine although the evidence is extremely limited [16]. Enteral pseudoephedrine has also been used successfully as an adjunctive therapy [16].

Current management guidelines dictate that mean arterial pressure (MAP) should be maintained above 85–90 mmHg for the first 5–7 days of therapy [19]. This resuscitation target has been questioned due to the lack of quality evidence showing a positive effect on outcomes [8]. Additionally, maintenance for 5–7 days may be insufficient because certain individuals benefit from longer management [4]. One study has shown that vasopressor therapy achieving the MAP goal is more likely to cause complications than to improve neurological outcomes, with dopamine leading in complications [20]. As such, the risk of vasopressors should be balanced against their benefits in each individual patient, and there should be clear goals for use in regard to improvement of the sensory and motor deficits vs. cardiovascular stabilization.

A recent study suggests that maintenance of a spinal cord perfusion pressure (mean arterial pressure – cerebral spinal fluid pressure) above 50 mmHg is a stronger predictor of neurologic recovery than systemic MAP and may also be useful in guiding management [21]. More studies with high quality evidence are needed to establish reasonable treatment goals that are linked to improved patient outcome.

6. Rehabilitation and recovery

Rehabilitation in patients with spinal cord injuries should be comprehensive, interdisciplinary, and patient-centered, with goals that are individualized and realistic. Interventions should not be delayed and complications need to be anticipated and promptly identified.

Neurogenic shock can persist for 1–6 weeks after the initial injury, certainly long enough to interfere with rehab in some cases [8, 22]. In additional to that, patients with spinal cord injuries are vulnerable to a number of cardiovascular complications which should be anticipated in the course of rehabilitation, and some with prolonged or severe bradycardia may require permanent pacemakers [16]. Cardiovascular complications are the leading causes of morbidity and mortality in patients in both the acute and chronic stages of spinal cord injury [17]. Common complications include autonomic dysreflexia, orthostatic hypotension, reduced cardiovascular reflexes and absence of cardiac pain during ischemia [18].

Independent of neurogenic shock, autonomic dysreflexia (AD) is a potentially fatal complication that occurs in 48–90% of patients with injuries above T6 [17]. It is caused by the loss of supraspinal sympathetic modulation and is characterized by sudden episodes of hypertension, headache, and tachycardia with prevailing reflex bradycardia [23, 24]. Additional sympathetic features include piloerection and cool extremities due to vasoconstriction below the level of injury [23]. In contrast to the sympathetic response below the level of injury, a parasympathetic response may predominate above the level of injury. A compensatory baroreceptor response leads to reflex bradycardia. Other features include flushing, sweating, and nasal congestion [24].

Stimuli that may induce an AD response include bladder distension, detrusor sphincter dyssynergia, kidney or bladder stones, or other painful stimuli such as ingrown toenails, pressure ulcers, infections, fecal impaction, musculoskeletal pain, and menstrual cramps [24]. Sequelae of untreated hypertension in the setting of autonomic dysreflexia include stroke, intracranial hemorrhage, seizures, cardiac arrest, hypertensive encephalopathy, and death [25]. An increase of 20–40 mmHg in systolic blood pressure in people with spinal cord injury should raise suspicion for AD, though the exact definition is not consistent across studies [25].

Primary treatment of AD includes sitting patients upright and lowering their legs, as well as removing or loosening tight clothing or accessories [26]. After that it becomes necessary to identify triggering noxious stimuli and address them. A distended bladder should be emptied with a catheter, a rectal exam may identify impaction, skin should be examined for pressure ulcers and more serious causes need to be suspected because they may not be obvious [26]. Medications that can be administered to help stabilize AD include the calcium channel blocker nifedipine, nitrates, and vasodilatory agents such as hydralazine [18, 23], although hypotension needs to be anticipated and patients will require appropriate hemodynamic monitoring.

Another cardiovascular consequence of spinal cord injury related both to neurogenic shock and autonomic dysreflexia is orthostatic hypotension (OH). It is defined by the American Autonomic Society as a reduction in systolic or diastolic blood pressure of ≥20/10 mmHg, within 3 min of standing upright [27]. Symptoms occur as a result of reduced cerebral perfusion pressure and include light-headedness, dizziness, syncope, pallor, nausea, fatigue, and sweating. Nevertheless, many patients do not report symptoms despite meeting the definition of OH, and some report symptoms in spite of not fully meeting that definition. Pharmacologic therapy may be used to treat OH but should be done carefully because of the already labile blood pressure in patients with spinal cord injury. The most common treatments are compression stockings, abdominal binders, midodrine, or fludrocortisone [23, 27].

Additional autonomic complications that occur after injury are the reduction of cardiovascular reflexes and the absence of cardiac pain. Cardiovascular reflexes regulate blood pressure, intravascular volume, and temperature [18]. The sensation of pain related to cardiac ischemia may be altered because cardiac pain fibers that travel with sympathetic afferent fibers (visceral sensory fibers) are disrupted in cervical or thoracic injuries above T4 [28]. As a consequence, spinal cord injury patients may have atypical presentations of cardiac ischemia including referred pain.

Other major components that are critical in spinal cord injury rehabilitation are bowel and bladder training, respiratory care, mobilization, as well as physical and occupational therapy. Not only should rehabilitation address the medical aspects of patient care, but the psychological impacts of spinal cord injury as well. A comprehensive approach treating the whole individual gives patients a better chance at achieving optimal functional recovery.

7. Conclusion

Neurogenic shock is a feared and difficult to treat complication of disruption of the sympathetic nervous system which most often occurs in the setting of a spinal cord injury. The refractory hypotension and bradycardia may be extremely dangerous for the patient, and may lead to cerebral anoxia, cardiac arrest, and more. Although there is no single accepted blood pressure and heart rate cutoff to define neurogenic shock, the signs are reasonably well established and definitive treatment is in line with current critical care management standards. Beyond the short term, neurogenic shock as well as autonomic dysreflexia, which may commonly accompany spinal injuries at the same level, can complicate the rehabilitation process. Hopefully future prospective studies will adopt standard ways of isolating and confirming neurogenic shock and establish treatment paradigms that improve patient outcomes.

Conflict of interest

The authors report no conflict of interest.

Author details

Anna Volski[1] and Daniel J. Ackerman[2*]

1 Lewis Katz School of Medicine at Temple University, St. Luke's University Health Network, Bethlehem, PA, USA

2 Department of Neurology, St. Luke's University Health Network, Bethlehem, PA, USA

*Address all correspondence to: daniel.ackerman@sluhn.org

References

[1] Millham FH. A brief history of shock. Surgery. 2010;**148**(5):1026-1037. DOI: 10.1016/j.surg.2010.02.014

[2] Blalock A. Peripheral circulatory failure. American Heart Journal. 1942;**23**(2):147-160

[3] Hagen EM. Acute complications of spinal cord injuries. World Journal of Orthopedics. 2015;**6**(1):17-12. DOI: 10.5312/wjo.v6.i1.17

[4] Ruiz I, Squair J, Phillips A, Lukac C, Huang D, Oxciano P, et al. Incidence and natural progression of neurogenic shock after traumatic spinal cord injury. Journal of Neurotrauma. 2018;**35**(3):461-466. DOI: 10.1089/neu.2016.4947

[5] Weaver L, Fleming J, Mathias C, Krassioukov A. Disordered cardiovascular control after spinal cord injury. Handbook of Clinical Neurology. 2012;**109**:213-233. DOI: 10.1016/B978-0-444-52137-8.00013-9

[6] Harrisson S. Penetrating ballistic spinal injury. In: Breeze J, Penn-Barwell J, Keene D, O'Reilly D, Jeyanathan J, Mahoney P, editors. Ballistic Trauma. Cham: Springer; 2017. pp. 201-214

[7] Ditunno J, Little J, Tessler A, Burns A. Spinal shock revisited: A four-phase model. Spinal Cord. 2004;**42**(7):383-395. DOI: 10.1038/sj.sc.3101603

[8] Casha S, Christie S. A systematic review of intensive cardiopulmonary management after spinal cord injury. Journal of Neurotrauma. 2011;**28**(8):1479-1495. DOI: 10.1089/neu.2009.1156

[9] Grigorean V, Sandu A, Popescu M, Iacobini M, Stoian R, Neascu C, et al. Cardiac dysfunctions following spinal cord injury. Journal of Medicine and Life. 2009;**2**(2):133-145

[10] Kandel E, Schwartz J, Jessell T, Principals of Neuroscience. 4th ed. New York: McGraw-Hill, Health Professions Division; 2000. p. 1414. ISBN 0-8385-7701-6

[11] Patten J. Neurological Differential Diagnosis. 2nd ed. Berlin Heidelberg New York: Springer-Verlag; 2004. ISBN 3-540-19937-3

[12] Taylor M, Wrenn P, O'Donnell A. Presentation of neurogenic shock within the emergency department. Emergency Medicine Journal. 2016;**34**:157-162. DOI: 10.1136/emermed-2016-205780

[13] Guly H, Bouamra O, Lecky F, on behalf of the Trauma Audit and Research Network. The incidence of neurogenic shock in patients with isolated spinal cord injury in the emergency department. Resuscitation. 2008;**76**:57-62. DOI: 10.1016/j.resuscitation.2007.06.008

[14] Asia Autonomic Standards Assessment Form [Internet]. 2016. Available from: https://asia-spinalinjury.org/wp-content/uploads/2016/02/Auto_Stan_Worksheet.pdf

[15] Consortium for Spinal Cord Medicine. Early acute management in adults with spinal cord injury: A clinical practice guideline for health-care professionals. Journal of Spinal Cord Medicine. 2008;**31**(4):403-479

[16] Wood GC, Boucher AB, Johnson JL, Wisniewski JN, Magnotti LJ, Croce MA, et al. Effectiveness of pseudoephedrine as adjunctive therapy for neurogenic shock after acute spinal cord injury: A case series. Journal of American College of Clinical Pharmacy. 2013;**34**(1):89-93. DOI: 10.1002/phar.1335

[17] Popa C, Popa F, Grigorean VT, Onose G, Sandu AM, Popescu M, et al. Vascular dysfunctions following spinal

cord injury. Journal of Medicine and Life. 2010;**3**(3):275-285

[18] Hagen EM, Rekand T, Gronning M, Faerestrand S. Cardiovascular complications of spinal cord injury. Tidsskrift for den Norske Lægeforening. 2012;**132**(9):1115-1120. DOI: 10.4045/tidsskr.11.0551

[19] Ryken TC, Hurlbert RJ, Hadley MN, Aarabi B, Dhall SS, Gelb DE, et al. The acute cardiopulmonary management of patients with cervical spinal cord injuries. Neurosurgery. 2013;**72**(2):84-92. DOI: 10.1227/NEU.0b013e318276ee16

[20] Readdy WJ, Saigal R, Whetstone WD, Mefford A, Ferguson AR, Talbott JF, et al. Failure of mean arterial pressure goals to improve outcomes following penetrating spinal cord injury. Neurosurgery. 2016;**79**(5):708-714. DOI: 10.1227/NEU.0000000000001249

[21] Squair JW, Bélanger LM, Tsang A, Ritchie L, Mac-Thiong JM, Parent S, et al. Spinal cord perfusion pressure predicts neurologic recovery in acute spinal cord injury. Neurology. 2017;**89**(16):1660-1667. DOI: 10.1212/ WNL.0000000000004519

[22] Lehmann KG, Lane JG, Piepmeier JM, Batsford WP. Cardiovascular abnormalities accompanying acute spinal cord injury in humans: Incidence, time course and severity. Journal of the American College of Cardiology. 1987;**10**(1):46-52

[23] Rabinstein A. Traumatic spinal cord injury. CONTINUUM: Lifelong Learning in Neurology. 2018;**24**(2):551-566

[24] Curt A, Nitsche B, Rodic B, et al. Assessment of autonomic dysreflexia in patients with spinal cord injury. Journal of Neurology, Neurosurgery, and Psychiatry. 1997;**62**(5):473-477. DOI: 10.1136/jnnp.62.5.473

[25] Eldahan KC, Rabchevsky AG. Autonomic dysreflexia after spinal cord injury: Systemic pathophysiology and methods of management. Autonomic Neuroscience. 2017;**209**:59-70. DOI: 10.1016/j.autneu.2017.05.002

[26] Kirshblum SC, Priebe MM, Ho CH, Scelza WM, Chiodo AE, Wuermser LA. Spinal cord injury medicine. 3. Rehabilitation phase after acute spinal cord injury. Archives of Physical Medicine and Rehabilitation. 2007;**88**(3 Suppl 1):S62-S70. DOI: 10.1016/ j.apmr.2006.12.003

[27] Wecht JM, William AB. Implication of altered autonomic control for orthostatic tolerance in SCI. Autonomic Neuroscience. 2018;**209**:51-58. DOI: 10.1016/j.autneu.2017.04.004

[28] Groah SL, Menter RR. Long term cardiac ischemia leading to coronary artery bypass grafting in a tetraplegic patient. Archives of Physical Medicine and Rehabilitation. 1998;**79**(9):1129-1132

Chapter 8

Spinal Shock: Differentiation from Neurogenic Shock and Key Management Approaches

Keith Conti, Vikas Yellapu, Joan Sweeney, Steven M. Falowski and Stanislaw P. Stawicki

Abstract

The conceptual differentiation of spinal and neurogenic shock tends to be misunderstood among clinicians. In order to better illustrate the differences in definition, presentation, and development of spinal shock (SS) from neurogenic and other forms of shock, we present herein a clinically relevant summary of typical characteristics of SS. First described in the eighteenth century, the continued investigation into the disease process and the response of neural structures to spinal cord trauma have led to a more complete description and understanding. We will begin in the first part of the chapter describing the etiology of SS, including a working definition, as it pertains to complete spinal cord injuries (SCIs). This is followed by the summary of pathophysiology and clinical presentations associated with each clinical phase of SS. Finally, we explore treatment options and considerations as they relate to incomplete SCI. We hope that by presenting a clear and well-delineated overview of SS, we will allow the clinician to better understand and more accurately predict the evolution of this process. This, in turn, should facilitate the ability to deliver better care for the patient.

Keywords: areflexia, clinical management, hyperreflexia, spinal injury, spinal shock, shock, trauma

1. Introduction and epidemiology

The specific definition of spinal shock (SS) has evolved over the past two centuries. Nonetheless, a significant level of ambiguity, controversy, and confusion still exists when differentiating between neurogenic shock (NS) and SS. Whytt first described this clinical entity in the 1750s without using the term "shock" and without the understanding of the underlying basic science and anatomy to accurately inform the definition. Rather, he focused on the observation that SS was associated with a loss of sensation accompanied by motor paralysis with initial loss but gradual recovery of reflexes [1]. The definition was then expanded over by Hall in the early 1840s, officially utilizing the terms "spinal shock" and "reflex arc" [2]. Another contributing factor to the previously elusive definition is the lack of uniform clinical presentation, manifestation, and duration of SS. Due to the substantial clinical variability and heterogeneity of presentations, we must first discuss the definitional aspect of SS so that the reader may have a clear idea and a

Phase	Timing	Neurological changes
1	0–1 day	1. Decreased spinal and supraspinal excitation 2. Loss of 5-HT production leading to loss of plateau potentials 3. Reduction of available synapses and dendrites
2	1–3 days	1. Increased postsynaptic sensitivity 2. Receptor upregulation due to decreased neurotransmitter activity
3	1–4 weeks	1. Increased neurotrophin activity allows for increased synaptic growth 2. Increased interneuron growth 3. Plateau potentials recovered in spinal neurons
4	1–12 months	1. Synapse growth in long axons

Table 1.
Four phases of spinal shock by Ditunno et al.

working model for our subsequent discussions of diagnosis, patient presentation, and treatment approaches.

Ditunno made a subtle point that the controversy surrounding the definition of SS could be attributed to observations made clinically. More specifically, he noted that not all reflexes are eradicated in a strictly binary on/off fashion. Some reflexes may only be depressed and yet still can be technically elicited. Finally, he noted that the resolution of SS does not occur in a binary fashion and often follows a prolonged course of weeks to months [3]. Similar observations by Illis suggested that the definition of SS cannot be comprehensive without including subcomponent definitions of clinical phases [4]. For the purposes of this chapter, we will utilize Ditunno's four-phase model of spinal shock, building upon the groundwork described by various pioneers such as Whytt and Hall [1, 3]. This model allows for clarification of the ambiguity surrounding the disease process while still retaining flexibility to appreciate the variability among clinical presentations. The details of Ditunno's four-phase model can be seen in **Table 1** [3].

The phases are organized according to post-injury time and the nervous system's response to insult. Of note, we will hold off on the discussion of each phase until the *Etiology and Pathophysiology* section as the separation of phases requires delving into how the neurons are responding to their environment as time progresses.

In 2007, there was an estimated global spinal cord injury (SCI) incidence of 2.3 cases/100,000 inhabitants [5]. It has been estimated 45% of SS cases are associated with motor vehicle collisions (MVC), 34% with domestic accidents, 15% with sporting accidents, and 6% with self-harm [6]. The incidence of SCI can vary across geographic, socioeconomic, and cultural factors, including the prevalence of contact sports and differences in primary transportation modality. All of the above factors are important determinants of the incidence of SCI. Finally, no discussion of the topic of SCI is complete without mentioning the tremendous human and economic cost associated with these injuries worldwide [7–9].

2. Spinal shock: etiology and pathophysiology

Spinal cord injuries (SCI) are typically divided into two subtypes, complete and incomplete. An SCI is considered incomplete if there is some degree of residual motor and/or sensory function below the neurologic level of injury that includes the lowest sacral segments, where the neurologic level of injury is defined as the most caudal level at which both motor and sensory modalities remain preserved [10]. It follows that patients affected by a complete SCI will not retain sensory or motor function in the lowest sacral segments.

Before directing our discussion to the management in incomplete SCI, additional information will be provided regarding complete SCIs, specifically in the context of SS. The understanding of key processes surrounding complete SCI is conceptually easier, especially when compared to the understanding of incomplete SCI. It is important to note that although severed neurons are separated from descending input—both excitatory and inhibitory—there remains synaptic contact with associated interneurons and reflex afferents, and even new synaptic connections can be established with sprouting neurons [11, 12]. Our subsequent discussion will describe the previously outlined "four phases" of spinal shock.

2.1 Phase I

As outlined in **Table 1**, **Phase I** of SS is marked by areflexia/hyporeflexia, a consequence of the loss of descending mediation. This phase occurs from 0 to 24 hours from time of injury. Under normal circumstances, both spinal motor neurons and interneurons receive certain baseline levels of background excitatory input from supraspinal axons. When an individual wishes to initiate voluntary movement, additional stimulus is superimposed above this "background activity." Supraspinal inputs mediating the background excitation of spinal motor neurons and interneurons are numerous and include vestibulospinal and reticulospinal pathways [13]. These two pathways will now be discussed in more detail.

The vestibulospinal pathway arises from first-order neurons located in Scarpa's ganglion which is situated in the distal part of the internal auditory meatus [14]. Afferents are sent from the ganglion through the vestibular part of the eighth cranial nerve before entering the brainstem at the pontomedullary junction. Upon entry, there are four second-order vestibular nuclei; however, we shall focus on the medial and lateral vestibulospinal tracts for the purposes of our current discussion. The medial and lateral vestibulospinal tracts arise from the medial and lateral vestibular nuclei, respectively [15, 16]. The latter descends the entire length of the spinal cord ipsilaterally and plays a crucial role in walking upright, while the former descends bilaterally in the medial longitudinal fasciculus and terminates at the mid-thoracic level, facilitating the integration of head and eye movements [17, 18].

The reticulospinal pathway arises from the brainstem, the pontine reticular formation, and the medullary reticular formation [19, 20]. Pontine reticular fibers traveling in the pontine reticulospinal tract remain uncrossed as they descend in the medial longitudinal fasciculus, terminating in axial and limb muscles involved in posture and gait stability [21]. At the level of the muscle, their effects are at least threefold: (a) facilitation of movement, (b) regulation of reflexes, and (c) contribution to muscle tone. The medullary reticular fibers traveling in the medullary reticulospinal tract serve a slightly different role [22–24]. First, the fibers originating from the medullary reticulospinal formation are located bilaterally in the reticulospinal tracts as they descend; however, most of the fibers remain uncrossed. As they terminate on axial and limb muscles, they serve an inhibitory role during the modulation of voluntary movement and reflexes.

In addition to supraspinal inputs, serotonergic (5-HT) neurons and noradrenergic (NE) neurons originating from the raphe nucleus and locus coeruleus, respectively, may also play a role in the background excitatory input as they influence spinal cord motor systems [25]. Mechanistically, this may involve the production of plateau potentials [26, 27]. The plateau potentials originate on dendrites, believed to be mediated through sustained activation of $Ca2^{+}$ channels, and provide amplification of excitatory inputs, with approximately sixfold "gain," thus allowing for prolonged neuronal firing with minimal excitatory input, as well as contributing to the background basal excitatory stimulation [28–30].

Baseline excitability in muscle spindles may also be handled in part by gamma-motor neurons [31, 32]. Upon SCI, gamma-motor neurons caudal to the injury may lose their ability to influence motor neurons via stretch reflex afferents as they lose their tonic descending facilitation. The loss of descending inhibition of inhibitory pathways within the spinal cord must also be considered, primarily because it likely contributes to decreased spinal reflexes [33, 34].

Finally, some of the more delayed developments involving the injured cord, both metabolic and structural, could contribute to the observed areflexia/hyporeflexia characteristics of SS. At the same time, the observed areflexia/hyporeflexia usually occurs immediately post-SCI, making any other pathophysiologic considerations secondary—rather than primary—factors [35, 36]. This "secondary factor" list includes (a) dendritic retraction and synaptic degeneration seen within 1–3 days post-SCI; (b) impaired delivery of metabolites and secretion of neurotrophins; and (c) the impact of growth factors caudal to the neurologic level of injury [36–38].

Upon traumatic injury resulting in complete SCI, the baseline excitation from supraspinal inputs will be lost, leading to hyperpolarization of the neurons [39]. This hyperpolarization leads to the neurons becoming less excitable and yields the clinical picture in **Phase I.**

2.2 Phase II

Appearing 1–3 days following the SCI, the return of cutaneous reflexes is observed [3]. It is still unknown whether this is due to replacement of synapses or to denervation supersensitivity. Morphological changes in the synapses have been documented within hours to days of SCI; however, these synapses may not become functional until weeks—or even months—have passed, making this an unlikely contributor to **Phase II** developments [40–45].

Denervation supersensitivity is defined as increased neuronal firing in response to a neurotransmitter [46]. This phenomenon has been shown to occur in both the peripheral (PNS) and central (CNS) nervous systems, including the brain and the spinal cord [47–51]. The proposed mechanisms involves upregulation of mRNA transcription and protein translation that begins within hours and peaks within days post-SCI, which is within the time scale of empirically observed changes [52]. More specifically, the overall process leads to increased synthesis and insertion of receptors into the postsynaptic membrane, altered synthesis and assembly of receptor subunits, decreased removal and/or degradation of receptor(s), and reduced excitatory neurotransmitter reuptake [52–55]. Mechanistically, NMDA glutamate receptors, serotonin 2A, and vanilloid VR1 receptors have been shown to increase either in association with mRNA synthesis or the observed density at the synapse [54, 56–58]. Hypoactivity of neurons has been shown to constitute a sufficient stimulus to increase production of the NMDA glutamate receptors [55]. Although the exact details are yet to be elucidated, neurotrophins, growth factors, and their respective receptors have been shown to stimulate an increase in transcription and translation [59–64]. Postulated downstream effects involve the modulation of NMDA receptors, resulting in increased excitability and/or decreasing GABA synaptic inhibition [65]. These effects seem to play a role in the development of SS during the initial period of 1–3 days post-SCI [3].

2.3 Phases III and IV

Stages III (1–4 weeks) and **IV (1–12 months)** of SS are often linked together and are best described through the lens of the human tibial H-reflex. The H-reflex has been used to model the recovery of reflexes caudal to SCI over time [66, 67].

In this context, an interesting phenomenon is observed beyond post-injury "day 3" temporal marker. More specifically, there is an increased reflex excitability observed at 2–4 weeks post-SCI with an increase in latency and another increase in reflex excitability at approximately 3–4 months post-SCI [3].

Overall, it has been shown that the 2–4-week mark increase in excitability can be attributed to axon-supplied synapse growth and/or disynaptic interneurons, while the increase in excitability at 3–4 months is mediated by primary afferents and/or soma-supplied synapse growth [3]. The timing of the observed changes in excitability suggests that there is an axon-length-dependent rate of synapse growth. Two mechanisms have been proposed to explain this phenomenon: (a) two periods of synaptic growth—early findings dependent on axonal synthesis and the later growth period dependent on somal synthesis and (b) disynaptic stretch reflex pathways, such as the Golgi tendon organ reflex, are preferentially hyperexcitable relative to the monosynaptic Ia afferents to motoneurons [3].

3. Diagnosis and clinical presentation

3.1 Phase I

Caudal to complete SCI within the first 24 hours, Phase I will present with flaccid, paralyzed muscles and deep tendon reflexes (DTRs) being initially absent. While the DTRs such as the ankle jerk (AJ) and knee jerk (KJ) are absent, a pathologic reflex, delayed plantar response (DPR), is often the first to return and should be observed within hours post-SCI [68]. Other cutaneous and polysynaptic reflexes such as the bulbocavernosus (BC), cremasteric (CM), and anal wink (AW) can also be seen to return during Phase I. Location of the lesion can be determined based on presenting symptoms. Lesions above the mid-pons will cause decerebrate rigidity, while those located below the mid-pons cause hyporeflexia [69]. In addition to skeletal motor and reflex findings during this time, there are autonomic findings that may be relevant if the lesion is in the cervical area. Findings include hypotension, atrioventricular conduction block, and bradyarrhythmia, and these can be continued through Phases II and III [3]. These findings are consistent with neurogenic shock, detailed in a separate chapter.

3.2 Phase II

One to 3 days post-SCI, the clinician should expect to see continued reflex return. Building upon Phase I, the cutaneous reflexes, BC, AW, and CM, become stronger [3]. Except for two patient populations, namely, the elderly and children, DTRs are still absent; however, the tibial H-reflex returns around the 24-hour marker [70, 71]. In the elderly, DTRs and the Babinski sign can occur during this phase [68]. Although not known for certain, the presence of pre-existing subclinical myelopathy might contribute to this early recovery as some animal studies have exhibited quicker recovery of DTRs in the setting of prior upper motor neuron lesions [68, 72, 73]. Children exhibit similar recovery, showing DTRs sometimes 3 days post-SCI, which might be attributable to their still developing descending supraspinal tracts, predisposing them to spinal hyperreflexia. The recovery of cutaneous reflexes during phase II is likely due to receptor plasticity [3].

3.3 Phase III

The third phase (days 4–30) is marked by early hyperreflexia. Excluding the two patient populations discussed in Phase II, almost all patients will regain DTRs during this period [3, 68]. The return of these reflexes is as follows: Babinski sign recovery will follow AJ recovery closely, with the AJ preceding the return of the KJ [3, 68, 74]. The clinician should expect to see most DTRs resolve during this phase with only 10% persisting beyond **Phase III** [3]. Ditunno discussed the variability of reflex return regarding the timing trend. There have been studies showing reduced tendon reflex excitability in certain trained populations, such as ballet dancers and power-trained athletes, relative to untrained or even endurance athletes [75–77]. There has also been evidence that pre-SCI experiences could influence the reflex excitability below an SCI [78, 79]. During this time the clinician will have to be aware of the developing autonomic functions. There is expected improvement in the bradyarrhythmia and hypotension described before; however, around this time autonomic dysreflexia can arise and is most commonly due to a distended bladder or bowel causing a massive sympathetic outflow below the neurologic level of injury [3]. Autonomic dysreflexia can lead to difficult-to-control hypertension and bradycardia and is most commonly seen in patients with SCI at or above T6 but has been seen as low as T10 [80].

3.4 Phase IV

One to 12 months post-injury, spasticity and hyperreflexia usually set in, characteristic of **Phase IV**. The remaining DTRs not extinguished during **Phase III** of SS should become absent during this period [3]. Minimal stimuli will elicit cutaneous reflexes, Babinski sign, and DTRs. It has been estimated that there will be detrusor paralysis recovery by 4–6 weeks [3]. The autonomic dysreflexia described in Phase III can also develop during Phase IV, including malignant hypertension, and following its emergence can become chronic/protracted.

4. Treatment

A detailed history is imperative for accurate diagnosis and treatment of spinal shock. As mentioned previously, prior patient life experiences (i.e., athletes, ballerinas, etc.) may play a role in the rate of hyperreflexia appearance [3]. Thus, a thorough history will help guide appropriate expectations of the clinical evolution of reflexes. The history will also help direct the clinician to what developments could be expected as these can depend on the type, severity, and timing of the incident. Certain substances and chemical mediators for reducing inflammatory processes, protecting neurons, and regenerating neural capacities have been investigated for efficacy in the management of SCI [6, 81–88]. Corticosteroids, specifically methylprednisolone, have been postulated to be part of a generalized recommendation to help alleviate inflammatory processes mediated by neutrophils and macrophages; however, clinical trials and non-randomized studies point to not having this as a general recommendation [81–85]. It has been recommended that a young patient, free of any underlying disease which could be influenced by corticosteroids, could be started on a short trial of methylprednisolone with a loading dose of 30 mg/kg with a maintenance dose of 5/mg/kg/h for the next 24 hours [6]. Symptomatic medications for autonomic dysfunction can include treatments for headaches, flushing, elevated blood pressure, orthostasis, and bladder and abdominal distension. Prompt attention to bowel and bladder hygiene, bladder catheterization, cautious use of bowel preparations, and anticholinergic medications may help with any associated hemodynamic instability. There are ongoing investigations into G-CSF and FGF-2, among others, as possessing neuroprotective qualities as well as stem cells of varying stages, olfactory ensheathing cells, and mesenchymal stromal cells that are possible candidates for regenerating neural capacities [86–88]. Consequently, the clinician should remain up to date on the current literature for therapeutic developments. Providers should also keep in mind that lesions above T6 can be accompanied by neurogenic shock, and we refer you to the neurogenic shock chapter for the diagnosis and management of that phenomenon.

Current guidelines and recommendation can be split up based on the location of SCI.

Cervical SCI:

1. Immediate immobilization through traction and alignment.
2. Identify if injury is above c5.
   a. Above C3: Immediate mechanical ventilation.
   b. C3–C5: Monitor closely for respiratory decompensation and ventilate if necessary.
   c. Maintain supportive care and ensure SBP > 90.
3. Neurosurgery consult to determine if neurosurgery is necessary [89].

Thoracolumbar SCI:

1. Stable fractures: Stabilization with brace from 6 to 12 weeks.
2. Unstable fractures: Surgical decompression [90].

Sacral SCI:

1. Unstable sacral fractures:
   a. Identify any active bleeds.
   b. Immediate reduction.
2. Stable sacral fracture:
   a. Reduction with brace for up to 4 months.
   b. Limit activity.

While it has been a standard practice to give high-dose methylprednisolone after spinal cord injury, recent studies have found that there is no advantage of steroids when considering neurological recovery [91, 92]. Given that SCI can result in long periods of immobility, it is important to consider antithrombotic prophylactic treatment. If patient is on bed rest, gastric and skin ulcer precautions must also be in place.

5. Considerations for incomplete SCI

Incomplete SCI can be classified using the American Spinal Injury Association (ASIA) into three broad categories. Grade A, B, and C injury designations are based on functions that are preserved. **Table 2** describes the preserved functions in all grades. Incomplete spinal cord injuries can be categorized into four types: central cord syndrome, anterior cord syndrome, posterior cord syndrome, and Brown-Sequard syndrome.

The incidence of incomplete SCI has reported range from 40 to 50% of all spinal injuries [93–95]. Central cord syndrome tends to be the most common injury with posterior cord being the rarest of the incomplete spinal injuries. We will start by exploring the central cord syndrome. Most cases of incomplete SCI are caused by motor vehicle accidents (MVA), falls, and swimming injuries [96, 97].

5.1 Central cord syndrome

Central cord syndrome (CCS) is seen primarily in patients in the fifth decade of life and beyond and is usually a result of hyperextension injury [95, 98]. In younger patients, CCS is usually due to high-velocity trauma. CCS in older patients tends to occur in the setting of pre-existing degenerative narrowing of the spinal canal; this narrowing combined with hyperextension can cause an expanding hematoma that exerts pressure on the spinal cord [99]. Depending on the location and severity, we see a different range of symptoms. Milder injuries can result in burning sensation of the upper extremities. Most presentations consist of weakness in all limbs, with upper extremities more affected than the lower extremities. Majority of central cord injuries are due to a lesion at the levels of C4–C6. Patients with the following history and signs should be evaluated for CCS [100].

1. Patients over 50 years of age: Hyperextension with a previous history of degenerative changes in the spinal canal.

2. Patients under 40 years of age: High velocity trauma (MVA, skiing, etc.).

3. Sensory Loss: Cape-like distribution (upper extremities and thorax with sacrum spared).

4. Motor loss: Weakness that is more prominent in the upper extremities than lower extremities.

5. Autonomic regulation: Loss of bowel and bladder. Orthostatic hypotension may also be seen [101].

Any patient that is being evaluated for incomplete SCI should have a high-resolution computed tomography (CT) to identify spinal fractures, dislocations,

Grade	Description
A	Complete spinal cord injury. No motor or sensory function
B	Motor function is lost, while sensory function is preserved
C	Sensory function is lost, with motor function spared at the sacral level
D	Sensory functions intact, and all motor functions are at least grade 3/5 (able to move against gravity, but not against active resistance)
E	No loss of function noted

Table 2.
American Spinal Injury Association (ASIA) classification for incomplete spinal cord injuries at level of injury.

and potential hematomas [100]. A magnetic resonance imaging (MRI) should be considered when CT is normal, but CCS is still suspected. In roughly 4–6% of individuals with CCS, it is possible that all imaging, with the exception of MRI, can show no abnormalities. Once the severity on the CCS is identified and classified using the American Spinal Injury Association (ASIA) scale (**Table 2**), management pathway can be selected [102]. The Congress of Neurological Surgeons recommends that patients receive immediate surgery in cases of fractures or dislocations [103, 104]. However, decompressive surgery in CCS is controversial as many studies looking at outcomes comparing surgical and nonsurgical management have been inconclusive. The use of steroids is not recommended as it has been shown no benefit when compared to observation [105–109].

It has been noted that 75–80% of patients can regain full neurological recovery [96, 110, 111]. Depending on the ASIA score that was determined during admission, one can begin determining prognostic considerations [112]. Usually younger patients with CCS from traumatic injuries tend to have the best prognosis [113]. The timeline for recovery can be up to 1 year after injury. Patients will usually regain functions in an ascending manner [99].

5.2 Brown-Sequard syndrome

Unlike CCS, the Brown-Sequard syndrome (BSS) is a rare type of incomplete SCI [114]. It is usually seen in penetrating trauma, including knife and gunshot wounds. It can also occur with the loss of vascular supply due to a herniation or edema to a hemisection [115–117]. BSS presents with ipsilateral loss of motor function, ipsilateral loss of sensation, and proprioception and contralateral loss of pain and temperature [114]. These symptoms are due to a lesion involving the corticospinal, dorsal column, and spinothalamic tracts, respectively. In some cases, there is loss of bowel and bladder function. BSS has the best prognosis of all the incomplete spinal cord injuries. Roughly 90–99% of patients gain back full function [99]. Diagnosis should be suspected based on a combination of physical examination/presenting signs and confirmed with an MRI. Management is similar to CCS, consisting of conservative approach with a strong focus on early rehabilitation. Surgery is indicated in the following scenarios [118–121]:

1. Lesion requiring decompression.

2. Presence of a tumor.

3. An abscess compressing the spinal cord.

Complete recovery following BSS can take up to 2 years. However, most patients regain full motor skills within the first 6 months. Pain and temperature sensations tend to recover before full motor function is regained [122, 123]. It is vital that patients receive immediate physical therapy following the acute treatment phase to maximize recovery. During the treatment and management phase of BSS, providers must be careful in completely addressing the underlying condition that lead to BSS, such as spinal cord herniation or a CSF leak through a dural tear, as these could lead to permanent loss of neurologic function [124, 125].

5.3 Anterior cord syndrome

Anterior cord syndrome (ACS) is a rare incomplete SCI that accounts for approximately 1–3% of spinal injuries [95]. It also has the worst prognosis of all the incomplete SCI, with only 10–20% of patients achieving some level of functional recovery [126]. ACS has two primary pathogenetic mechanisms. In about 90% of cases, it is caused by decreased vascular perfusion to the anterior spinal artery which supplies the anterior 2/3 of the spinal cord [95, 126]. Another possible cause is from increased direct pressure on the spinal cord caused by compression trauma or "over-flexion" [127]. The first signs of ACS include bilateral loss of motor function, pain, and temperature sensation. These findings are more dominant in the lower extremities. Patients also tend to present with loss of bladder and bowel function [126]. Presentation of ACS is usually acute with severe back pain and loss of neurologic function mentioned. The best confirmatory test is a spinal MRI; however, computed tomography angiography (CTA) may be used for faster diagnosis. Emergent surgical management may be required depending on the underlying pathology responsible for the ACS (e.g., aortic aneurysm). Once the underlying condition is treated, management of ACS is similar to other SCIs and consists of physical and occupational therapy. While the patient may never regain the lost motor and sensory function, it is vital that physical therapy is provided on a regular basis to prevent contractions and spastic paralysis [128].

5.4 Posterior cord syndrome

Posterior cord syndrome (PCS) has an incidence of roughly <1% [95, 99]. Like ACS it carries a very poor prognosis. The causes of PCS include vascular compromise to the posterior spinal artery, trauma, multiple sclerosis (MS), vitamin B12 deficiency, and syphilis. Since PCS affects the posterior aspect of the spinal cord containing dorsal column fibers, one typically sees presentations that involve loss of proprioception and vibratory sensation with motor function being preserved. Patients occasionally will have sensation of "electric shocks" running down their spine, which is known as Lhermitte's sign and can indicate MS or a metabolic deficiency [121, 128]. CTA might allow for rapid diagnosis of vascular comprise/threat and allow for emergent treatment. However, MRI imaging showing infarctions is the most reliable method of confirming the diagnosis [99]. Once the underlying pathology is treated, PCS management will require rigorous physical and occupational rehabilitation course [121].

6. Conclusions

It is important to distinguish the differences between spinal shock and neurogenic shock, both in terms of definitions and clinical manifestations. Spinal shock encompasses a diverse set of injuries involving various parts of the spinal

	Spinal shock	**Neurogenic shock**
Damage location	Different areas of the spinal cord	Sympathetic pathways—above T6 vertebral level
Systemic hypotension	Possible, depending on the location and severity of injury	Always
Onset time	Sudden to days	Sudden
Time to resolution	Weeks to months	Hours to days

Table 3.
Spinal shock versus neurogenic shock.

cord, whereas neurogenic shock tends to be a result of spinal injuries above the level of T6. Spinal shock occurs in phases (I–IV) that are temporally distributed over a period of weeks to months, whereas neurogenic shock tends to have sudden onset that requires more urgent management. **Table 3** outlines the key differences between spinal and neurogenic shock. Patients with SS and injuries above the level of T6 should always be evaluated for neurogenic shock symptoms, such as

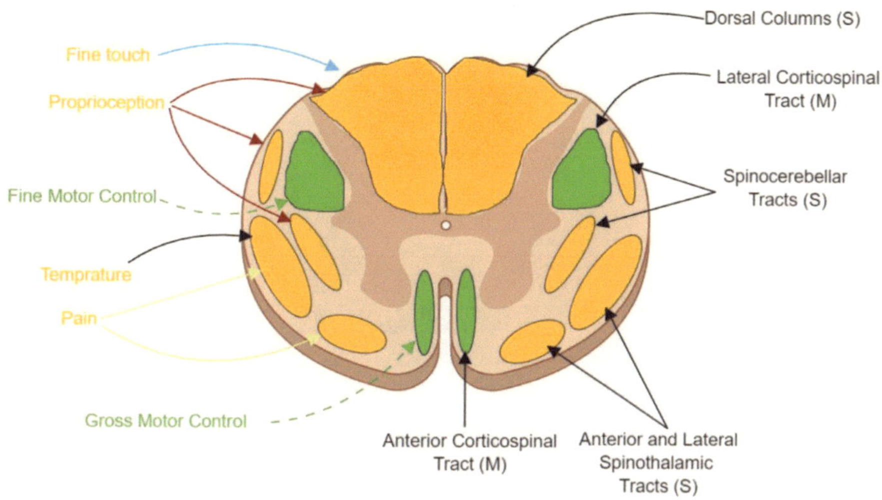

Figure 1.
This represents the different tracts on a T8 spinal cross section. The sensory pathways (S) and motor pathways (M) are identified with specific characteristics depicted on the right. This image was created using Biorender and is used here based on the terms and conditions of Biorender®.

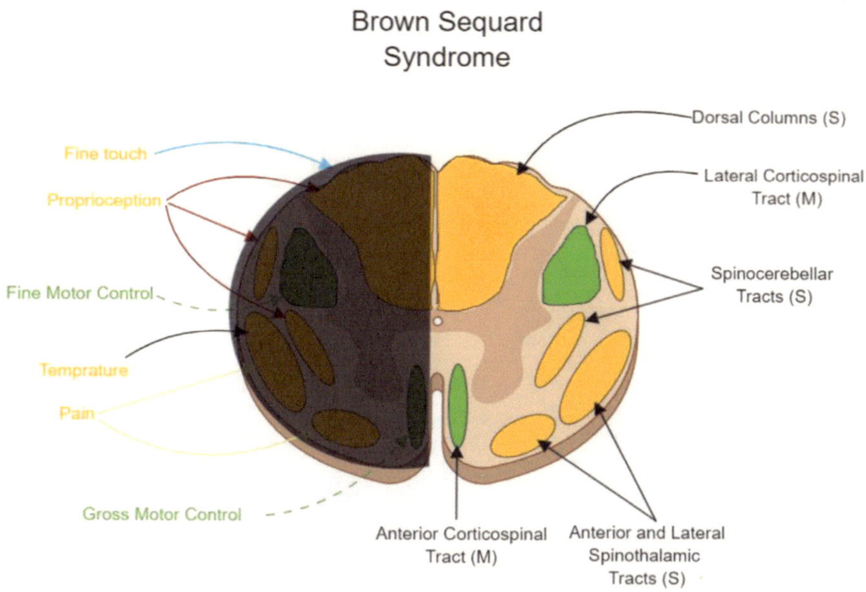

Figure 2.
Image representing lesion that would be considered Brown-Sequard and the pathways involved in the hemisection injury. This image was created using Biorender and is used here based on the terms and conditions of Biorender®.

hypotension, hypothermia, and bradycardia. Both complete and incomplete SS injuries can develop hypotension but will not develop systemic vasodilation (as would be seen in the event of neurogenic shock). Accurately differentiating neurogenic and spinal shock is important because it will help clinicians in determining important management decisions in patients with SCI (**Figures 1–5**).

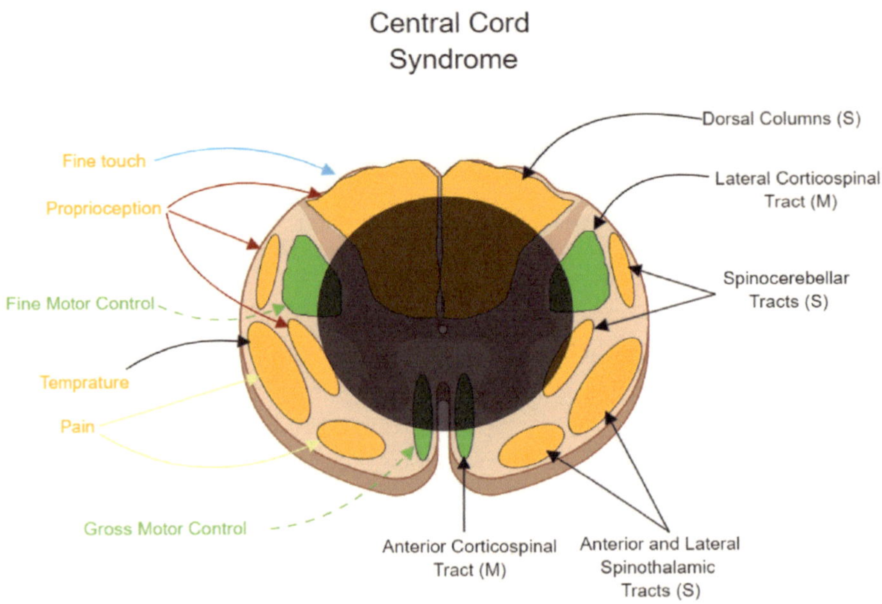

Figure 3.
Image represents central cord injury and the pathways involved. This image was created using Biorender and is used here based on the terms and conditions of Biorender®.

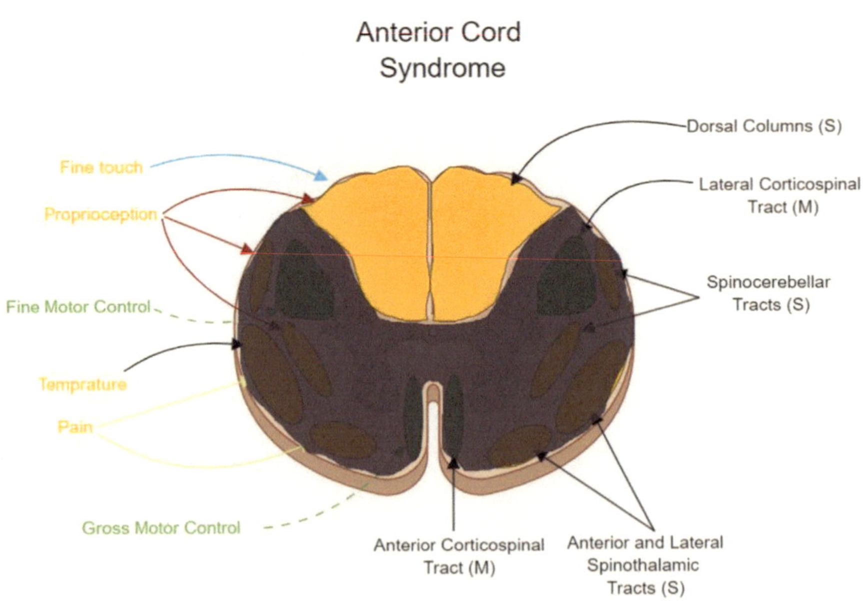

Figure 4.
Image represents anterior cord injury and the pathways involved. This image was created using Biorender and is used here based on the terms and conditions of Biorender®.

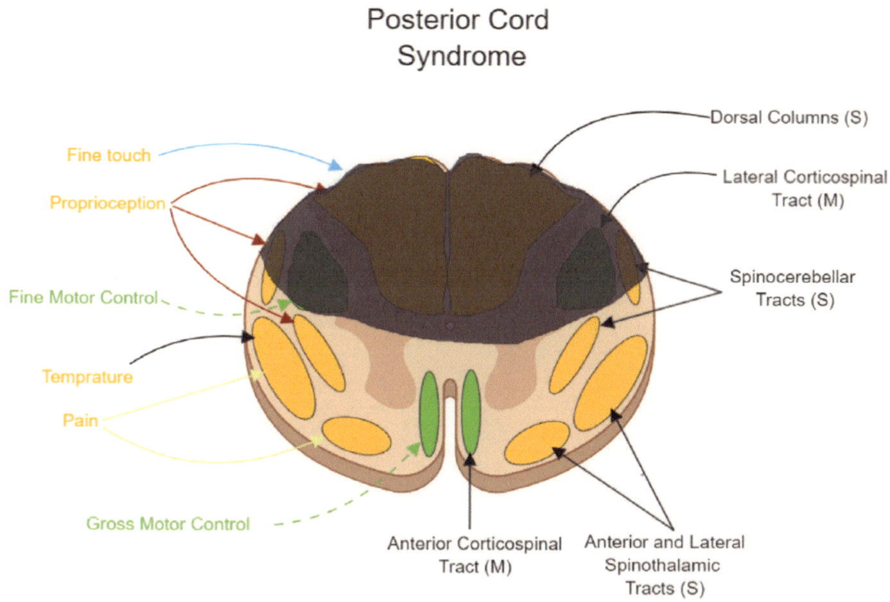

Figure 5.
Image represents posterior cord injury and the pathways involved. This image was created using Biorender and is used here based on the terms and conditions of Biorender®.

Glossary

SS	spinal shock
SCI	spinal cord injury
DTR	deep tendon reflex
DPR	deep plantar reflex
CM	cremasteric
KJ	knee jerk
BC	bulbocavernosus
AJ	ankle jerk
AW	anal wink
CCS	central cord syndrome
BSS	Brown-Sequard syndrome
ACS	anterior cord syndrome
PCS	posterior cord syndrome
CSF	cerebrospinal fluid

Author details

Keith Conti[1], Vikas Yellapu[2]*, Joan Sweeney[3], Steven M. Falowski[4] and Stanislaw P. Stawicki[2]

1 Medical School of Temple University/St. Luke's University Health Network, Bethlehem, Pennsylvania, USA

2 Department of Research and Innovation, St. Luke's University Health Network, EW-2 Research Administration, Bethlehem, Pennsylvania, USA

3 Center for Neurosciences, St. Luke's University Health Network, Bethlehem, Pennsylvania, USA

4 Department of Neurosurgery, St. Luke's University Health Network, Bethlehem, Pennsylvania, USA

*Address all correspondence to: vikas.yellapu@sluhn.org

References

[1] Levine DN. "Sherrington's" the integrative action of the nervous system: A centennial appraisal. Journal of the Neurological Sciences. New York. 2007;**253**(1-2):1-6

[2] Hall M. A synopsis of the diastaltic nervous system: Being the Croonian Lectures, delivered at the Royal College of Physicians. The Lancet. 1850;**55**(1392):521-522

[3] Ditunno J et al. Spinal shock revisited: A four-phase model. Spinal Cord. 2004;**42**(7):383

[4] Illis LS. Clinical evaluation and pathophysiology of the spinal cord in the chronic phase. In: Spinal Cord Dysfunction. New York: Oxford University Press; 1988. pp. 107-128

[5] Lee B et al. The global map for traumatic spinal cord injury epidemiology: Update 2011, global incidence rate. Spinal Cord. 2014;**52**(2):110

[6] Ziu E, Mesfin FB. Spinal Shock. StatPearls Publishing; 2019

[7] DeVivo MJ et al. Comparison of statistical methods for calculating life expectancy after spinal cord injury. Spinal Cord. 2018;**56**(7):666-667

[8] Mitchell R et al. Health outcomes and costs of acute traumatic spinal injury in New South Wales, Australia. The Spine Journal. 2018;**18**(7):1172-1179

[9] Hall OT et al. The burden of traumatic spinal cord injury in the United States: Disability-adjusted life years. Archives of Physical Medicine and Rehabilitation. 2019;**100**(1):95-100

[10] Ho CH et al. Spinal cord injury medicine. 1. Epidemiology and classification. Archives of Physical Medicine and Rehabilitation. 2007;**88**(3):S49-S54

[11] Goldberger ME, Murray M. Patterns of sprouting and implications for recovery of function. Advances in Neurology. 1988;**47**:361-385

[12] Murray M, Goldberger ME. Restitution of function and collateral sprouting in the cat spinal cord: The partially hemisected animal. Journal of Comparative Neurology. 1974;**158**(1):19-36

[13] Pierrot-Deseilligny E, David B. The Circuitry of the Human Spinal Cord: Spinal and Corticospinal Mechanisms of Movement. Cambridge: Cambridge University Press; 2012

[14] Murofushi T, Kimitaka K. Vestibular Evoked Myogenic Potential: Its Basics and Clinical Applications. Tokoyo: Springer Science & Business Media; 2009

[15] Boyle R, Goldberg J, Highstein S. Inputs from regularly and irregularly discharging vestibular nerve afferents to secondary neurons in squirrel monkey vestibular nuclei. III. Correlation with vestibulospinal and vestibuloocular output pathways. Journal of Neurophysiology. 1992;**68**(2):471-484

[16] Gacek RR. Neuroanatomical correlates of vestibular function. The Annals of Otology, Rhinology, and Laryngology. 1980;**89**(1):2-5

[17] Stack B, Sims A, et al. Cranio. 2009;**27**(4):248-260

[18] Konrad HR, Girardi M, Helfert R. Balance and aging. The Laryngoscope. 1999;**109**(9):1454-1460

[19] Matsuyama K et al. Locomotor role of the corticoreticular–reticulospinal–spinal interneuronal system. In:

Progress in Brain Research. Vol. 143. Amsterdam: Elsevier; 2004. pp. 239-249

[20] Peterson B, Pitts N, Fukushima K. Reticulospinal connections with limb and axial motoneurons. Experimental Brain Research. 1979;**36**(1):1-20

[21] MacKinnon CD. Sensorimotor anatomy of gait, balance, and falls. In: Handbook of Clinical Neurology. Vol. 159. Amsterdam: Elsevier; 2018. pp. 3-26

[22] Takakusaki K et al. Role of basal ganglia–brainstem systems in the control of postural muscle tone and locomotion. In: Progress in Brain Research. Amsterdam: Elsevier; 2004. pp. 231-237

[23] Takakusaki K. Neurophysiology of gait: From the spinal cord to the frontal lobe. Movement Disorders. 2013;**28**(11):1483-1491

[24] Takakusaki K et al. Basal ganglia efferents to the brainstem centers controlling postural muscle tone and locomotion: A new concept for understanding motor disorders in basal ganglia dysfunction. Neuroscience. 2003;**119**(1):293-308

[25] Svirskis G, Gutman A, Hounsgaard J. Electrotonic structure of motoneurons in the spinal cord of the turtle: Inferences for the mechanisms of bistability. Journal of Neurophysiology. 2001;**85**(1):391-398

[26] Machacek D et al. Serotonin 5-HT2 receptor activation induces a long-lasting amplification of spinal reflex actions in the rat. The Journal of Physiology. 2001;**537**(1):201-207

[27] Alaburda A, Perrier J-F, Hounsgaard J. Mechanisms causing plateau potentials in spinal motoneurones. In: Sensorimotor Control of Movement and Posture. New York: Springer; 2002. pp. 219-226

[28] Miller J et al. Restoration of extensor excitability in the acute spinal cat by the 5-HT2 agonist DOI. Journal of Neurophysiology. 1996;**75**(2):620-628

[29] Lee RH, Heckman CJ. Adjustable amplification of synaptic input in the dendrites of spinal motoneurons in vivo. Journal of Neuroscience. 2000;**20**(17):6734-6740

[30] Binder MD, Heckman C, Powers RK. Relative strengths and distributions of different sources of synaptic input to the motoneurone pool. In: Sensorimotor Control of Movement and Posture. New York: Springer; 2002. pp. 207-212

[31] Weaver RA, Landau WM, Higgins JF. Fusimotor function: Part II. Evidence of fusimotor depression in human spinal shock. Archives of Neurology. 1963;**9**(2):127-132

[32] Zapata P. Peripheral and central factors in the pathophysiology of spinal shock. Acta Physiologica Latino Americana. 1966;**16**(3):266

[33] Ashby P, Verrier M, Lightfoot E. Segmental reflex pathways in spinal shock and spinal spasticity in man. Journal of Neurology, Neurosurgery & Psychiatry. 1974;**37**(12):1352-1360

[34] Chen XY et al. Short-term and medium-term effects of spinal cord tract transections on soleus H-reflex in freely moving rats. Journal of Neurotrauma. 2001;**18**(3):313-327

[35] Simpson RK Jr, Robertson CS, Goodman JC. The role of glycine in spinal shock. The Journal of Spinal Cord Medicine. 1996;**19**(4):215-224

[36] Schwartzman RJ et al. Regional metabolic changes in the spinal cord related to spinal shock and later hyperreflexia in monkeys. Annals of Neurology: Official Journal of the

American Neurological Association and the Child Neurology Society. 1983;**14**(1):33-37

[37] Illis L. The motor neuron surface and spinal shock. Modern Trends in Neurology. 1967;**4**:53-68

[38] Llewellyn-Smith IJ, Weaver LC. Changes in synaptic inputs to sympathetic preganglionic neurons after spinal cord injury. Journal of Comparative Neurology. 2001;**435**(2):226-240

[39] Hiersemenzel L-P, Curt A, Dietz V. From spinal shock to spasticity neuronal adaptations to a spinal cord injury. Neurology. 2000;**54**(8):1574-1582

[40] Goshgarian HG, Yu XJ, Rafols JA. Neuronal and glial changes in the rat phrenic nucleus occurring within hours after spinal cord injury. Journal of Comparative Neurology. 1989;**284**(4):519-533

[41] Beattie MS, Leedy MG, Bresnahan JC. Evidence for alterations of synaptic inputs to sacral spinal reflex circuits after spinal cord transection in the cat. Experimental Neurology. 1993;**123**(1):35-50

[42] Masliah E et al. Reactive synaptogenesis assessed by synaptophysin immunoreactivity is associated with GAP-43 in the dentate gyrus of the adult rat. Experimental Neurology. 1991;**113**(2):131-142

[43] Matthews DA, Cotman C, Lynch G. An electron microscopic study of lesion-induced synaptogenesis in the dentate gyrus of the adult rat. I. Magnitude and time course of degeneration. Brain Research. 1976;**115**(1):1-21

[44] Reeves TM, Smith DC. Reinnervation of the dentate gyrus and recovery of alternation behavior following entorhinal cortex lesions. Behavioral Neuroscience. 1987;**101**(2):179

[45] Stroemer RP, Kent TA, Hulsebosch CE. Enhanced neocortical neural sprouting, synaptogenesis, and behavioral recovery with D-amphetamine therapy after neocortical infarction in rats. Stroke. 1998;**29**(11):2381-2395

[46] Turrigiano GG, Nelson SB. Homeostatic plasticity in the developing nervous system. Nature Reviews Neuroscience. 2004;**5**(2):97

[47] Vita G et al. Autoradiographic localization of substance P receptors in rat spinal cord: Effects of experimental spinal transection. Functional Neurology. 1987;**2**(4):421-426

[48] Brown LM et al. Alterations in serotonin binding sites after 5, 7-dihydroxytryptamine treatment in the rat spinal cord. Neuroscience Letters. 1989;**102**(1):103-107

[49] Kroin JS, Bianchi GD, Penn RD. Spinal cord transection produces a long-term increase in GABAB binding in the rat substantia gelatinosa. Synapse. 1993;**14**(4):263-267

[50] Roudet C et al. Normal distribution of alpha 2-adrenoceptors in the rat spinal cord and its modification after noradrenergic denervation: A quantitative autoradiographic study. Journal of Neuroscience Research. 1994;**39**(3):319-329

[51] Sawynok J, Reid A. Spinal supersensitivity to 5-HT1, 5-HT2 and 5-HT3 receptor agonists following 5, 7-dihydroxytryptamine. European Journal of Pharmacology. 1994;**264**(3):249-257

[52] Ehlers MD. Activity level controls postsynaptic composition and signaling via the ubiquitin-proteasome system. Nature Neuroscience. 2003;**6**(3):231

[53] Barry MF, Ziff EB. Receptor trafficking and the plasticity of excitatory synapses. Current Opinion in Neurobiology. 2002;**12**(3):279-286

[54] Grossman S, Rosenberg L, Wrathall J. Relationship of altered glutamate receptor subunit mRNA expression to acute cell loss after spinal cord contusion. Experimental Neurology. 2001;**168**(2):283-289

[55] Grossman SD, Wrathall JR. The role of activity blockade on glutamate receptor subunit expression in the spinal cord. Brain Research. 2000;**880**(1-2):183-186

[56] Grossman SD et al. Changes in NMDA receptor subunit expression in response to contusive spinal cord injury. Journal of Neurochemistry. 2000;**75**(1):174-184

[57] Basura GJ et al. Distribution of serotonin 2A and 2C receptor mRNA expression in the cervical ventral horn and phrenic motoneurons following spinal cord hemisection. Experimental Neurology. 2001;**169**(2):255-263

[58] Zhou Y et al. Change of vanilloid receptor 1 following neuromodulation in rats with spinal cord injury. Journal of Surgical Research. 2002;**107**(1):140-144

[59] Ikeda O et al. Acute up-regulation of brain-derived neurotrophic factor expression resulting from experimentally induced injury in the rat spinal cord. Acta Neuropathologica. 2001;**102**(3):239-245

[60] Widenfalk J et al. Neurotrophic factors and receptors in the immature and adult spinal cord after mechanical injury or kainic acid. Journal of Neuroscience. 2001;**21**(10):3457-3475

[61] Oyesiku NM, Wilcox JN, Wigston DJ. Changes in expression of ciliary neurotrophic factor (CNTF) and CNTF-receptor α after spinal cord injury. Journal of Neurobiology. 1997;**32**(3):251-261

[62] Hayashi M et al. Sequential mRNA expression for immediate early genes, cytokines, and neurotrophins in spinal cord injury. Journal of Neurotrauma. 2000;**17**(3):203-218

[63] Nakamura M, Bregman BS. Differences in neurotrophic factor gene expression profiles between neonate and adult rat spinal cord after injury. Experimental Neurology. 2001;**169**(2):407-415

[64] King V et al. Changes in truncated trkB and p75 receptor expression in the rat spinal cord following spinal cord hemisection and spinal cord hemisection plus neurotrophin treatment. Experimental Neurology. 2000;**165**(2):327-341

[65] Schinder AF, Poo M-M. The neurotrophin hypothesis for synaptic plasticity. Trends in Neurosciences. 2000;**23**(12):639-645

[66] Sayenko DG et al. Acute effects of whole body vibration during passive standing on soleus H-reflex in subjects with and without spinal cord injury. Neuroscience Letters. 2010;**482**(1):66-70

[67] Little JW et al. Incomplete spinal cord injury: Neuronal mechanisms of motor recovery and hyperreflexia. Archives of Physical Medicine and Rehabilitation. 1999;**80**(5):587-599

[68] Ko H et al. The pattern of reflex recovery during spinal shock. Spinal Cord. 1999;**37**(6):402

[69] Ditunno JF et al. Spinal shock revisited: A four-phase model. Spinal Cord. 2004;**42**(7):383-395

[70] Cadilhac J et al. Somatosensory evoked potentials and Hoffmann reflex in acute spinal cord lesions;

physiopathological and prognostic aspects. Electroencephalography and Clinical Neurophysiology. 1977;**43**(2):160-167

[71] Leis A et al. Behavior of the H-reflex in humans following mechanical perturbation or injury to rostral spinal cord. Muscle & Nerve: Official Journal of the American Association of Electrodiagnostic Medicine. 1996;**19**(11):1373-1382

[72] Liu CN, Chambers W, McCouch G. Reflexes in the spinal monkey (*Macaca mulatta*). Brain. 1966;**89**(2):349-358

[73] Riddoch G. The reflex functions of the completely divided spinal cord in man, compared with those associated with less severe lesions. Brain. 1917;**40**(2-3):264-402

[74] Guttmann L. Spinal shock. Handbook of Clinical Neurology. 1976;**26**:243-262

[75] Casabona A, Polizzi M, Perciavalle V. Differences in H-reflex between athletes trained for explosive contractions and non-trained subjects. European Journal of Applied Physiology and Occupational Physiology. 1990;**61**(1-2):26-32

[76] Nielsen J, Crone C, Hultborn H. H-reflexes are smaller in dancers from the Royal Danish Ballet than in well-trained athletes. European Journal of Applied Physiology and Occupational Physiology. 1993;**66**(2):116-121

[77] Maffiuletti NA et al. Electrical and mechanical Hmax-to-Mmaxratio in power-and endurance-trained athletes. Journal of Applied Physiology. 2001;**90**(1):3-9

[78] Steinmetz JE et al. Long-term retention of a peripherally induced flexor reflex alteration in rats. Brain Research. 1985;**327**(1-2):312-315

[79] Kauppila T, Kontinen VK, Pertovaara A. Influence of spinalization on spinal withdrawal reflex responses varies depending on the submodality of the test stimulus and the experimental pathophysiological condition in the rat. Brain Research. 1998;**797**(2):234-242

[80] Valles M et al. Cerebral hemorrhage due to autonomic dysreflexia in a spinal cord injury patient. Spinal Cord. 2005;**43**(12):738

[81] Bracken MB et al. Administration of methylprednisolone for 24 or 48 hours or tirilazad mesylate for 48 hours in the treatment of acute spinal cord injury: Results of the Third National Acute Spinal Cord Injury Randomized Controlled Trial. JAMA. 1997;**277**(20):1597-1604

[82] Bracken MB et al. A randomized, controlled trial of methylprednisolone or naloxone in the treatment of acute spinal-cord injury: Results of the second national acute spinal cord injury study. New England Journal of Medicine. 1990;**322**(20):1405-1411

[83] Petitjean ME et al. Medical Treatment of Spinal Cord Injury in the Acute Stage. Vol. 17. No. 2. Annales Francaises D'anesthesie et de Reanimation (Anaesthesia: Critical Care & Pain Medicine); 1998

[84] Hurlbert RJ et al. Pharmacological therapy for acute spinal cord injury. Neurosurgery. 2015;**76**(suppl_1):S71-S83

[85] Suberviola B et al. Early complications of high-dose methylprednisolone in acute spinal cord injury patients. Injury. 2008;**39**(7):748-752

[86] Vaquero J et al. An approach to personalized cell therapy in chronic complete paraplegia: The Puerta de Hierro phase I/II clinical trial. Cytotherapy. 2016;**18**(8):1025-1036

[87] Siddiqui AM, Khazaei M, Fehlings MG. Translating mechanisms of neuroprotection, regeneration, and repair to treatment of spinal cord injury. In: Progress in Brain Research. Elsevier; 2015. pp. 15-54

[88] Ahuja CS, Fehlings M. Concise review: Bridging the gap: Novel neuroregenerative and neuroprotective strategies in spinal cord injury. Stem Cells Translational Medicine. 2016;**5**(7):914-924

[89] Bonner S, Smith C. Initial management of acute spinal cord injury. Continuing Education in Anaesthesia Critical Care & Pain. 2013;**13**(6):224-231

[90] Riccio AR et al. Management of thoracic spine injuries part I: Thoracic spine anatomy and stability. Contemporary Neurosurgery. 2016;**38**(10):1-6

[91] Liu Z et al. High-dose methylprednisolone for acute traumatic spinal cord injury. Neurology. 2019;**93**(9):e841

[92] Fehlings MG et al. A clinical practice guideline for the management of patients with acute spinal cord injury: Recommendations on the use of methylprednisolone sodium succinate. Global Spine Journal. 2017;7(3_suppl):203S-211S

[93] Jensen MP et al. Symptom burden in persons with spinal cord injury. Archives of Physical Medicine and Rehabilitation. 2007;**88**(5):638-645

[94] Wyndaele M, Wyndaele JJ. Incidence, prevalence and epidemiology of spinal cord injury: What learns a worldwide literature survey? Spinal Cord. 2006;**44**:523

[95] McKinley W et al. Incidence and outcomes of spinal cord injury clinical syndromes. The Journal of Spinal Cord Medicine. 2007;**30**(3):215-224

[96] Ishida Y, Tominaga T. Predictors of neurologic recovery in acute central cervical cord injury with only upper extremity impairment. Spine. 2002;**27**(15):1652-1657

[97] Harrop JS, Sharan A, Ratliff J. Central cord injury: Pathophysiology, management, and outcomes. The Spine Journal. 2006;**6**(6 Supplement): S198-S206

[98] Corbo S, Doty CI. Vertebral column and spinal cord trauma. In: Stone CK, Humphries RL, editors. Current Diagnosis and Treatment: Emergency Medicine. 8th ed. New York, NY: McGraw-Hill Education; 2017

[99] Tay BKB et al. Chapter 4. Disorders, diseases, and injuries of the spine. In: Skinner HB, McMahon PJ, editors. Current Diagnosis and Treatment in Orthopedics. 5th ed. New York, NY: The McGraw-Hill Companies; 2014

[100] Ropper AH et al. Diseases of the spinal cord. In: Adams and Victor's Principles of Neurology. 11th ed. New York, NY: McGraw-Hill Education; 2019

[101] Claydon VE, Steeves JD, Krassioukov A. Orthostatic hypotension following spinal cord injury: Understanding clinical pathophysiology. Spinal Cord. 2006;**44**(6):341-351

[102] Gossman W, Stobart MA, Gilis CC. Central Cord Syndrome. StatPearls [Internet]. StatPearls Publishing; 2019

[103] Theodore N et al. The diagnosis and management of traumatic atlanto-occipital dislocation injuries. Neurosurgery. 2013;**72**(Suppl 2):114-126

[104] James G et al. Traumatic central cord syndrome: Results of surgical management. Journal of Neurosurgery: Spine. 2002;**97**(1):25-32

[105] Aarabi B et al. Management of acute traumatic central cord syndrome (ATCCS). Neurosurgery. 2013;**72**(suppl_3):195-204

[106] Bose B et al. Reanalysis of central cervical cord injury management. Neurosurgery. 1984;**15**(3):367-372

[107] Carlson GD et al. Sustained spinal cord compression: Part I: Time-dependent effect on long-term pathophysiology. JBJS. 2003;**85**(1):86-94

[108] Papadopoulos SM et al. Immediate spinal cord decompression for cervical spinal cord injury: Feasibility and outcome. Journal of Trauma and Acute Care Surgery. 2002;**52**(2):323-332

[109] McKinley W et al. Outcomes of early surgical management versus late or no surgical intervention after acute spinal cord injury. Archives of Physical Medicine and Rehabilitation. 2004;**85**(11):1818-1825

[110] Dvorak MF et al. Factors predicting motor recovery and functional outcome after traumatic central cord syndrome: A long-term follow-up. Spine. 2005;**30**(20):2303-2311

[111] Aito S et al. Neurological and functional outcome in traumatic central cord syndrome. Spinal Cord. 2007;**45**(4):292

[112] Fehlings MG et al. Essentials of Spinal Cord Injury : From Basic Research to Clinical Practice. New York, United States: Thieme Medical Publishers, Incorporated; 2012

[113] Ahuja CS et al. Traumatic spinal cord injury. Nature Reviews. Disease Primers. 2017;**3**:17018

[114] Waxman SG. The spinal cord. In: Clinical Neuroanatomy. 28th ed. New York, NY: McGraw-Hill Education; 2017

[115] Lipper MH, Goldstein JH, Do HM. Brown-Séquard syndrome of the cervical spinal cord after chiropractic manipulation. American Journal of Neuroradiology. 1998;**19**(7):1349-1352

[116] Lim E et al. Traumatic atypical Brown-Sequard syndrome: Case report and literature review. Clinical Neurology and Neurosurgery. 2003;**105**(2):143-145

[117] Moskowitz E, Schroeppel T. Brown-Sequard syndrome. Trauma Surgery & Acute Care Open. 2018;**3**(1):e000169

[118] Rath N, Balain B. Spinal cord injury-the role of surgical treatment for neurological improvement. Journal of Clinical Orthopaedics and Trauma. 2017;**8**(2):99-102

[119] Steinmetz MP, Mekhail A, Benzel EC. Management of metastatic tumors of the spine: Strategies and operative indications. Neurosurgical Focus. 2001;**11**(6):1-6

[120] Schmidt RD, Markovchick V. Nontraumatic spinal cord compression. The Journal of Emergency Medicine. 1992;**10**(2):189-199

[121] Kupfer M et al. Spinal cord injury. In: Maitin IB, Cruz E, editors. Current Diagnosis and Treatment: Physical Medicine and Rehabilitation. New York, NY: McGraw-Hill Education; 2015

[122] Abouhashem S et al. Management of Brown-Sequard syndrome in cervical disc diseases. Turkish Neurosurgery. 2013;**23**(4):470-475

[123] Keenan MAE, Mehta S, McMahon PJ. Chapter 12. Rehabilitation. In: Skinner HB, McMahon PJ, editors. Current Diagnosis and Treatment in Orthopedics. 5th ed. New York, NY: The McGraw-Hill Companies; 2014

[124] Inoue T, Cohen-Gadol AA, Krauss WE. Low-pressure headaches and spinal cord herniation: Case report. Journal of Neurosurgery: Spine. 2003;**98**(1):93-95

[125] Kim J-M et al. Idiopathic spinal cord herniation as a treatable cause of progressive Brown-Sequard syndrome. Journal of Clinical Neurology. 2007;**3**(4):204-207

[126] Pandey AS, Thompson BG. Neurosurgery. In: Doherty GM, editor. Current Diagnosis and Treatment: Surgery. 14th ed. New York, NY: McGraw-Hill Education; 2015

[127] Go S. Spine trauma. In: Tintinalli JE et al., editors. Tintinalli's Emergency Medicine: A Comprehensive Study Guide. 8th ed. New York, NY: McGraw-Hill Education; 2016

[128] Ropper AH et al. Disorders of non-painful somatic sensation. In: Adams and Victor's Principles of Neurology. 11th ed. New York, NY: McGraw-Hill Education; 2019

Chapter 9

Amniotic Fluid Embolism

Neesaytee Boulden, Joseph Bell, Jose Rojas-Suarez and Jorge E. Tolosa

Abstract

Amniotic fluid embolism (AFE) is a rare complication of pregnancy often resulting in catastrophic maternal and fetal outcomes. Given the rarity of this condition, there is a wide variation in reported incidence of amniotic fluid embolism. The pathophysiology of AFE is not completely understood. It is thought to be the result of a breach of the maternal-fetal barrier resulting in an abnormal maternal proinflammatory response. AFE presents as a sudden onset of hypoxia, hypotension, and coagulopathy during labor and delivery or in the immediate postpartum period. Abnormalities in the fetal heart tracing are almost always present. Risk factors often include advanced maternal age, induction of labor, cesarean delivery, operative vaginal delivery, placenta previa, and placental abruption. The diagnosis of amniotic fluid embolism is made based on clinical presentation. There are no laboratory tests that confirm the diagnosis of AFE; however, serum tryptase levels, complement levels, zinc coproporphyrin, and serum sialyl Tn (STn) may support the diagnosis. Management of women with AES is supportive and most often requires admission to an intensive care unit. Although maternal morbidity and mortality remain high, advances in medical technology and improvements in obstetrical critical care and early diagnosis of AFE have improved outcomes.

Keywords: amniotic fluid embolism, maternal mortality, DIC, pregnancy, hypoxia, shock, hypotension

1. Introduction

Amniotic fluid embolism (AFE) is a rare pregnancy complication often resulting in significant maternal and fetal/neonatal morbidity and mortality. AFE is one of the leading causes of maternal mortality in developed countries and is most often diagnosed at the time of delivery or in the immediate postpartum period. The term amniotic fluid embolism developed from a theory based on a small subset of patients who were deemed to have died as result of an embolic event associated with amniotic fluid. This theory has largely been discredited by a growing body of evidence that suggests AFE is most likely the result of an abnormal proinflammatory response in the host [1]. Given the rarity of this syndrome, the reported incidence varies greatly from 1.9 per 100,000 in the United Kingdom to as high as 6.1 per 100,000 in Australia [1, 2]. However, even with prompt diagnosis and timely treatment, maternal mortality rates remain high.

IntechOpen

2. Pathophysiology

AFE was first described in the 1920s by J.R. Meyer. It was later recognized as a syndrome in 1941 when Steiner and Lushbaugh reported autopsy findings of 32 women who died suddenly during childbirth. The common histopathological finding among these women was the presence of amniotic fluid debris in the pulmonary vasculature [1]. Therefore, the historical hypothesis was based on an obstruction of the pulmonary arteries from amniotic fluid or fetal debris [1, 3]. Medical advancements in the 1980s allowed for more frequent use of the pulmonary artery catheter to obtain arterial histologic specimens from living patients [1]. There were several reports of pathologic findings that were previously thought to be diagnostic of AFE found in pregnant women that did not have AFE. These findings called into question previous cases diagnosed as AFE that were based solely on pathologic findings.

The second and more commonly accepted theory is that AFE results from a complex sequence of reactions involving an abnormal activation of proinflammatory mediators in the host leading to an immunologic response [1–7]. This response is similar to the systemic inflammatory response syndrome (SIRS). Amniotic fluid contains several procoagulant factors including platelet-activating factor, leukotrienes, bradykinin, cytokines, thromboxane, and arachidonic acid, which aids in the understanding of why disseminated intravascular coagulation (DIC) is observed in 80% or more of women diagnosed with AFE [1, 7, 8]. In conjunction with these responses, a profound hemodynamic change leads to the maternal collapse and death in patients with AFE. Thus, during the first minutes, a sudden increase in pulmonary vascular resistance as a result of an inflammatory/anaphylactoid vasoconstriction leads to a right ventricular dysfunction with dilation of the right ventricular chambers, with a left shift of the interventricular septum and a decrease of the left ventricular filling pressures, with hypotension and cardiovascular collapse [9]. This severe pulmonary vasoconstriction produces an oxygen shunt, with ventilation-perfusion mismatching and severe hypoxia. Finally, left ventricular failure may be present as a consequence of myocardial injury secondary to some inflammatory mediators or myocardial ischemia [10].

Complement activation is thought by some to play a role in the pathophysiology of AFE. Virtually all patients diagnosed with AFE develop some degree of acute respiratory distress syndrome (ARDS). Various case series evaluating serum complement levels in patients with AFE have noted significantly decreased levels of C3 and C4 compared to a control group of normal laboring patients who all had complement levels within the normal range [7]. Decreased levels of C3 are thought to be consistent with complement activation.

3. Incidence and risk factors

3.1 Incidence

The true incidence of amniotic fluid embolism is unknown. Discrepancies in diagnosis as well as inconsistencies in reporting practices lead to a wide range of estimates. AFE incidence ranges between 1 in 8000 and 1 in 80,000 pregnancies [8, 11, 12]. In 2012, Knight et al. reviewed available data sources from Australia, Canada, the Netherlands, the United Kingdom, and the United States to investigate incidence rates and identify variations in methodology in diagnosis of AFE. Their analysis found a reported incidence of AFE ranging from 1.9 cases per 100,000 in the United Kingdom to 6.1 cases per 100,000 cases in Australia. Differences in the reported incidence were attributed to a lack of internationally accepted diagnostic criteria for nonfatal cases of AFE as well as variance in methodology.

3.2 Risk factors

Review of various data registries reveals a wide range of conflicting data regarding identifiable risk factors for AFE. Historically, risk factors associated with AFE included situations where there was an increased likelihood of exchange of maternal and fetal components [1, 2, 13]. Events such as cesarean delivery, operative vaginal delivery, cervical trauma, placenta previa, and abruption were frequently reported [9, 13–16].

Knight et al. in 2012 reviewed data sources on incidence of AFE in Australia, Canada, the Netherlands, the United Kingdom, and the United States. Where data was available, they also examined risk factors associated with AFE. There were only two associations that were consistent across all five countries: induction of labor and maternal age [2]. In the Netherlands the association with age was not statistically significant. This may be a result of the limited power of the study given that all reported cases occurred in women who were 29 years of age or older. The data from Canada showed an association between AFE and all methods of medical induction of labor, while in the United Kingdom, there was only a statistically significant association with induction of labor using vaginal prostaglandins [2]. In the United States, all methods of induction of labor showed an increased odds ratio; however, this was not statistically significant [2]. Increased odds of AFE associated with placental previa and placental abruption was also observed. In the United Kingdom there was a statistically significant association between cesarean section when the amniotic fluid embolism occurred after delivery. There was no association with forceps or vacuum delivery; however, only a small subset of women underwent an operative vaginal delivery, so there is limited power to detect this association [2].

Another group of researchers who conducted a population-based cohort study on 3 million birth records in the United States from 1999 to 2003 found AFE was associated with maternal age greater than 35 (OR 2.2, 95% CI 1.5–2.1). However, they did not find that AFE was significantly associated with induction of labor. They also reported an association of placenta previa (OR 30.4, 95% CI 15.4–60.1) and cesarean delivery (OR 5.7, 95% CI 3.7–8.7) [16].

Maternal risk factors [1, 3, 5, 6, 8, 9, 11, 13–16]:

- Advanced maternal age, >35
- Multiparity
- Diabetes
- Ethnic minority

Fetal risk factors [15, 16]:

- Male fetus
- Multifetal gestation
- Fetal distress
- Polyhydramnios
- Intrauterine death

Obstetrical factors [1, 3, 5, 6, 8, 9, 11, 13–16]:

- Induction or augmentation of labor
- Cesarean section
- Cervical or abdominal trauma
- Premature rupture of membranes
- Operative vaginal delivery
- Placenta previa/accreta
- Placental abruption
- Eclampsia

4. Diagnosis

There should be a high level of suspicion of AFE for a pregnant or postpartum woman with an acute onset of cardiopulmonary compromise, DIC, and altered mental status. The diagnosis of AFE is one of exclusion and is based upon clinical findings of sudden onset of hypoxia, cardiovascular compromise, and/or coagulopathy. The differential diagnosis of AFE includes, but is not limited to, pulmonary embolism, anaphylaxis, placental abruption, myocardial infarction, eclampsia, aspiration, and septic shock [1, 4, 5]. To date there are no specific laboratory tests available to diagnosis AFE. Some recent publications have suggested an insulin-like growth factor binding protein-1 as a useful biomarker for AFE diagnosis, with high sensitivity and specificity; however, this is not extensively used [6].

The Society of Maternal-Fetal Medicine (SMFM) and the Amniotic Fluid Embolism Foundation proposed a definition of AFE based on four diagnostic criteria, which are all required to be present. This definition was specifically developed for research purposes.

1. "Sudden onset of cardiorespiratory arrest, or both hypotension (systolic blood pressure < 90 mm Hg) and respiratory compromise (dyspnea, cyanosis, or peripheral capillary oxygen saturation < 90%)

2. Documentation of overt DIC after appearance of these initial signs or symptoms, using this scoring system of the Scientific and Standardization Committee on DIC of the International Society on Thrombosis and Hemostasis (ISTH), modified for pregnancy. Coagulopathy must be detected before loss of sufficient blood to itself account for *dilutional* or shock-related consumptive coagulopathy

3. Clinical onset during labor or within 30 minutes of delivery of placenta

4. Absence of fever (≥38°C) during labor" [6, 14].

Although there are no specific tests that are currently recommended to confirm the diagnosis of amniotic fluid embolism, there are test that may help to support the diagnosis. Initial evaluation should always include assessment of arterial blood gas to determine the degree of hypoxemia. In addition to arterial blood gas measurements, serial complete blood counts and coagulation studies should be trended in order to detect early coagulopathy [9]. These studies can aid in the early identification of DIC. Abnormalities often include a prolonged prothrombin time (PT) which is due to consumption of clotting factors as well as a decreased fibrinogen. Intervention is often indicated if the PT is 1.5 times the normal limit. Activated partial thromboplastin time may not be as helpful as values may be within normal reference range.

Additional laboratory tests proposed include various markers of C3 and C4 complement activation, serum tryptase, insulin-like growth factor binding protein-1, urinary histamine, and arachidonic acid metabolites [1, 4, 9]. Tryptase is a serine protease that has a half-life of several hours and has been useful in the diagnosis of anaphylaxis. Given the similarities of the reported pathophysiology of AEF and anaphylaxis, elevated levels of serum tryptase may aid in diagnosis. There have been reports of the use of immunostaining techniques of the monoclonal TKH-2 antibodies in maternal serum and lung tissue. Although data is limited, there are a few studies that have evaluated the use of serum sialyl Tn (STn) which is a fetal antigen in meconium as well as amniotic fluid that can be detected with TKH-2 monoclonal antibodies. TKH-2 reacts with fetal components (meconium and mucin) which stain the lung tissue of women with AFE [4, 5, 9]. Researchers found that serum levels of sialyl Tn greater than 50 U/ml had a sensitivity between 78 and 100% and a specificity between 97 and 99% [9]. Another biomarker of interest is zinc coproporphyrin, which is also a component of amniotic fluid found in maternal serum and can be elevated in women with AFE [1, 4, 9].

Radiographic findings are nonspecific and not diagnostic. The most common radiographic abnormalities in AFE are bilateral interstitial and alveolar infiltrates with areas of increased opacity which is indistinguishable from pulmonary edema [4, 9]. The use of bedside transesophageal echocardiography may aid in early identification of acute pulmonary vasoconstriction or left heart failure precipitating earlier intervention [4, 9].

5. Clinical presentation

The classic presentation of AFE is often described as an acute onset of respiratory distress, hypoxia, hypotension (including cardiac arrest), seizures, and DIC either during labor, during delivery, or in the immediate postpartum period. If AFE occurs during labor, electronic fetal heart tracings frequently demonstrate acute changes characteristic of fetal hypoxia. There is often a rapid progression from the time of onset of the initial signs and symptoms to end organ damage and death. Severe consumptive coagulopathy is seen in only two obstetric conditions, AFE and massive placental abruption [4]. DIC is present in approximately 80% of patients with AFE and may develop at any time; however, half of affected patients develop coagulopathy within 4 hours of initial symptoms [2].

6. Management

The management of women diagnosed with AFE is centered on supportive care. Unfortunately, even with prompt recognition and appropriate treatment, maternal morbidity and mortality remain high. The Society for Maternal-Fetal Medicine (SMFM) recommends a multidisciplinary team approach consisting of anesthesiology, critical care medicine, respiratory therapy, and maternal-fetal medicine [6]. Treatment is initially focused on maternal cardiopulmonary stabilization with a goal to limit end organ damage [2]. Intravenous access with two large bore IVs should be obtained in anticipation of the need for aggressive fluid resuscitation. Hypotension is corrected with optimization of preload via rapid infusion of isotonic crystalloid and colloid solutions [4, 8, 9]. Transthoracic or transesophageal echocardiography is helpful to guide fluid therapy [4–6, 9]. Placement of an arterial line and pulmonary catheter if feasible is also useful. In addition to IVF resuscitation, transfusions of packed red blood cells are necessary to aid in hypotension as well as restoration of oxygen carrying capacity. The use of vasopressors and or inotropic support is often necessary. A central line should be placed for infusion of vasopressors as well as monitoring. Following stabilization of the patient, admission to an intensive care unit is recommended for close monitoring. Initial laboratory testing should include a CBC, arterial blood gas, electrolytes, and a coagulation panel.

6.1 Hypoxia

Acute hypoxia is frequently the first sign of AFE and has been reported to be present in >90% of patients according to the AFE National Registry [2]. Maternal oxygenation should be monitored by pulse oximetry. The degree of respiratory compromise will determine the approach for oxygen delivery. Regardless of the route of delivery, oxygen should be administered immediately and judiciously. Intubation is often necessary but may not be required in all cases.

6.2 Cardiac arrest

The early phase of AFE often consists of right ventricular failure which can be identified with the use of transthoracic or transesophageal echocardiography [9, 13]. Findings of echocardiography may include a dilated right ventricle and a collapsed left ventricle with leftward deviation of the interventricular septum [9, 13]. Cardiopulmonary resuscitation (CPR) should be initiated immediately with priority given to high-quality chest compressions before rescue breaths [6]. Standard basic life support (BLS) and advanced cardiac life support (ACLS) protocols should also be initiated [1, 6]. If the fetus is undelivered and has reached a gestational age of potential viability (≥23 weeks), immediate delivery is indicated [1, 2, 6]. Preparation for a perimortem cesarean section should occur simultaneously with the initiation of CPR [1, 10]. The undelivered patient should be placed in a left lateral tilt that displaces the uterus to avoid compression of the aorta and IVC [2, 6]. Patients that progress to cardiac arrest have a dismal prognosis compared to their counterparts with AFE that do not develop cardiac arrest.

6.3 Coagulopathy

Hemorrhage with DIC requires initiation of a massive transfusion protocol. Correcting the coagulopathy may require aggressive repletion of red blood cells and blood products, fresh frozen plasma, platelets, and/or cryoprecipitate. Consideration should be given to arterial catheterization if possible, which allows for accurate blood pressure monitoring as well as blood sampling [5]. The use of recombinant factor VIIa has been reported in the literature, though data on its use is limited and conflicting. Research suggests that the use of recombinant factor VIIa most likely should be reserved for cases where conventional resuscitative measures fail [1]. Increasing evidence suggests the use of thrombelastometry for early identification of patients with AFE but also to guide management, providing a point of care for monitoring during the hemorrhagic phase of AFE [17].

Additional approaches to treatment of amniotic fluid embolism reported in the literature include extracorporeal membrane oxygenation (ECMO), plasma exchange transfusions, cardiopulmonary bypass, uterine artery embolization, continuous hemofiltration, pulmonary artery thromboembolectomy, intra-aortic balloon pump with ECMO, high-dose corticosteroids, C1 esterase inhibitors, and serum protease inhibitor therapy. There are no high-quality data available for many of the treatment approaches mentioned.

Aprotinin is a single-chain polypeptide derived from bovine tissues and is an inhibitor of proteolytic enzymes [9]. It is used in the treatment of hemorrhage associated with raised plasma concentrations of plasmin and may be effective for hemorrhage associated with AFE. Other fibrinolytic agents like tranexamic acid and aminocaproic acid are used in the management of hemorrhage and may be useful. Hysterectomy is necessary in individuals when uterine hemorrhage persists despite more conservative measures.

7. Outcomes

Mortality associated with amniotic fluid embolism appears to have declined which is likely associated with early diagnosis as well as improvements in critical care [4, 5, 9]. Disease severity (i.e., the presence or absence of cardiac arrest) is closely related to prognosis. Mortality rates vary greatly depending upon criteria used for diagnosis of AFE but have been reported as high as 60–70% [1, 9, 14]. The use of population-based studies appears to provide the best available evidence of the mortality rate associated with AFE. Analysis of a collection of 9 population-based studies published since 1999 which included more than 17 million births in 8 countries and 751 cases of amniotic fluid embolism revealed an overall mortality rate of 20.3% [7]. Morbidity, however, remains extremely high and can include serious neurologic impairment, renal failure, cardiac failure, arrhythmias, and myocardial infarction [5, 9].

Although limited data is available, neonatal survival rates are reported in the range of 70% [4, 5, 9]. Survival is dependent upon timing of delivery relative to onset of symptoms. Neonates delivered prior to onset of symptoms or soon after onset of symptoms have lower rates of morbidity and mortality.

There is no data to suggest that survivors of AFE have an increased risk of recurrence in a subsequent pregnancy. However, the risk of recurrence is unknown. There have been published case reports of successful pregnancies following an AFE.

8. Summary

Amniotic fluid embolism remains an elusive disease with catastrophic outcomes. The pathophysiology remains unclear even with new research developments over the last 10 years. However, the theory that the syndrome may be caused by an abnormal maternal proinflammatory response incited by fetal components is promising. The variation in maternal response to fetal and amniotic components present in the maternal circulation may provide useful information and requires further investigation. Various laboratory tests and biomarkers have been proposed that may aid in diagnosis of an AFE; however, there is no gold standard diagnostic test available at this time. AFE remains a diagnosis of exclusion and relies on clinical judgment. A high level of suspicion in laboring or postpartum women with acute cardiopulmonary compromise or coagulopathy is required for optimal maternal and fetal outcomes.

Methodology

A literature search was performed using PubMed. The term "amniotic fluid embolism" was used to search the database. The search was further narrowed using year of publication. Articles from 2005 to the present were selected. A combination of case reports, case series, population-based cohort studies, case control analysis, and review articles were included for review.

Author details

Neesaytee Boulden[1], Joseph Bell[2], Jose Rojas-Suarez[3] and Jorge E. Tolosa[2,4,5,6*]

1 Department of Obstetrics and Gynecology, St. Luke's University Hospital, Bethlehem, PA, United States

2 Department of Obstetrics and Gynecology, Maternal Fetal Medicine, St. Luke's University Hospital, Bethlehem, PA, United States

3 Intensive Care and Obstetric Research Group (GRICIO), Universidad de Cartagena, Cartagena de Indias, Colombia

4 Oregon Health and Science University, Portland, OR, United States

5 Departamento de Obstetricia y Ginecología, Universidad de Antioquia, Medellín, Colombia

6 FUNDARED-MATERNA, Bogotá, Colombia

*Address all correspondence to: jorge.tolosa@sluhn.org

References

[1] Clark S. Amniotic fluid embolism. Obstetrics and Gynecology. 2014;**123**:337-348. DOI: 10.1097/AOG.0000000000000107

[2] Knight M, Berg C, Brocklehurst P, Kramer M, Lewis G, Oats J, et al. Amniotic fluid embolism incidence, risk factors and outcomes: A review and recommendations. BMC Pregnancy and Childbirth. 2012;**12**:7

[3] Tamura N, Farhana M, Tomoaki O, Hiroaki I, Naohiro K. Amniotic fluid embolus: Pathophysiology from the perspective of pathology. The Journal of Obstetrics and Gynaecology Research. 2017;**43**:627-632. DOI: 10.1111/jog.13284

[4] Moore J, Baldisseri M. Amniotic fluid embolism. Critical Care Medicine. 2005;**33**:S279-S285. DOI: 10.1097/01.CCM.0000183158.71311.28

[5] Kaur K, Bhardwaj M, Kumar SS, Singh T, Hooda S. Amniotic fluid embolism. Journal of Anesthesiology Clinical Pharmacology. 2016;**32**:153-159

[6] Society for Maternal-Fetal Medicine (SMFM) with the assistance of Pacheco LD, Saade G, et al. Amniotic fluid embolism: Diagnosis and management. American Journal of Obstetrics and Gynecology. 2016;**215**:B16-B24

[7] Benson M. Current concepts of immunology and diagnosis in amniotic fluid embolism. Clinical & Developmental Immunology. 2012;**2012**:946576

[8] Knight M, Tuffnell D, Brocklehurst P, Spark P, Kurinczuk J. Incidence and risk factors for amniotic fluid embolism. Obstetrics and Gynecology. 2010;**115**:910-917

[9] Stanten RD, Iverson LI, Daugharty TM, Lovett SM, Terry C, Blumenstock E. Amniotic fluid embolism causing catastrophic pulmonary vasoconstriction: Diagnosis by transesophageal echocardiogram and treatment by cardiopulmonary bypass. Obstetrics and Gynecology. 2003;**102**:496-498

[10] James CF, Feinglass NG, Menke DM, Grinton SF, Papadimos TJ. Massive amniotic fluid embolism: Diagnosis aided by emergency transesophageal echocardiography. International Journal of Obstetric Anesthesia. 2004;**13**:279-283

[11] Clark S. Amniotic fluid embolism. Clinical Obstetrics and Gynecology. 2010;**53**:322-328. DOI: 10.1097/GRF.ob013e3181e0ead2

[12] Davies S. Amniotic fluid embolism: A review of the literature. Canadian Journal of Anaesthesia. 2000;**48**:88-98

[13] Shamshirsaz AS, Clark S. Amniotic fluid embolism. Obstetrics and Gynecology Clinics of North America. 2016;**43**:779-790

[14] Bonnet MP, Zlotnik D, Saucedo M, Chassard D, Bouvier-Colle M, Deneux-Tharaux C. Maternal death due to amniotic fluid embolism; a national study in France. Obstetric Anesthesiology. 2018;**126**(1):175-181

[15] Sultan P, Seligman K, Carvalho B.Amniotic fluid embolism: update and review. Current Opinion in Anesthesiology. 2016;**29**:288-296

[16] Abenhaim HA, Azoulay L, Kramer MS, Leduc L. Incidence and risk factors of amniotic fluid embolisms: a population based study on 3 million births in the United States. A J Obstet Gynecol 2008;**199**:49e1-49e8

[17] Annecke T, Geisenberger T, Kürzl R, Penning R, Heindl B. Algorithmbased coagulation management of catastrophic amniotic fluid embolism. Blood Coagulation & Fibrinolysis. 2010;**21**(1):95-100

Chapter 10

Burn Shock and Resuscitation: Many Priorities, One Goal

John Sojka, Andrew C. Krakowski and Stanislaw P. Stawicki

Abstract

Burn injuries come in a wide variety of presentations, depending on the size and depth of the thermal insult, concurrent traumatic or inhalation injury, as well as the associated physiological response of the burn victim. To minimize patient morbidity and reduce mortality, prompt recognition and tailored treatment strategies are critically important. As the percentage of total body surface area (TBSA) burned increases so do the body's physiologic response and the associated complexity of management. Understanding the pathophysiology of burn injury allows the practitioner to optimize and individualize burn patient management—a component of care critical to limiting wound progression and improving outcomes. Burn patient care starts with an accurate and thorough burn patient evaluation conducted in person by an experienced provider. For burns >10–15% TBSA, prompt initiation of fluid resuscitation greatly impacts clinical outcomes. Several formulae have been published to guide crystalloid and/or colloid fluid resuscitation in the setting of burn shock. Other important considerations include ambient temperature control, early enteral nutritional support, vitamin and mineral supplementation, assessment for inhalation injury, glycemic control, early recognition of potential complications of large volume resuscitation, potential need for cardiovascular support, and early wound excision and coverage. Burn patients often require multidisciplinary teams to manage the physical, social, and psychological effects associated with their injury. Dedicated burn centers are the ideal places for meeting the complex needs of each burn patient.

Keywords: burn injury, shock, resuscitation, traumatic injury, Parkland formula, West Penn formula, dermato-surgical considerations

1. Introduction

Burns are among the most challenging and physiologically complex injuries and can be associated with the development of early hemodynamic collapse and shock [1, 2]. Patients who have sustained significant burns are at risk of rapidly developing "burn shock" due to the simultaneous presence of local and systemic inflammatory response to injury that most closely resembles hypovolemic shock [3, 4]. While burns themselves have the potential to be the primary source of shock, the presence of large burns should not distract the vigilant provider from ruling out additional injuries during their assessment of a trauma patient [5, 6]. After addressing any immediate airway threat during the initial trauma evaluation, it is of utmost importance to promptly determine the presence of other potentially life-threatening non-burn injuries. Once other life-threatening injuries are ruled out, the resuscitating team's focus can be directed toward managing the burn. Rapid initiation of therapy tailored to each burn patient during the initial 48 h from the time of burn injury is critical for preventing burn shock, secondary injuries, and other downstream sequelae [3]. In this chapter, we will discuss the fundamentals of burn shock, starting with pathophysiologic and mechanistic considerations and concluding with clinical management pearls.

2. Overview of mechanistic considerations

Burn management begins with a complete history and physical examination, known as the "burn patient evaluation" (BPE), which is intended to quantify and classify the thermal injury [7, 8]. Burns are typically described and classified by etiologic cause, extent of body surface area involved, and depth [9–11]. There are three broad categories of etiologies associated with burn injuries—thermal, chemical, and electrical [12–14]. Thermal mechanisms can be further broken down into flame burns, scald burns, contact burns, steam burns, or flash burns [15, 16]. This chapter focuses primarily on thermal injuries, although many of the concepts discussed herein also apply to other burn types.

The understanding of mechanistic considerations and associated tissue injury patterns is of critical importance when evaluating and treating burn victims [17, 18]. For example, thermal injury causes coagulative necrosis of the affected tissue, and the depth of injury is directly dependent on temperature and duration of exposure, which will vary widely across different types of thermal exposures and injured tissue characteristics [19, 20]. The extent of chemical-induced tissue injury will vary with substance type (acids, alkalis, or hydrocarbon-based organic solvents), concentration, and duration of exposure, but all require expedited clinical management and lavage (when appropriate) of affected areas [21–25]. Electrical injuries will vary in nature between high and low voltage exposure, and depending on exact circumstances, involved victims may be at an increased risk of presenting with cardiovascular and neurologic manifestations, as well as associated traumatic injuries from falling or violent muscle contractions [26–30].

3. Pathophysiology of burn injury

The skin plays a crucial role in maintaining physiologic homeostasis through thermal regulation, sensory reception, synthesis of vitamins and hormones, maintaining fluid/electrolyte balance, and providing barrier protection to underlying tissues [31–34]. When exposed to excessive heat, human tissues develop clinical burn injury [35]. During thermal insult, the epidermis and dermis are able to limit the direct transfer of energy to underlying tissues [19]. Various pathophysiologic derangements occur including denaturation of macromolecular structures, cell membrane dysfunction or destruction, cytokine release, arrest of local blood flow, and eventually cell/tissue death [35]. Following the initial insult, the final depth of irreversible tissue injury may increase depending on how local tissues respond to the complex microvascular and inflammatory environment in their immediate surroundings [35–38]. Morphologically, the tissue environment at the location of burn injury has three physiologically distinct zones. Based on the immediate proximity (e.g., distance or depth) from the primary burn site, these zones are the zone of coagulation, zone of stasis, and zone of hyperemia (**Figure 1**) [12, 38].

The zone of coagulation refers to the area of tissue that has been irreversibly damaged at the time of injury and has undergone coagulative necrosis [39, 40].

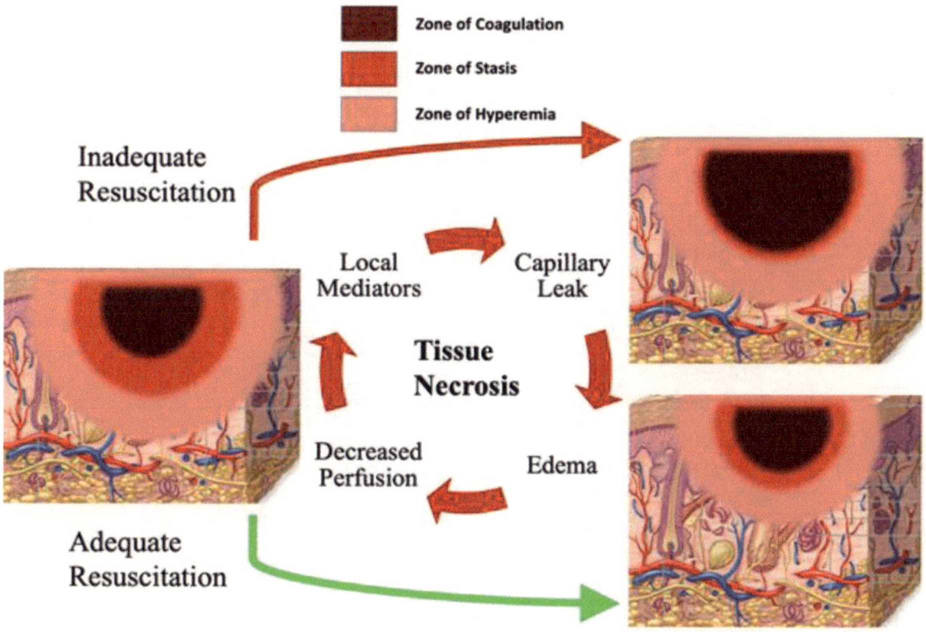

Figure 1.
This schematic displays how resuscitation interacts with the pathophysiologic changes associated with burn injury.

The zone of stasis, also known as the "watershed" region, represents the area of tissue injury that may be reversible under optimal resuscitative circumstances [40, 41]. This zone is characterized by vascular injury, capillary leakage, and high concentrations of thromboxane A_2—a potent vasoconstrictor produced locally by platelets [1]. Catecholamines and serotonin also play an important role in modulating tissue responses within this zone [1]. The end effect is impaired tissue perfusion, and thus elevated risk of propagating the area of tissue necrosis during the initial 24–48 h following the index injury [1, 36, 42]. The zone of stasis is the area where early intervention with therapy directed at reducing vasoconstriction, optimizing perfusion, and controlling local inflammation may have the greatest effect at limiting the depth of injury. The zone of hyperemia is the most remote zone of cutaneous injury (relative to the primary burn site) where vasodilation is noted in viable tissue undergoing the healing process. This vasodilation is multifactorial and likely mediated through a combination of histamine- and kinin-related mechanisms [1, 43].

Accurate determination of burn wound depth is crucial for guiding clinical management (**Table 1**) [9, 44]. Some superficially limited burns may heal with local treatment alone, while deeper burns are more likely to require operative intervention. Although various tools are available to assist in this assessment [44–49], burn depth is usually determined during BPE through visual inspection by an experienced practitioner who then goes on to classify his or her findings in accordance to pre-established "degrees of injury severity" outlined below:

1. Superficial—commonly referred to as "first degree"—burns are generally limited to the epidermis. The burned skin is characterized by the presence of blanching erythema that tends to appear dry (without blistering) and is very tender on exam due to the proximity of sensory nerve endings. Common examples include sunburns or mild scalding from hot water [50]. Management of these burns is directed at reducing further injury, pain control, and provision of comfort measures. Within the first hour, exposing the injury to cool

Depth/ degree	Etiology	Tissue layer	Appearance	Pain	Healing time
Superficial I°	Sunlight exposure, hot liquids with low viscosity and short exposure	Epidermis only	Pink to red, moist, no blisters	Moderate–severe	3–7 days
Superficial partial IIa°	Hot liquids, chemical burns with weak acid or alkali, flash	Superficial (papillary) dermis	Blister, red, moist, intact epidermal appendages, blanching on pressure	Severe	1–3 weeks, long-term pigment changes may occur
Deep partial IIb°	Flame, chemical, electrical, hot liquids with high viscosity	Deeper layer (reticular) dermis	Dry, white, non-blanching, loss of all epidermal appendages	Minimal	3–6 weeks, with scars
Deep III°	Flame, electrical, chemical, blast, self-immolation	Full skin thickness with extension into subcutaneous tissues	Leathery, dry, white or red with visibly thrombosed vessels	No	Does not heal by primary intention, requires skin graft
IV°	Mostly prolonged flame exposure	Involves tendon, muscle, or bone	Skeletonizing of tissue, charring	No	Extensive reconstructive, limb salvage versus amputation

Table 1.
Description of clinical characteristics of burn wounds of various depths.

water or applying a cold compress can help stop the burning process and relieve pain. Topical steroids, with their vasoconstrictive effects, are often considered "first-line" treatment for acute sunburn; however, their true efficacy remains controversial [51]. Topical applications such as menthol, camphor, pramoxine, lidocaine, and diclofenac gel, if available, may be useful for reducing pain, erythema, and edema. Soothing remedies such as aloe lotion (especially when refrigerated prior to application), baking soda, and oatmeal may provide additional relief. Oral nonsteroidal anti-inflammatory drugs (NSAIDs) help provide analgesia and may assist in reducing sunburn erythema. Healing of superficial burns occurs typically over a period of 3–7 days and will not result in scar formation [50, 52]. Of note, these burns are usually not included when estimating the total body surface area (TBSA) during the BPE, mainly because burns limited to the epidermis tend not to cause significant fluid shifts or losses.

2. Moderate partial thickness burns—also referred to as "superficial second degree" injuries—by definition involve the superficial layers of the dermis [50]. Partial thickness burns are further divided into two subtypes—superficial (focus of the current paragraph) and deep (discussed in next paragraph). Superficial partial thickness burns have similar appearance to first degree

burns but will additionally appear weepy and blistered [53]. Increased exposure of dermal nerve endings for pain, touch, temperature, and pressure contributes to these burns being very painful [54, 55]. Dermal blood vessels that carry oxygen and nutrients to the skin while removing metabolic waste products are also exposed giving the wound a blanching erythematous appearance. Exposure of sweat and sebaceous glands contributes to the wound's weepy appearance and the increase in evaporative losses [56]. Hair follicles, sweat glands, and rete ridges are typically spared allowing for reepithelialization to occur over the following 1–2 weeks post injury; however, alteration in cellular milieu at the site of the injury may result in permanent skin discoloration [56–58]. Finally, the risk of scarring is increased at this injury severity level, as is the overall risk of infection.

3. Deep partial thickness burns—also known as "deep second degree burns"—extend deeper into the dermis, resulting in a wound that appears pale and mottled [59, 60]. Since not all nerve endings have been destroyed in this type of burn, there may be considerable amounts of associated pain. Coagulative necrosis of the dermis from deep partial thickness burns is considered to have extended beyond the rete ridges, thus leaving behind only hair follicles and sweat glands to contribute to reepithelialization [61]. Without the rete ridges, the healing process is significantly slower and may result in more severe scarring. Ablative fractional laser resurfacing, excision, and skin grafting can improve both the healing time and scar quality. Consequently, the boundaries of clinical management tend to become blurry when approaching deep partial thickness and full thickness burns (discussed in next paragraph).

4. Full thickness burns—also known as "third degree burns"—extend beyond the epidermal and dermal tissues and into the subcutaneous fat [62, 63]. Full thickness burns are associated with complete destruction of all nerve endings, dermal glands, and hair follicles. In addition, thermal damage to superficial veins causes thrombosis [64, 65]. As a result of the above changes, the burn area is insensate and may appear charred, brown, and leathery, or at times white and waxy. Only the wound edges have retained the necessary components for reepithelialization of the wound, which is why full thickness burns also require excision and grafting in order to heal [50, 66].

5. Fourth degree burns are defined as thermal injuries that involve tissues and structures deep to subcutaneous layer. This includes damage to muscle, tendon, or bone [67]. Patients who suffer from survivable fourth degree burns may require extensive limb-sparing efforts and reconstructive surgery to avoid amputation [67, 68].

Determining the size, or total body surface area, of a burn is the cornerstone of the BPE and provides fundamental information to guide subsequent clinical management. Properly conducted BPE also provides insight into the burn victim's physiologic state and resuscitative fluid needs, as well as general prognostic information. It is important to remember that burn injuries have the potential to quickly evolve and progress if resuscitative conditions are not optimal [69, 70]. In other words, superficial and partial thickness burns can become deep partial thickness burns, and deep partial thickness burns have the potential to become full thickness burns. Optimizing the resuscitation effort can mitigate the tissue loss by enhancing perfusion and limiting secondary injury.

4. The burn patient evaluation (BPE)

When performing the BPE, the "rule of nines" is a quick way to get an approximate estimate of burn size in the field in order to properly communicate the state of a patient over the radio to the accepting facility and initiate early goal directed therapy. When calculating TBSA of partial and full thickness burns on adults, the following body surface percentages are assigned to the corresponding anatomic regions (**Figure 2**):

- Entire head is 9%
- Neck is 1%
- Anterior trunk is 18%
- Posterior trunk is 18%
- Each upper extremity is 9%
- Each lower extremity is 18%

When compared to adults, children have disproportionately larger heads [71], thus requiring an adjusted allotment of body surface area per anatomic region (**Figure 2**). Consequently, the adjusted percentages for TBSA evaluation in a child are:

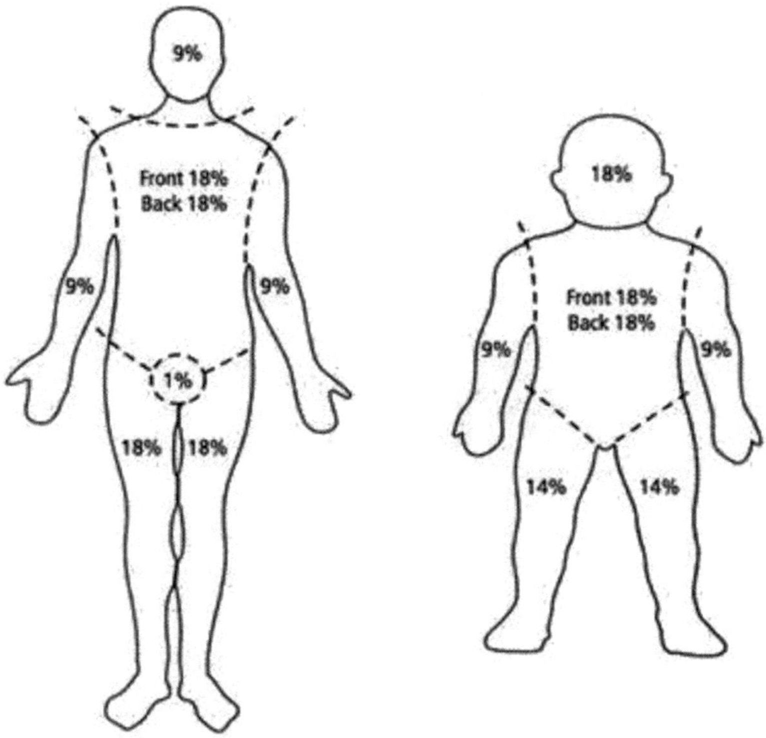

Figure 2.
(A) Left, diagram showing body surface area allocations for adult burn patients; (B) right, schematic representation of body surface area allocations for pediatric burn patients.

- Heads and neck combined are 18%
- Anterior trunk is 18%
- Posterior trunk is 18%
- Each upper extremity is 9%
- Each lower extremity is 14%

Another quick TBSA estimation technique is to use an area equal to the patient's own palm (with extended fingers) as an equivalent of approximately 1% TBSA. This measuring standard is then applied to each burned area and is especially useful in cases of patchy injury distribution [72, 73].

During the secondary BPE, especially after full exposure is completed, a better estimation of TBSA can be obtained to more precisely direct further hemodynamic and fluid resuscitation. In the 1940s, Lund and Browder introduced a seminal paper on estimating burn size and provided a simple chart that breaks down TBSA of smaller areas of the body for different age groups [71, 74]. This method is

Area	0–1 years	1–4 years	5–9 years	10–14 years	15 years	Adult	%2°	%3°	%TBSA
Head	19	17	13	11	9	7			
Neck	2	2	2	2	2	2			
Ant trunk	13	13	13	13	13	13			
Post trunk	13	13	13	13	13	13			
R buttock	2.5	2.5	2.5	2.5	2.5	2.5			
L buttock	2.5	2.5	2.5	2.5	2.5	2.5			
Genitalia	1	1	1	1	1	1			
R arm	4	4	4	4	4	4			
L arm	4	4	4	4	4	4			
R forearm	3	3	3	3	3	3			
L forearm	3	3	3	3	3	3			
R hand	2.5	2.5	2.5	2.5	2.5	2.5			
L hand	2.5	2.5	2.5	2.5	2.5	2.5			
R thigh	5.5	6	6.5	8	8.5	9			
L thigh	5.5	6	6.5	8	8.5	9			
R leg	5	5	5.5	6	6.5	7			
L leg	5	5	5.5	6	6.5	7			
R foot	3.5	3.5	3.5	3.5	3.5	3.5			
L foot	3.5	3.5	3.5	3.5	3.5	3.5			
Total									

Table 2.
Lund and Browder's chart for calculating %TBSA of varying age groups, with sufficient granularity to provide adequate accounting of the size and depth of the patient's burns, categorized by anatomic area.

considered to be the most accurate and reliable method of determining TBSA, with only a few caveats. More specifically, patient populations that may not be accurately represented by Lund and Browder's chart include the morbidly obese, amputees, women with large breasts, and gravid women (**Table 2**) [71, 75].

5. Burn shock

When burns cover <10% of the TBSA, the associated inflammatory response and vascular leakage tend to remain localized within the immediate proximity of the injured tissue. However, as the TBSA approaches 15–20%, the overall quantity of cytokines released systemically into the circulatory system increases dramatically, contributing to systemic inflammatory response whereby uninjured anatomically distant body regions experience various deleterious downstream manifestations such as vasoactive changes, increased capillary permeability, and tissue edema [3, 76, 77]. In the setting of such more severe burns, abrupt fluid shifts from vasculature into the interstitial space quickly lead to clinically apparent hypovolemic shock. In the setting of severe burn injury, this type of shock is appropriately termed "burn shock" [78, 79]. The state of hypovolemic shock during the acute, or "ebb," phase can be further exacerbated by the copresence of low cardiac output from decreased effective circulating blood volume, increased blood viscosity, and depressed cardiac contractility [77, 79, 80]. Most severely affected patients may experience multisystem organ failure (MOF) [81].

From a clinical management standpoint, the initiation of appropriate fluid resuscitation immediately upon the completion of BPE is imperative to providing (and maintaining) the necessary cardiovascular support. Every additional hour from time of injury that resuscitative fluid administration is delayed increases the risk of mortality [82]. Under resuscitation can lead to tissue hypoperfusion, acute renal injury, and death. Over-resuscitating, however, can cause increased tissue edema, compartment syndromes, acute respiratory distress syndrome (ARDS), infections (e.g., pneumonia), and MOF [83–85]. Therefore, proper resuscitation of burn patients requires individually tailored fluid administration and close monitoring in order to prevent secondary, mostly iatrogenic injuries.

Initiating appropriate intravenous fluid resuscitation requires establishing and maintaining dependable vascular access [3]. Short, large bore peripheral intravenous catheters placed through unburned skin are ideal because this approach avoids potentially thrombosed superficial veins underlying full thickness burn areas. That said, venous access through burned skin is preferred over no venous access, and in most situations may be more rapidly available then central venous access. Central venous access is reliable but comes with increased risk of complications compared to other available options such as saphenous venous cut-down or intraosseous route [86, 87]. Once adequate vascular access is established, fluid resuscitation should be initiated immediately. Optimally, a protocol-driven approach to fluid administration is preferred [88, 89].

The rate of clinical failure (defined as patient deterioration or mortality) with prompt and adequate resuscitation is relatively low (e.g., <5% even for patients with burned TBSA >85%) [90]. As a general guideline, patients who benefit the most from formula-based, calculated fluid resuscitation include adults between 15 and 50 years of age with ≥20% TBSA involving second and third degree burns; children ≤15 years old and adults ≥50 years of age with ≥ 10% TBSA involving second and third degree burns. In practice, many institutions will consider initiating resuscitative fluids when adult burn victim presents with injuries involving ≥15% TBSA [91]. A significant body of research regarding modern fluid resuscitation protocols demonstrates that systemic capillary leakage during the initial 24-h period after injury permits movement of large molecules into the interstitial space [92, 93]. For this reason, colloids are generally considered to provide little added benefit to crystalloid administration in the first 24 h. The topic is somewhat controversial, however, as some researchers argue that capillary permeability may begin returning to normal as early as 6–8 h after injury [90, 94, 95]. Consequently, the latter group advocates that earlier colloid addition may reduce the total amount of fluid necessary to achieve hemodynamic resuscitation and intravascular volume restoration.

5.1 The Parkland formula

The Parkland formula is among the most widely used and studied burn patient resuscitation paradigms [91, 96–98]. When originally published, this resuscitation approach advocated total crystalloid infusion of 4 mL/kg for each percent of body surface area burned [96–98]. The equation estimates the total amount of Ringer's lactate to be given in the initial 24-h post-burn period. Half of the calculated total fluid amount is to be given in the first 8 h and the remaining over the following 16 h [91, 98]. At the same time, certain limitations inherent to formula-based resuscitative approaches do exist. For example, the Parkland formula has been noted to underestimate the total volume of Ringer's lactate needed during the first 24 h in severe burns (>40% TBSA) [91, 99]. This tendency to need larger than estimated fluid volume is referred to as "fluid creep" [84, 100]. Although the exact factors responsible for this phenomenon are still being debated, one effective way of addressing it involves frequent urine output monitoring with hourly adjustments in fluid rates [84]. Goal urine output for adults is 0.5 mL/kg/h and for children ≤30 kg is 1 mL/kg/h. Some institutions have developed protocols that incorporate hourly fluid infusion rate adjustments of 10–30% depending on whether urine output is above or below goal [84]. As an example, we will consider using an hourly rate adjustment of 20% in an adult burn victim. In such scenario, if urine output decreased to <0.5 mL/kg/h, then the current fluid rate would be increased by 20%. If urine output was maintained at 0.5–1 mL/kg/h, then no rate adjustments are made. Finally, if urine output was measured to be >1 mL/kg/h, then the current fluid rate would be reduced by 20%.

5.2 The Galveston formula

Children have larger surface/volume ratios compared to adults, which translates to disproportionately higher infusion rates. The Galveston formula is designed to account for this difference, whereby during the first 24 h, patients receive fluids based on 5000 mL/m^2 × %TBSA +2000 mL/m^2 daily maintenance [101]. Similar to Parkland formula, half of the calculated total is given in the first 8 h and the rest over the remaining 16 h [102]. Children have lower glycogen stores than adults and consequently should have 5% dextrose added to the primary resuscitative crystalloid solution [103, 104]. As the formula indicates, children require greater amount of resuscitation fluid per kilogram than adults. Unfortunately, children also have lower physiologic reserves, which may predispose them to side effects of more aggressive fluid resuscitation approaches [105]. For example, it has been shown that the cardiac output of pediatric burn victims may not return to pre-burn levels for 24–48 h post-injury, even with complete intravascular status restoration. Furthermore, excessive secretion of antidiuretic hormone may lead to oliguria that extends beyond 48–72 h post-burn [105]. Taking the above parameters into consideration, it is recommended that urine output surveillance and fluid rate adjustments be made on a more frequent basis than adults.

5.3 Post-acute resuscitation period

Following the initial 24 h of resuscitation, both Parkland and Galveston and some derived formulae provide for a transition to reflect the changing vascular environment as hemodynamic and vascular homeostasis returns. The so-called Baxter formula—a derivation of the Parkland method—introduces a fourth "8-h period" during which plasma is given at 0.3–0.5 mL/kg/%TBSA in order to complete resuscitation [106]. The Galveston formula for pediatric patients calls for Ringer's lactate with dextrose at a rate of 3750 mL/m^2 burned area + 1500 mL/m^2 total area over a 24-h period [107]. It is important to remember that these formulae, like the many other proposed paradigms, should be considered within the overall context of a multifaceted approach to manage the burn patient. Once appropriate initial resuscitation has been completed, subsequent fluid administration should be tailored to maintain post-resuscitation stability while avoiding any secondary/iatrogenic injury.

An important question arises regarding the course of action in cases where resuscitation formulae are followed appropriately yet the patient fails to meet the intended resuscitation endpoints. Such an occurrence may indicate that a secondary diagnosis (or a complication) is present, including inhalation injury, infection/sepsis, compartment syndrome, or an acute cardiovascular event (e.g., pulmonary embolism) [108]. There is no single perfect marker for determining when a patient is adequately resuscitated. Traditionally, monitoring urine output has been considered as the gold standard for ongoing assessment of resuscitative adequacy. This is because it is a convenient, practical, and inexpensive way to determine if tissues are being adequately perfused in near real-time [109]. The ability to maintain urine output of ≥ 0.5 mL/kg/h in adults and older children (>50 kg) may guide appropriate resuscitation in most patients, but relying on urine output alone can be both challenging and potentially misleading. For example, a recent systematic review showed that when compared to hourly urine output measurements, hemodynamic monitoring appeared to provide some degree of survival benefit, with no associated effect on renal failure [109]. At the same time, heterogeneity of data quality within that same review was problematic, and when only randomized controlled trials were examined in isolation, the mortality benefit of hemodynamic monitoring over hourly urine outputs was no longer present [109].

In practice, a patient whose cumulative fluid resuscitation approaches 250 mL/kg during the initial 24 h post-injury period should place the treating clinician on high alert for complications related to excessive or over-resuscitation [100, 108]. Careful evaluation of the patient's extremities for signs and symptoms of compartment syndrome should be performed. In particular, burned extremities in which escharotomies may not have been indicated initially may develop the need for escharotomy as increased tissue edema underlying the burned skin further exacerbates venous flow disruption and eventually leads to compromised arterial flow [3]. The emergence of compartment syndrome may be associated with the symptoms of numbness, tingling, or pain with passive movement of the involved extremity [110]. Assessment of capillary refill as well as Doppler signals of digital arteries, palmar arches, and plantar arches of affected limbs should be performed frequently as part of clinical surveillance [50, 111]. Finally, tissue pressure measurements can be checked, and if found to be >30–40 mmHg, this would also be an indication for urgent escharotomy [112, 113]. Burn care providers must remember that the determination to perform an escharotomy can (and often should) be made using clinical exam as the primary decision tool.

When performing escharotomy, areas of constrictive eschar are incised longitudinally along medial and lateral aspects of the affected body region/extremity

[114, 115]. Even after escharotomy, severely injured limbs continue to be at risk for developing compartment syndrome requiring fasciotomy [116]. Although uncommon, sudden restoration of perfusion to muscle compartments after prolonged ischemia can potentiate the swelling within an already edematous muscle tissue and cause limb-threatening compartment pressure elevations [117, 118].

Intraabdominal organs and tissues are not excluded from the widespread edema resulting from the combination of physiologic changes due to initial injury and subsequent resuscitation. Development of abdominal compartment syndrome in a burn patient undergoing massive fluid resuscitation can be difficult to identify [119, 120]. Due to high sensitivity of the renal system to increased intraabdominal pressures, decreased urine output from diminished kidney perfusion is one of the earlier signs of abdominal compartment syndrome [121–123]. Of note, in a burn patient undergoing massive fluid resuscitation, observed decrease in urine output may be erroneously interpreted as insufficient resuscitation, thus prompting the clinician to inappropriately increase fluid administration [124, 125]. One important consideration is the performance of relevant clinical cross-checks, where additional clinical variables are examined concurrently, including elevated peak airway pressures and decreased tidal volumes in mechanically ventilated patients. Patients who develop abdominal compartment syndrome will become increasingly difficult to ventilate due to increased abdominal pressures being transmitted across the diaphragms into the thoracic cavity.

When indicated, abdominal compartment pressures are fairly easy to measure. Abdominal compartment pressures are most accurately obtained in patients who are ventilated, sedated, and paralyzed (however, this is rarely the case). Placed in the supine position, the patient should be completely flat and level with the ground. Through a Foley catheter, approximately 50–100 mL of normal saline is instilled into the empty bladder, and a pressure transducer is connected to the port at the proximal end of the catheter [126, 127]. Patients with abdominal pressures approaching 30 mmHg in the setting of end organ dysfunction should be considered for decompressive laparotomy [126].

In the absence of chronic kidney disease and abdominal compartment syndrome, low urine output and depressed cardiac indices, especially in the setting of large volume fluid administration could indicate ongoing under-resuscitation and/or the presence of cardiac dysfunction. Key factors associated with the presence of clinical under-resuscitation include significant delays in initiating resuscitative fluids, underestimation of partial and full thickness burn %TBSA, or concurrent lung injury requiring mechanical ventilation [85, 88, 128]. Burn injuries have been shown to increase cardiac stress and cause myocardial dysfunction [1, 129]. Myocardial dysfunction, in turn, leads to decreased contractility and cardiac output [130]. Dedicated evaluation consisting of a clinical exam, an electrocardiogram (EKG), and bedside echocardiography may be indicated. Advanced hemodynamic monitoring may be of benefit in selected cases [99, 131, 132].

Overly aggressive intravenous fluid resuscitation has also been reported to lead to abnormal intraocular pressure elevations [84, 133]. Similar to other "compartment syndromes," sustained intraocular pressures of ≥20–30 mmHg may lead to permanent injury and vision loss [133–135]. Any unexpected or unexplained symptoms of vision changes or ocular pain should prompt a thorough reevaluation for changes in the patient's clinical exam, fluid balance, and any other aforementioned complications.

Colloid-based resuscitation. If the patient appears to be under-resuscitated despite ongoing administration of large volumes of crystalloids, the resuscitating provider should strongly consider transitioning the resuscitative efforts to incorporate colloid-based fluid administration [83, 136]. Although there is still some controversy regarding the optimal application and timing of various colloids during burn patient resuscitation, especially in the setting of severe burns, there is clear evidence in support of colloid use in general [83, 136, 137]. Research suggests that the use of colloids in resuscitation of severe burns (>40% TBSA or > 30% TBSA with inhalation injury) may decrease the total resuscitation volume, reduce the incidence of abdominal compartment syndrome, number of days spent on a ventilator, and potentially even mortality [138–140]. The majority of historically important formulae include some form of colloids administered at various timeframes within the first 48 h post-burn. The presence of this general theme throughout the literature corroborates the importance of colloids for resuscitation of severe burns, especially in the management of burn shock in the most severely injured population. Despite this, definitive evidence regarding the efficacy of either approach continues to be elusive.

The Parkland formula does not call for the transition to colloids prior to the first 24-h mark. If earlier administration of colloids is desired, one might consider transitioning to the Brooke Formula or West Penn formula [88, 93]. During the initial 24-h post-burn period, the Brooke Formula can be delivered as a combination of crystalloid and colloid fluids, including 1.5 mL/kg/%TBSA of Ringer's lactate plus 0.5 mL/kg/%TBSA of a colloid and 2000 mL of 5% dextrose in water [81, 141, 142]. After the first 24-h period, the formula mandates reducing the crystalloid and colloid fluid rates by 50–75% and repeating the 2000 mL of 5% dextrose in water [81, 141, 142]. The West Penn formula—first published in the early 1990s—is the most recently proposed derivation of colloid-based burn resuscitation formulae. The West Penn formula calls for Ringer's lactate at a set rate of 83 mL/h and fresh frozen plasma (FFP) at an initial rate of 75 mL/kg/36 h. The rate of FFP administration is then titrated on an hourly basis to a urine output of 0.5–1 mL/kg/h and both fluids are continued for until the 48-h mark after burn injury is reached [88, 143].

6. Ambient temperature control

Over the past several decades, major advances have been made in our understanding of the complex physiologic changes that occur as a result of severe burn injury. While burn shock, as outlined in previous sections of this chapter, is historically compartmentalized as a form of "hypovolemic shock," we now know that "fluids alone do not cure burn shock" [143]. Consequently, there are various strategies that may be employed to help counteract or "blunt" the cascading physiologic response to burn injury. For example, even simple measures such as increasing the ambient temperature (up to 33°C) have been shown to reduce the hypermetabolic response focused on maintaining elevated body core temperatures during the acute injury phase [144].

7. Nutritional support

Delays in nutritional support can have devastating effects on patient outcomes [145]. The post-burn hypermetabolic state that begins immediately after injury can approach 200% of normal resting energy expenditure [146]. This can naturally lead to rapid depletion of energy stores, loss of muscle tissue, and further worsening of any pre-existing or acquired malnutrition. Malnutrition itself contributes to alterations in cell membrane transport, organ dysfunction, immune compromise, and delayed/abnormal wound healing [147]. Ideally, nutritional support is initiated within 6 h of injury. Due to the tremendous increase in metabolic demand, severely burned patients are simply unable to fully meet the caloric demands on their own accord. For this reason, it is recommended that a post-pyloric feeding access be placed on admission, with prompt (preferably protocol-driven) initiation of tube feeding formulae specifically tailored to meet individual patient requirements [148, 149]. For gastric tube feeds, the choice of continuous versus bolus administration may be a secondary consideration [150]. For post-pyloric feeding, continuous administration requires the presence of intact intestinal function.

Unfortunately, the gastrointestinal tract itself is affected adversely by severe burn injury, and varied degrees of ileus may develop in the acute post-burn timeframe [151]. In the setting of complete intolerance to enteral feeding, total parenteral nutrition may be considered on highly selective basis [152]. Total parenteral nutrition is generally not recommended due to associated increases in rates of complications and mortality compared to enteral feeding, and the latter should be started as soon as the gastrointestinal dysfunction resolves [152]. A commonly used formula for calculating caloric requirements is the Curreri formula (including its variants) which calls for 25 kcal/kg/day maintenance plus additional 40 kcal/%TBSA/day [153–155].

Adequate and prompt nutritional support is critical to the overall management of burn patients, and its importance parallels the severity (e.g., %TBSA) and complexity (e.g., inhalation component) of the injury [148, 156, 157]. In addition to ensuring adequate caloric provision, it may be important to consider supplementing the patient's enteral intake with specific vitamins and minerals. For example, there has been increasing support in the literature for administration of high dose vitamin C (a.k.a., ascorbic acid) during the acute phase of burn injury [158, 159]. Cellular oxidative stress from reactive oxygen species generated immediately after burn injury appears to play a significant role in cardiovascular dysfunction of burn shock. Vitamin C is a powerful antioxidant, and it has been suggested that high dose ascorbic acid administration during the acute phase of burn shock may be protective to microvascular circulation, beneficial to cardiac output, help optimize fluid resuscitation, and may enhance wound healing [159, 160]. Other proposed components of the so-called "pharmacological" nutritional supplementation after burn injury include glutamine, arginine, n-3 (polyunsaturated) fatty acids, as well as various other vitamins and trace minerals [149, 161].

8. Special hemodynamic considerations

Patients who develop burn shock and remain hemodynamically labile despite large volume resuscitation may require additional cardiovascular support. Low cardiac output during the acute post-injury phase is a common component of early "burn shock" [162, 163] and may be more pronounced among geriatric patients [164]. In some cases, inotropic support with dobutamine may be required to maintain adequate systemic perfusion [165, 166]. Vasopressors should be avoided if possible as their vasoconstrictive properties can lead to decreased end-organ perfusion, including skin (and thus elevated risk of the propagation of primary injury or impaired healing of skin grafts) and bowel (e.g., contribution to potential bowel ischemia). This is especially applicable to patients with initial low cardiac output and early multiple organ dysfunction [167]. Patients who do require vasopressor support should undergo close hemodynamic monitoring (MAP, CVP, echocardiography, SvO_2). As the patient transitions from the "ebb phase" to the "flow phase" (typically around the 48–72 h mark) of the post-burn state, hemodynamic behavior evolves toward the hyperdynamic profile [168]. As the hyperdynamic phase begins, cardiac output may exceed 1.5 times that of a normal baseline. Increases in cardiac output entail much greater cardiac work and overall energy expenditure. For these reasons, propranolol is highly efficacious during acute care in burn patients [169]. In fact, long-term propranolol administration initiated in the acute setting decreases cardiac work, decreases lipolysis, improves nitrogen balance, helps restore insulin sensitivity, and mitigates post-traumatic stress disorder [170–173].

9. The importance of endocrine system, including glycemic control

As part of the hypermetabolic response to burn injury, significant increases in catecholamines, glucagon, and cortisol stimulate rapid glycolysis-gluconeogenesis cycle gyrations [174]. The result is the appearance of hyperglycemia and a concurrent state of insulin resistance. The magnitude of the overall effect appears to be dependent on the severity and size of the burn injury [175]. The administration of insulin to maintain a serum glucose goal of ≤120 mg/dL has proven to be effective in attenuating some of the hypermetabolic changes that take place immediately after injury [176]. Insulin administration has been shown to improve muscle protein synthesis, normalize mitochondrial function, reduce oxidative stress, limit lean muscle mass loss, accelerate healing time, and improve long-term rehabilitation [176–179]. In addition to the normalization of serum glucose levels, the reduction in glycemic variability may be equally important [180, 181]. Other beneficial effects of goal-directed insulin therapy have been identified, including potential reductions in mortality, infections, sepsis, acute kidney injury, multiple organ failure, days on a ventilator, and hospital length of stay [177, 178, 182].

Although beyond the scope of the current chapter, various other endocrine system components are affected—both acutely and chronically—following burn injury [178, 183–188]. This includes the thyroid hormone metabolism [183, 184], the hypothalamic–pituitary axis [185], the renin-angiotensin system [185, 187], the reproductive system [185], among others [186]. Additional important endocrine considerations include the effects of exogenous hormone therapies, such as oxandrolone, recombinant human growth hormone, and incretin analogs [188]. Readers are referred to the primary sources listed above for further information.

10. Comment on inhalation injury

Inhalation injury requiring mechanical ventilation is associated with increased mortality and greater volume of fluid resuscitation [189–191]. Carbonaceous debris in or around the mouth, facial burns, and singed facial or nasal hair are often cited as important clues during the BPE with respect to the presence of inhalation injury [192, 193]. However, the history of closed space smoke exposure is perhaps the most important clue as to whether or not a patient might have sustained an inhalation injury. Unlike burn injuries to the skin and subdermal tissues, which are primarily thermal in nature, inhalation injury is primarily a result of chemical exposure of tracheo-bronchial and pulmonary tissues to toxic products of combustion [191, 194, 195]. Primary thermal injury to the airway is often limited to the supraglottic region [195]. Diagnosis of lung injury is graded on a standardized scale from 0 to 4 based on bronchoscopic findings of airway edema, inflammation, mucosal necrosis, tissue sloughing, and presence of soot and carbonaceous material in the airway (see **Table 3**) [195].

Inhalation injury grading scale		
Grade 0	No injury	Normal mucosa, absence of carbonaceous material
Grade 1	Mild	Minor or patchy areas of erythema, carbonaceous deposits in bronchi
Grade 2	Moderate	Moderate degree of erythema, carbonaceous deposits, bronchorrhea, with or without bronchial compromise
Grade 3	Severe	Severe inflammation with friability, copious carbonaceous deposits, bronchorrhea, bronchial obstruction
Grade 4	Massive	Mucosal sloughing, necrosis, endoluminal obliteration

Endorf and Gamelli [190].

Table 3.
Description of inhalation injury severity grading based on bronchoscopic evaluation.

If there is any concern for inhalation injury based on the initial or subsequent BPE, patient should be placed on 100% oxygen via non-rebreather mask and undergo measurements of blood carboxyhemoglobin and cyanide levels [196, 197]. In patients with early evidence of upper airway edema or impending respiratory failure as suggested by oxygen saturations below 92% and the simultaneous presence of tachypnea with hypercapnia, intubation should be expeditious [128, 198, 199]. Ventilator management for these patients is similar to ARDS using low tidal volumes and pressure control ventilation with permissive hypercapnia (as high as $PaCO_2$ of 60 mmHg) [200, 201]. Additionally, sloughing of the injured pulmonary lining requires aggressive pulmonary toilet, chest physiotherapy, frequent suctioning, bronchoscopic removal of casts, and nebulizer therapy [128, 202, 203]. Various nebulizer combinations and frequencies of albuterol, heparin, acetylcysteine, hypertonic saline, and racemic epinephrine should be considered on a case by case basis depending on injury severity and clinical progression [128]. Patients should be closely monitored for development of ventilator-assisted pneumonia considering their primary injury has induced a transient immunosuppressed state—a factor that is further exacerbated by the presence of inhalation injury [204, 205]. Finally, for patients with very severe inhalation injury who continue to worsen despite maximal traditional mechanical ventilatory support, the use of high-frequency oscillatory ventilation may be indicated [206, 207].

11. Special topics and dermato-surgical considerations in burn management

11.1 Dermato-surgical considerations

When excisional burn debridement is indicated, it is recommended that it be completed within the first 24–48 h after injury [208, 209]. Early debridement can help decrease the ongoing systemic response to inflammation stemming from the persistence of devitalized tissue [210, 211]. Removal of deep partial or full-thickness burn tissue with grafting and coverage with either permanent (preferred) or temporary graft can substantially decrease the daily rate of evaporative losses [212, 213]. Institution of aggressive operative management of burns, combined with optimization of non-surgical aspects of burn care, can result in a significant decline in mortality rates. More recent developments in this particular area include the introduction of selective enzymatic debridement agent designed specifically for burn wounds [214].

11.2 Dermatologic conditions that require burn center management

Historically, the spheres of the dermatologist and the burn surgeon have failed to overlap as much as the associated anatomic and physiologic considerations might lead one to believe they should. Reasons for this lack of collegiality and collaboration have included training bias (i.e., an "elixir" versus "cold steel" approach), lack of awareness of the other's expertise, and good old fashioned egos and turf wars. Thankfully, a new era of cooperation between these specialties has begun to emerge based on large part around the understanding that a multimodal, multidisciplinary approach may lead to more optimal clinical outcomes. The intersection of these two specialties may perhaps be best illustrated through several devastating dermatological conditions that involve the acute and extensive necrosis of cutaneous tissue, leading to catastrophic deterioration of the affected patient and a clinical picture that closely resembles a large thermal burn.

11.3 Toxic epidermal necrolysis (TEN)

TEN is a severe, life-threatening disorder (with a mortality rate approaching 40%) characterized by generalized loss of epidermis and mucosa (**Figure 3**), typically involving more than 30% of the skin [215]. A tell-tale clinical finding that is almost always present in TEN is the phenomenon in which intact superficial epidermis can, via a pushing or shearing force, be dislodged and slid over underlying layers of skin; this indicates a plane of cleavage in the skin at the epidermal-dermal junction and is referred to as Nikolsky's sign [216]. TEN is almost always medication-induced and involves a cytotoxic T-cell reaction with apoptosis of keratinocytes mediated by Fas ligand [217]. Consequently, the first step in treatment is similar to that of a burn injury—stop the underlying causative agent (i.e., discontinue all medications that are not essential). The next step is to confirm the diagnosis through a careful medication history and skin biopsy with frozen section. The finding of full-thickness epidermal involvement distinguishes TEN from other conditions such as staphylococcal scalded skin syndrome (see

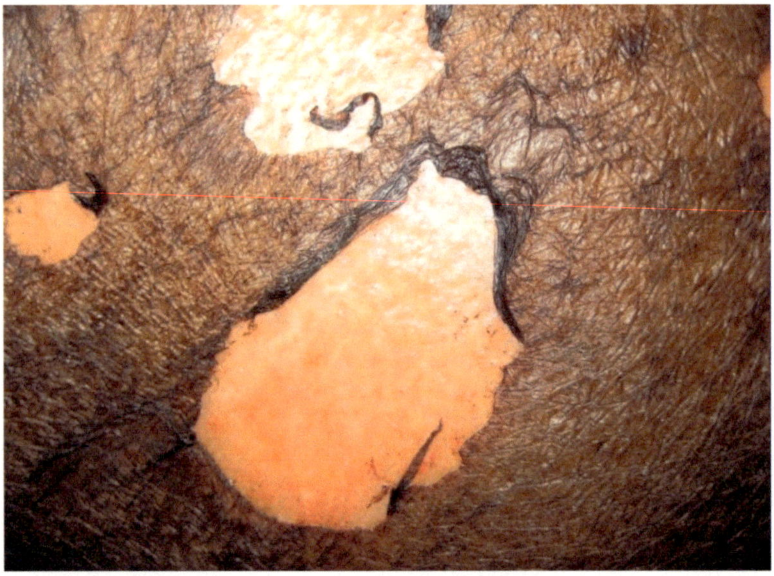

Figure 3.
Typical appearance of toxic epidermal necrolysis (TEN).

below), which may appear similar but are treated very differently. In addition to the more controversial therapeutic roles that systemic steroids, intravenous immunoglobulins, and plasmapheresis may play, the mainstay clinical TEN management is excellent "burn care," ideally in a burn center with careful attention to pain management, electrolyte balance, topical disinfection, access to burn beds and nonadherent dressings, and prompt treatment of secondary infections. An ophthalmologic consultation is also required because of the risk of corneal erosions and scarring [218].

11.4 Staphylococcal scalded skin syndrome (SSSS)

The SSSS is typically characterized by fever and rapid onset of diffuse, painful erythema progressing to widespread formation of thin-walled, easily ruptured, fluid-filled vesicles and bullae (**Figure 4**). Newborns and small infants tend to be most susceptible, though adults may certainly be affected. Nikolsky's sign is almost always present [216]. The clinical presentation of SSSS is the result of specific exotoxins that cleave desmoglein-1 (i.e., disrupt the connection between keratinocytes) and cause cellular detachment within the epidermis. While exotoxins are released by S. aureus, cultures to isolate these bacteria, however, are often negative. More helpful is a skin biopsy with frozen section that should demonstrate a very superficial epidermal split (in contrast to TEN where there is full-thickness epidermal necrosis). Differentiating SSSS from similar clinical presentations is critical because treatment typically involves the addition of medications (i.e., antibiotics) rather than the cessation of them. SSSS patients may require topical disinfection and careful placement on a burn bed covered with nonadherent sheeting. Attention to fluid replacement, pain management, electrolyte balance, and temperature and humidity control are paramount. Less urgent but just as important, the diagnosis of SSSS should prompt a search for staphylococcal "carriers" among close contacts of the affected patient. Healing is usually rapid with correct therapy and vigilant wound care [219].

11.5 Necrotizing fasciitis

Necrotizing fasciitis refers to the severe and rapid destruction of skin, subcutaneous fat, and muscle caused by bacterial infection (e.g., group A streptococci,

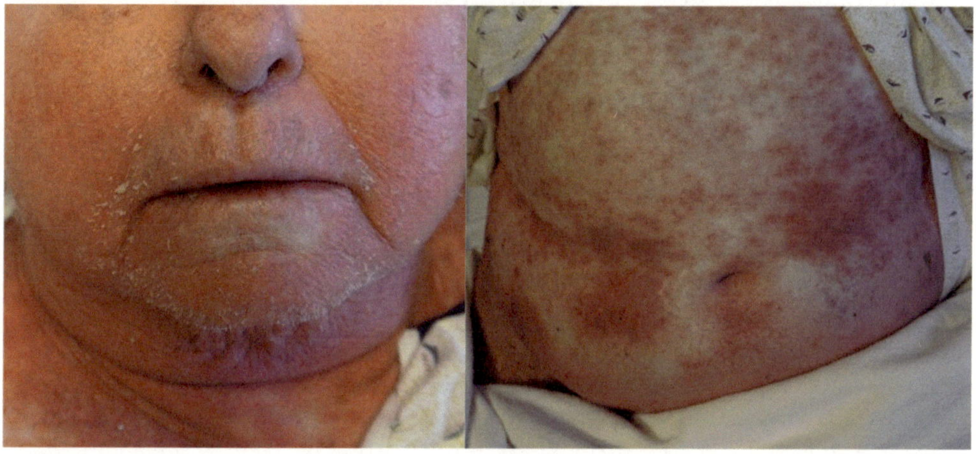

Figure 4.
Typical appearance of staphylococcal scalded skin syndrome (SSSS). Left—face; right—abdomen.

community-based methicillin-resistant *Staphylococcus aureus*, Gram-negative bacteria, mixed infection, etc.) [220, 221]. It is characterized by widespread dermal necrosis, vessel thrombosis, and a massive, destructive inflammatory reaction. Mortality rate without surgical involvement may approach 100%. Similar to burn wounds, surgical management of this condition may include extensive debridement and management of the associated compartment syndrome. Also similar to burns, successful treatment depends on careful fluid replacement, broad-spectrum antibiotic coverage (including for Gram-negative organisms), specialized surgical dressings, and vigilant monitoring for signs of shock [222, 223]. Eventual skin grafting and/or tissue flaps may be required to cover large soft tissue defects.

Directly relevant to the theme of the current chapter, all three of the above dermatological conditions (and many others) are subject to the same general complications and considerations, and their final prognosis is directly proportional to the extent of their skin injuries and the level of expert care they urgently receive.

12. The evolving burn scar paradigm

Irreversible scarring has long been thought to be the unavoidable, aggregated response to gross tissue injury after a severe burn. From the historical "tooth and claw" injury perspective, such a clinical endpoint made perfect sense: the inflammatory cascade would effectively help plug hemorrhage, prevent infection, and patch up the wounded enough so that they could get back into action. In the context of modern medicine, however, scarring is no longer necessarily ideal. When one considers the phenomenon of the burn survivor's paradox—in which severely burned patients are living longer through more extreme injuries but are consequently forced to deal with the physical, psychosocial, and financial implications associated with their survival—it is clear that a disfiguring or function-limiting scar no longer confers the same advantages it did in pre-historic times. Consequently, a relatively new field of dermato-surgical medicine is evolving to address this new perspective with a focus on scar prevention, mitigation, rehabilitation, and an overall goal to reintegrate the burn survivor to "normalcy."

Many animals (e.g., starfish, salamanders, lizards, etc.) have long been known to be able to regenerate tissue; however, it was not until relatively recently, in 2012, that researchers demonstrated the phenomenon of skin shedding and tissue regeneration in an adult mammal population, using the African spiny mouse as a model [224]. Coupling this discovery with the fact that fetal wounds heal without a scar early in human gestation and that adult humans retain the capacity to heal micro-wounds (e.g., bee stings, venipuncture, or facial rejuvenation with a fractional carbon dioxide laser, etc.) without scarring, we can now start to imagine that the door to scarless burn wound healing may not be as permanently closed to us as we once believed.

12.1 Skin copying and epidermal micrografting

Prevention of scarring might be as simple as ensuring that normal skin replaces the major wound defect [225, 226]. In essence, that is what full-thickness skin grafting seeks to accomplish, allowing the surgeon to bring in hair follicles, sweat glands, reticular dermis, subcutaneous fat, and other deep structures and relocating them to the wound bed. Unfortunately, it does so by creating another full-thickness skin wound at the donor site, a fact that limits this strategy to small wounds. Additionally, for a full-thickness graft to properly "take," it must connect successfully to the wound bed's underlying blood supply or the grafted tissue may die. Recently, an autologous micrografting device came to market offering to deliver the benefits of a full-thickness skin graft without the limitations. In this technique, the proprietary device (CelluTome™ Epidermal Harvesting System, KCI, an Acelity Company, San Antonio, TX) uses suction and heat to homogenously harvest hundreds of exceedingly small columns (700 μm diameter) of full-thickness skin without the need for anesthesia [227, 228]. The micrografts are then manually transferred directly to the recipient area. Donor sites reepithelialize within days and with little to no evidence of scarring. The recipient sites appear to demonstrate accelerated reepithelialization and seem to heal without the "fish-net" patterning associated with split-thickness skin grafts. While this novel technology is promising, long-term, prospective studies are needed to evaluate the true efficacy and clinical outcomes of this approach [227–230].

12.2 Stem cell therapy

The "holy grail" of employing stem cell therapy to improve—or even perfect!—desired wound healing after burn injury has long attracted the attention of burn surgeons. Combined gene delivery with stem cell therapy remains particularly promising. This process involves inserting a gene into recipient cells with the goal of delivering a concoction of growth factor genes at critical time points in the wound healing process [231]. This could be accomplished through any number of techniques including viral transfection, high pressure injection, liposomal vectors, naked DNA application, and it even introduces a new potential role for laser-assisted drug delivery (see below) [232]. Optimized culture conditions, preconditioning cell treatments, and the development of ideal scaffolds or matrices to optimize cell mobilization, homing, adhesion, and differentiation remain elusive but may be just over the horizon.

12.3 Cell culture autografting

In burn patients where the injuries are so extensive that donor site availability is limited or not practical, the notion of culturing human keratinocytes remains a still hopeful approach. From a general perspective, this technique is accomplished by, first, taking a small sample of the patient's own healthy skin [233]. Next, the cells within the epidermis are separated, and the keratinocytes are grown, a process that involves providing the cells with specific nutrients. The resulting cultured skin is then applied to cover the burn wound, thus reducing the amount of healthy skin that must be removed for traditional burn wound grafting. Several companies are developing competing technologies to accomplish this goal, with one company receiving FDA approval, in 2018, for its proprietary "spray-on skin" system [234].

12.4 Laser surgery

Multiple laser and energy-based devices are now employed within the burn scar management algorithm in an effort to better "rehabilitate" the injured skin. This armamentarium includes, primarily, the vascular-specific pulsed dye laser (PDL), which helps to reduce erythema and hypertrophic scar formation, and the technique of ablative or non-ablative fractional laser resurfacing, which helps to normalize scar texture, thickness, and stiffness of the scars.

The pulsed dye laser (PDL) was the first laser to be specifically developed to treat port wine birthmarks with the principle of "selective photothermolysis" in mind [235]. First-generation PDL devices utilized a yellow light emitting at wavelength 577 nm to target oxyhemoglobin, a chromophore with absorption peaks located around 418, 542, and 577 nm. Through diffusion of heat, this laser caused selective thermal damage of the abnormally dilated blood vessels with minimal to no collateral damage of surrounding cutaneous structures. Eventually, 585 and 595 nm wavelength PDL devices were developed to allow slightly deeper penetration through the skin (to a depth of around 1.2 mm) while still maintaining precise absorption. The development of surface cooling devices has, subsequently, afforded the use of higher energy fluences with larger spot sizes and improved treatment in darker skin surfaces. When applied to hypertrophic burn scars, PDL causes selective photothermolysis that induces coagulation necrosis of capillaries within the scar itself [236]. Because hypertrophic burn scars are characterized by pathologic neovascularization, PDL devices help to mitigate inflammation and collagen production and reduce the overall hypervascular response. From a patient perspective, PDL is also useful for helping to improve overall burn scar texture, pruritus, pain, and pliability [237].

Laser resurfacing has long been used for cosmetic indications such as treatment of fine rhytids of the eyelids and mouth, treatment of photoaging, and management of dyspigmentation. Original "fully ablative" devices, such as the carbon dioxide laser, target intracellular water as the main chromophore. Because of the abundance of water in human tissue, this process leads to non-selective and near-immediate vaporization of treated skin and a denaturation of surrounding extracellular proteins. In contrast to ablative devices, nonablative approaches induce coagulation as their primary mechanism of action without directly destroying tissue or exposing dermis to the external environment. The concept of "fractional photothermolysis" was fairly recently introduced and describes treatment of the target tissue with the generation of a precise array of evenly spaced areas of injury known as microscopic treatment zones (MTZ) [238]. Clinically, this technique results in untreated areas between the MTZs, containing significant amounts of intact epidermis and dermis available as a reservoir for a more rapid micro-healing response. With ablative fractional resurfacing (AFR) technologies, such as the fractional carbon dioxide (CO_2) and Erbium-YAG lasers, the operating surgeon may change device parameters to adjust for desired depth of treatment (to a maximum of about 3.5–4.0 mm with current devices) and accurately control the total ablated surface area within a treated area. The general rule for AFR is to decrease density (i.e., total ablated surface area) while increasing fluence (i.e., energy). How repeated pixelated thermal injuries to a burn scar could result in subjective and objective improvements is not entirely understood; however, the technique has consistently demonstrated the ability to facilitate rapid reepithelialization and a vigorous scar remodeling process while maintaining excellent safety margins [239–243]. Perhaps most notably, long-term, persistent gains in pliability, resulting in improved function and quality of life, most likely occur from a gradual process of diffuse dermal remodeling and a relative rehabilitation of dysfunctional scar tissue [244].

The varied nature of individual burn scars, the heterogeneity of burn patients, small sample sizes, a lack of treatment controls, and the cost of the devices themselves have been major limitations to research surrounding the use of lasers in the treatment of burn scars. Thankfully, several large, prospective studies are currently underway to investigate the utility of these devices, including in the pediatric population.

12.5 Laser-assisted drug delivery

The notion that certain medications or agents could be delivered topically through burn scar tissue has three potential advantages over oral administration of the same agent: directed therapy to the targeted tissue, limited systemic toxicity and side effects, and avoidance of first-pass metabolism. To this end, various chemical, biochemical, and physical strategies have attempted to enhance topical drug delivery into burn scar tissue. It is only relatively recently that AFR devices have been utilized for this purpose [245]. In a process referred to as "laser-assisted drug delivery," AFR devices create vertical columns of ablated tissue in the MTZs that then serve as conduits or channels for delivery of specific topical medications or agents. Pairing the delivery of topical agents temporally with AFR therapy is believed to allow for increased penetration and absorption of the applied agents, an approach that is particularly helpful in the treatment of burn scar tissue given its variable and fibrotic nature. Corticosteroids, 5-fluorouracil (5-FU), imiquimod, methotrexate, and other immunomodulators have all been used for this purpose with varying degrees of success. Overall, laser-assisted drug delivery is a promising intervention for burn scar treatment. Investigation of the optimal channel depth and channel density continues and will likely depend on each individual drug or agent's chemical structure and the desired clinical target. Likewise, many drugs and agents have not been designed to be delivered to their target tissues in this manner, so larger prospective studies to determine safety and efficacy of this procedure will be critical.

13. Conclusion

The primary goal of clinical management of burns is to prevent the development of "burn shock." Early classification of burns by depth and size is critical to goal-directed treatment strategies, with subsequent approaches guided by the post-injury physiological and metabolic demands. Appropriate anticipation and proactive, multimodality support of the patient, through fluid resuscitation, nutritional supplementation, and pharmacologic therapy is required for optimizing patient outcomes. Additionally, clinicians should closely monitor the patient for the development of secondary adverse events, such as infections and under- or over-resuscitation. Management of burns is complex and requires specialized facilities, teams of experienced burn surgeons, dedicated burn nurses, social workers, nutritionists, physical therapists, occupational therapists, pharmacists, respiratory interventionists, pain specialists, dermatologists, and psychologists [246, 247].

Burn center referral criteria	
1	Partial thickness burns >10% TBSA
2	Burns involving the face, hands, feet, genitalia, perineum, or major joints
3	Third degree burns in any age group
4	Electrical burns, lightning injury
5	Chemical burns
6	Inhalation injury
7	Burn injury in patients with preexisting medical disorders that could complicate management, prolong recovery, or affect mortality
8	Any patient with burns and traumatic injury wherein the burn poses the greatest risk of morbidity/mortality. When a traumatic injury poses the greatest risk, adequate stabilization of the patient at a trauma center may be necessary prior to transport
9	Burned children in hospitals lacking the qualified personnel/equipment necessary to care for children
10	Burn injury to patients who require special social, emotional, or rehabilitative intervention

Excerpted from Guidelines for the Operation of Burn Centers (pp. 79–86), Resources for Optimal Care of the Injured Patient 2006, Committee on Trauma, American College of Surgeons.

Table 4.
Summary of burn center referral criteria; Legend: TBSA = Total body surface area.

The tremendous amount of progress in treatment of thermal injuries over the past several decades was possible because of the continuous evolution of trauma systems and burn centers, along with the development of state-of-the-art resuscitative and procedural approaches.

The critical timeline for thermal injury management occurs in the first 48 h from time of initial burn. Early burn classification should determine need for referral to a designated burn center (**Table 4**). The American Burn Association (ABA) list criteria for burn injuries that warrant referral to a designated burn center including: partial thickness burns of greater than 10% TBSA, burns involving the face, hands, feet, genitalia, or major joints, any third degree burns, electrical burns, chemical burns, inhalation injuries, burn injury to patients with significant pre-existing medical conditions, burns with additional traumatic injury, burns in children, or any burn injury to patients who may require special social, emotional, or rehabilitative assistance.

Author details

John Sojka[1], Andrew C. Krakowski[2] and Stanislaw P. Stawicki[3]*

1 Department of Surgery, St. Luke's University Health Network, University Hospital Campus, Bethlehem, Pennsylvania, USA

2 Department of Dermatology, St. Luke's University Health Network, Anderson Campus, Easton, Pennsylvania, USA

3 Department of Research and Innovation, St. Luke's University Health Network, Bethlehem, Pennsylvania, USA

*Address all correspondence to: stawicki.ace@gmail.com

References

[1] Kramer GC, Lund T, Beckum OK. Pathophysiology of burn shock. In: Total Burn Care. Philadelphia, Pennsylvania: Saunders Elsevier; 2007. p. 93

[2] Ipaktchi K, Arbabi S. Advances in burn critical care. Critical Care Medicine. 2006;**34**(9):S239-S244

[3] Latenser BA. Critical care of the burn patient: The first 48 hours. Critical Care Medicine. 2009;**37**(10):2819-2826

[4] Bittner EA et al. Acute and perioperative care of the burn-injured patient. Anesthesiology: The Journal of the American Society of Anesthesiologists. 2015;**122**(2):448-464

[5] Santaniello JM et al. Ten year experience of burn, trauma, and combined burn/trauma injuries comparing outcomes. Journal of Trauma and Acute Care Surgery. 2004;**57**(4):696-701

[6] Hawkins A et al. The impact of combined trauma and burns on patient mortality. Journal of Trauma and Acute Care Surgery. 2005;**58**(2):284-288

[7] Richard R, Staley M. Burn patient evaluation and treatment planning. In: Burn Care and Rehabilitation: Principles and Practice. Philadelphia: FA Davis; 1994. pp. 201-218

[8] Luterman A. Burn injuries. Initial evaluation and treatment. Cutis. 1978;**22**(4):437-442

[9] Jaskille AD et al. Critical review of burn depth assessment techniques: Part I. Historical review. Journal of Burn Care & Research. 2009;**30**(6):937-947

[10] Griglak M. Thermal injury. Emergency Medicine Clinics of North America. 1992;**10**(2):369-383

[11] Baxter CR, Waeckerle JF. Emergency treatment of burn injury. Annals of Emergency Medicine. 1988;**17**(12):1305-1315

[12] Hettiaratchy S, Dziewulski P. ABC of burns: Pathophysiology and types of burns. British Medical Journal. 2004;**328**(7453):1427

[13] Palao R et al. Chemical burns: Pathophysiology and treatment. Burns. 2010;**36**(3):295-304

[14] Zubair M, Besner GE. Pediatric electrical burns: Management strategies. Burns. 1997;**23**(5):413-420

[15] Xu F et al. Quantification and the underlying mechanism of skin thermal damage: A review. Journal of Mechanics in Medicine and Biology. 2010;**10**(03):373-400

[16] Cooper PN. Burn injury. In: Essentials of Autopsy Practice. London, England: Springer; 2006. pp. 215-232

[17] Jeschke MG. The hepatic acute phase response to thermal injury. In: Acute Phase Proteins-Regulation and Functions of Acute Phase Proteins. England: IntechOpen; 2011

[18] Jeschke MG et al. The pathophysiologic response to severe burn injury. Annals of Surgery. 2008;**248**(3):387

[19] Moritz AR, Henriques F Jr. Studies of thermal injury: II. The relative importance of time and surface temperature in the causation of cutaneous burns. The American Journal of Pathology. 1947;**23**(5):695

[20] Pearce J, Thomsen S. Rate process analysis of thermal damage. In: Optical-Thermal Response of Laser-Irradiated Tissue. Boston, Massachusetts: Springer; 1995. pp. 561-606

[21] Harchelroad F, Rottinghaus D. Chemical burns. In: Emergency

Medicine: A Comprehensive Study Guide. 6th ed. New York, NY: McGraw-Hill; 2004. pp. 1226-1230

[22] Edlich R et al. Modern concepts of treatment and prevention of chemical injuries. Journal of Long-Term Effects of Medical Implants. 2005;**15**(3)

[23] Seth R, Chester D, Moiemen N. A review of chemical burns. Trauma. 2007;**9**(2):81-94

[24] Hall AH, Maibach HI. Water decontamination of chemical skin/eye splashes: A critical review. Cutaneous and Ocular Toxicology. 2006;**25**(2):67-83

[25] Levine MD, Zane R. Chemical injuries. In: Rosen's Emergency Medicine. 8th ed. Philadelphia, PA: Elsevier/Saunders; 2014. pp. 818-827

[26] Cooper MA. Emergent care of lightning and electrical injuries. In: Seminars in Neurology. New York, NY: Thieme Medical Publishers, Inc.; 1995. pp. 268-278

[27] Baxter CR. Present concepts in the management of major electrical injury. Surgical Clinics of North America. 1970;**50**(6):1401-1418

[28] Ten Duis HJ. Acute electrical burns. In: Seminars in Neurology. New York, NY: Thieme Medical Publishers, Inc.; 1995. pp. 381-386

[29] Koumbourlis AC. Electrical injuries. Critical Care Medicine. 2002;**30**(11):S424-S430

[30] Solem L, Fischer RP, Strate RG. The natural history of electrical injury. The Journal of Trauma. 1977;**17**(7):487-492

[31] Nadel ER, Bullard RW, Stolwijk J. Importance of skin temperature in the regulation of sweating. Journal of Applied Physiology. 1971;**31**(1):80-87

[32] Holick MF et al. Vitamin D and skin physiology: AD-lightful story. Journal of Bone and Mineral Research. 2007;**22**(S2):V28-V33

[33] Proksch E, Brandner JM, Jensen JM. The skin: An indispensable barrier. Experimental Dermatology. 2008;**17**(12):1063-1072

[34] Langer K. On the anatomy and physiology of the skin: III. The elasticity of the cutis. British Journal of Plastic Surgery. 1978;**31**(3):185-199

[35] Orgill DP, Porter SA, Taylor HO. Heat injury to cells in perfused systems. Annals of the New York Academy of Sciences. 2006;**1066**(1):106-118

[36] Keck M et al. Pathophysiology of burns. Wiener Medizinische Wochenschrift. 2009;**159**(13-14):327-336

[37] Shupp JW et al. A review of the local pathophysiologic bases of burn wound progression. Journal of Burn Care & Research. 2010;**31**(6):849-873

[38] Singh V et al. The pathogenesis of burn wound conversion. Annals of Plastic Surgery. 2007;**59**(1):109-115

[39] Singer AJ et al. Apoptosis and necrosis in the ischemic zone adjacent to third degree burns. Academic Emergency Medicine. 2008;**15**(6):549-554

[40] Choi M, Ehrlich HP. U75412E, a lazaroid, prevents progressive burn ischemia in a rat burn model. The American Journal of Pathology. 1993;**142**(2):519

[41] Kim D et al. Microvascular assessment of burn depth conversion during varying resuscitation conditions. The Journal of Burn Care & Rehabilitation. 2001;**22**(6):406-416

[42] Rose LF, Chan RK. The burn wound microenvironment. Advances in Wound Care. 2016;**5**(3):106-118

[43] Arturson MG. The pathophysiology of severe thermal injury. The Journal of Burn Care & Rehabilitation. 1985;**6**(2):129-146

[44] Monstrey S et al. Assessment of burn depth and burn wound healing potential. Burns. 2008;**34**(6): 761-769

[45] Hansen GL et al. Wound status evaluation using color image processing. IEEE Transactions on Medical Imaging. 1997;**16**(1):78-86

[46] Anselmo VJ, Zawacki BE. Multispectral photographic analysis a new quantitative tool to assist in the early diagnosis of thermal burn depth. Annals of Biomedical Engineering. 1977;**5**(2):179-193

[47] Green HA et al. Burn depth estimation using indocyanine green fluorescence. Archives of Dermatology. 1992;**128**(1):43-49

[48] Medina-Preciado JD et al. Noninvasive determination of burn depth in children by digital infrared thermal imaging. Journal of Biomedical Optics. 2012;**18**(6):061204

[49] Leonardi L et al. Visible-Near Infrared Spectroscopy in Burn Injury Assessment. 2010. Google Patents

[50] Panasci K. Burns and wounds. In: Acute Care Handbook for Physical Therapists. Vol. 7. St. Louis, Missouri: Elsevier Saunders; 2013. p. 283

[51] Faurschou A, Wulf HC. Topical corticosteroids in the treatment of acute sunburn: a randomized, double-blind clinical trial. Archives of Dermatology. 2008;**144**(5):620-624

[52] Gallagher G, Rae CP, Kinsella J. Treatment of pain in severe burns. American Journal of Clinical Dermatology. 2000;**1**(6):329-335

[53] Hartford CE, Kealey GP. Care of outpatient burns. In: Total Burn Care. Vol. 3. 2007. pp. 67-80

[54] Summer GJ et al. Burn injury pain: The continuing challenge. The Journal of Pain. 2007;**8**(7):533-548

[55] Connor-Ballard PA. Understanding and managing burn pain: Part 1. The American Journal of Nursing. 2009;**109**(4):48-56

[56] Rittié L et al. Eccrine sweat glands are major contributors to reepithelialization of human wounds. The American Journal of Pathology. 2013;**182**(1):163-171

[57] Finnerty CC et al. Hypertrophic scarring: the greatest unmet challenge after burn injury. The Lancet. 2016;**388**(10052):1427-1436

[58] Grover R, Morgan B. Management of hypopigmentation following burn injury. Burns. 1996;**22**(8):627-630

[59] Sittig K, Richardson K. Acute burn management. In: Wound Healing: Evidence-Based Management. Philadelphia, Pennsylvania: F. A. Davis Company; 2010. p. 333

[60] Dunne JA, Rawlins JM. Management of burns. Surgery (Oxford). 2014;**32**(9):477-484

[61] Costagliola M, Agrosi M. Second-degree burns: A comparative, multicenter, randomized trial of hyaluronic acid plus silver sulfadiazine vs. silver sulfadiazine alone. Current Medical Research and Opinion. 2005;**21**(8):1235-1240

[62] Orgill DP. Excision and skin grafting of thermal burns. New England Journal of Medicine. 2009;**360**(9):893-901

[63] Sheridan RL. Comprehensive treatment of burns. Current Problems in Surgery. 2001;**38**(9):657-756

[64] Altintas M, Vogt P. Burn Injury. In: General Trauma Care and Related Aspects. Berlin, Heidelberg: Springer; 2014. pp. 169-176

[65] Hawkins HK, Jay J, Finnerty CC. Pathophysiology of the burn scar. In: Total Burn Care. Elsevier; 2018. pp. 466-475.e3

[66] Pereira C, Gold W, Herndon D. Burn coverage technologies: Current concepts and future directions. Journal of Biomaterials Applications. 2007;**22**(2):101-121

[67] Parrett BM et al. Fourth-degree burns to the lower extremity with exposed tendon and bone: A ten-year experience. Journal of Burn Care & Research. 2006;**27**(1):34-39

[68] De Lorenzi F, Van der Hulst R, Boeckx W. Free flaps in burn reconstruction. Burns. 2001;**27**(6):603-612

[69] Baxter CR, Marvin JA, Curreri PW. Early management of thermal burns. Postgraduate Medicine. 1974;**55**(1):131-139

[70] Williams C. Successful assessment and management of burn injuries. Nursing Standard. 2009;**23**(32):53-62

[71] Minimas D. A critical evaluation of the Lund and Browder chart. Wounds UK. 2007;**3**(3):58

[72] Agarwal P, Sahu S. Determination of hand and palm area as a ratio of body surface area in Indian population. Indian Journal of Plastic Surgery: Official Publication of the Association of Plastic Surgeons of India. 2010;**43**(1):49

[73] Malic C et al. Resuscitation burn card—A useful tool for burn injury assessment. Burns. 2007;**33**(2):195-199

[74] Lund CC. The estimation of areas of burns. Surgery, Gynecology & Obstetrics. 1944;**79**:352-358

[75] Wang C. Assessment and physiology of Burns. In: Anesthesia for Trauma. New York, NY: Springer; 2014. pp. 271-289

[76] Knighton J, Jako M. Nursing management of the burn-injured person. In: Handbook of Burns. Vienna, Austria: Springer; 2012. pp. 387-430

[77] Evers LH, Bhavsar D, Mailänder P. The biology of burn injury. Experimental Dermatology. 2010;**19**(9):777-783

[78] Robins EV. Burn shock. Critical Care Nursing Clinics. 1990;**2**(2):299-307

[79] Pham TN, Cancio LC, Gibran NS. American Burn Association practice guidelines burn shock resuscitation. Journal of Burn Care & Research. 2008;**29**(1):257-266

[80] Holm C et al. A clinical randomized study on the effects of invasive monitoring on burn shock resuscitation. Burns. 2004;**30**(8):798-807

[81] Nguyen TT et al. Current treatment of severely burned patients. Annals of Surgery. 1996;**223**(1):14

[82] Wolf SE et al. Mortality determinants in massive pediatric burns. An analysis of 103 children with > or = 80% TBSA burns (> or = 70% full-thickness). Annals of Surgery. 1997;**225**(5):554

[83] Lawrence A et al. Colloid administration normalizes resuscitation ratio and ameliorates "fluid creep". Journal of Burn Care & Research. 2010;**31**(1):40-47

[84] Saffle JR. The phenomenon of "fluid creep" in acute burn resuscitation. Journal of Burn Care & Research. 2007;**28**(3):382-395

[85] Chung KK et al. Resuscitation of severely burned military casualties:

Fluid begets more fluid. Journal of Trauma and Acute Care Surgery. 2009;**67**(2):231-237

[86] Kornbau C et al. Central line complications. International Journal of Critical Illness and Injury Science. 2015;**5**(3):170

[87] Leidel BA et al. Comparison of intraosseous versus central venous vascular access in adults under resuscitation in the emergency department with inaccessible peripheral veins. Resuscitation. 2012;**83**(1):40-45

[88] Mayer CL, Werman HA, Springer BL. Management of Burn Injuries. Trauma Reports. 2019;**20**:1

[89] Spelten O et al. Estimation of substitution volume after burn trauma. Systematic review of published formulae. Der Anaesthetist. 2011;**60**(4):303-311

[90] Warden GD. Burn shock resuscitation. World Journal of Surgery. 1992;**16**(1):16-23

[91] Cartotto RC et al. How well does the Parkland formula estimate actual fluid resuscitation volumes? The Journal of Burn Care & Rehabilitation. 2002;**23**(4):258-265

[92] Cartotto R. Fluid resuscitation of the thermally injured patient. Clinics in Plastic Surgery. 2009;**36**(4):569-581

[93] Cartotto R, Greenhalgh D. Colloids in acute burn resuscitation. Critical Care Clinics. 2016;**32**(4):507-523

[94] Diver AJ. The evolution of burn fluid resuscitation. International Journal of Surgery. 2008;**6**(4):345-350

[95] Holm C. Resuscitation in shock associated with burns. Tradition or evidence-based medicine? Resuscitation. 2000;**44**(3):157-164

[96] Branski LK et al. Emerging infections in burns. Surgical Infections. 2009;**10**(5):389-397

[97] Carleton S. Cardiac problems associated with burns. Cardiology Clinics. 1995;**13**(2):257-262

[98] Hettiaratchy S, Papini R. ABC of burns: Initial management of a major burn: II—Assessment and resuscitation. British Medical Journal. 2004;**329**(7457):101

[99] Papp A et al. Myocardial function and haemodynamics in extensive burn trauma: evaluation by clinical signs, invasive monitoring, echocardiography and cytokine concentrations. A prospective clinical study. Acta Anaesthesiologica Scandinavica. 2003;**47**(10):1257-1263

[100] Atiyeh B et al. Acute burn resuscitation and fluid creep: It is time for colloid rehabilitation. Annals of Burns and Fire Disasters. 2012;**25**(2):59

[101] Fairbrother H. Optimizing emergency management to reduce morbidity and mortality in pediatric burn patients. Pediatric Emergency Medicine Practice. 2015;**12**(5):1-23

[102] Rose J, Herndon D. Advances in the treatment of burn patients. Burns. 1997;**23**:S19-S26

[103] Morehouse JD et al. Resuscitation of the thermally injured patient. Critical Care Clinics. 1992;**8**(2):355-365

[104] Gomez R, Cancio LC. Management of burn wounds in the emergency department. Emergency Medicine Clinics of North America. 2007;**25**(1):135-146

[105] Carvajal HF. Fluid resuscitation of pediatric burn victims: A critical appraisal. Pediatric Nephrology. 1994;**8**(3):357-366

[106] Baxter CR, Shires T. Physiological response to crystalloid resuscitation of severe burns. Annals of the New York Academy of Sciences. 1968;**150**(3):874-894

[107] Schiller WR. Burn management in children. Pediatric Annals. 1996;**25**(8):431-438

[108] Bratland B. Fluid resuscitation in treatment of burn shock. 2010. Available online at: https://dspace.cuni.cz/bitstream/handle/20.500.11956/31350/DPTX_2008_1_11120_0_44413_0_64919.pdf?sequence=1 [Last access date: 24 May 2019]

[109] Paratz JD et al. Burn resuscitation—hourly urine output versus alternative endpoints: A systematic review. Shock. 2014;**42**(4):295-306

[110] Matsen FA III. Compartmental syndromes. Hospital Practice. 1980;**15**(2):113-117

[111] Singh S et al. Burns and thermal injuries. Journal of Orthopedics, Traumatology and Rehabilitation. 2013;**6**(1):47

[112] Burd A et al. Decompression not escharotomy in acute burns. Burns. 2006;**32**(3):284-292

[113] de Barros MEPM et al. Revisiting escharotomy in patients with burns in extremities. Journal of Burn Care & Research. 2017;**38**(4):e691-e698

[114] Durrant C, Simpson A, Williams G. Thermal injury–The first 24 h. Current Anaesthesia & Critical Care. 2008;**19**(5-6):256-263

[115] Cancio LC, Lundy JB, Sheridan RL. Evolving Changes in the Management of Burns and Environmental Injuries. Fort Sam Houston, TX: Army Inst. of Surgical Research; 2012

[116] Brown RL et al. The adequacy of limb escharotomies-fasciotomies after referral to a major burn center. The Journal of Trauma. 1994;**37**(6):916-920

[117] Orgill DP, Piccolo N. Escharotomy and decompressive therapies in burns. Journal of Burn Care & Research. 2009;**30**(5):759-768

[118] Li X, Liang D, Liu X. Compartment syndrome in burn patients: A report of five cases. Burns. 2002;**28**(8):787-789

[119] Oda J et al. Resuscitation fluid volume and abdominal compartment syndrome in patients with major burns. Burns. 2006;**32**(2):151-154

[120] Azzopardi EA et al. Fluid resuscitation in adults with severe burns at risk of secondary abdominal compartment syndrome—An evidence based systematic review. Burns. 2009;**35**(7):911-920

[121] Stawicki SP, Cipolla J, Bria C. Comparison of open abdomens in nontrauma and trauma patients: A retrospective study. International Journal of Academic Medicine. 2016;**2**(3):51

[122] Stawicki SP et al. The concept of damage control: Extending the paradigm to emergency general surgery. Injury. 2008;**39**(1):93-101

[123] Ivy ME et al. Intra-abdominal hypertension and abdominal compartment syndrome in burn patients. Journal of Trauma and Acute Care Surgery. 2000;**49**(3):387-391

[124] American Burn Association. Advanced Burn Life Support Course. Chicago, Illinois: American Burn Association; 2011

[125] Oliver R, Spain D, Stadelmann W. Burns, resuscitation and early management. 2004. Available online at: http://www.nhsfife.org/weborgs/nhs/

uploadfiles/publications/c64_Burns.doc [Last access date: 24 May 2019]

[126] Smith BP et al. Review of abdominal damage control and open abdomens: Focus on gastrointestinal complications. Journal of Gastrointestinal & Liver Diseases. 2010;**19**(4)

[127] Fusco MA, Martin RS, Chang MC. Estimation of intra-abdominal pressure by bladder pressure measurement: Validity and methodology. Journal of Trauma and Acute Care Surgery. 2001;**50**(2):297-302

[128] ve Tedavisi İYT et al. Diagnosis and treatment of the inhalation injuries: Review of the literature. KÜ Tıp Fak Derg. 2013;**15**(3):23-39

[129] Horton JW. Left ventricular contractile dysfunction as a complication of thermal injury. Shock. 2004;**22**(6):495-507

[130] Giroir BP et al. Inhibition of tumor necrosis factor prevents myocardial dysfunction during burn shock. American Journal of Physiology-Heart and Circulatory Physiology. 1994;**267**(1):H118-H124

[131] Bernard F et al. Prognostic significance of early cardiac index measurements in severely burned patients. Burns. 1994;**20**(6):529-531

[132] Bak Z et al. Cardiac dysfunction after burns. Burns. 2008;**34**(5):603-609

[133] Sullivan SR et al. Elevated orbital pressure: Another untoward effect of massive resuscitation after burn injury. Journal of Trauma and Acute Care Surgery. 2006;**60**(1):72-76

[134] Malbrain ML et al. The polycompartment syndrome: A concise state-of-the-art review. Anaesthesiology Intensive Therapy. 2014;**46**(5):433-450

[135] Singh CN et al. Orbital compartment syndrome in burn patients. Ophthalmic Plastic & Reconstructive Surgery. 2008;**24**(2):102-106

[136] O'mara MS et al. A prospective, randomized evaluation of intra-abdominal pressures with crystalloid and colloid resuscitation in burn patients. Journal of Trauma and Acute Care Surgery. 2005;**58**(5):1011-1018

[137] Faraklas I et al. Colloid normalizes resuscitation ratio in pediatric burns. Journal of Burn Care & Research. 2011;**32**(1):91-97

[138] Hershberger RC et al. Abdominal compartment syndrome in the severely burned patient. Journal of Burn Care & Research. 2007;**28**(5):708-714

[139] Park SH, Hemmila MR, Wahl WL. Early albumin use improves mortality in difficult to resuscitate burn patients. Journal of Trauma and Acute Care Surgery. 2012;**73**(5):1294-1297

[140] Tricklebank S. Modern trends in fluid therapy for burns. Burns. 2009;**35**(6):757-767

[141] Ullmann Y et al. Evaluation of the validity of the Haifa formula for fluid resuscitation in burn patients at the Rambam Medical Centre. Annals of Burns and Fire Disasters. 2000;**13**(4):206-212

[142] Molyneux K. Fluid resuscitation in burn patients: Above and beyond baxter. School of Physician Assistant Studies. 2008. p. 182

[143] Jones L et al. Burn resuscitation with fresh frozen plasma: 5 years of experience with the West Penn formula. Austin Journal of Emergency and Critical Care Medicine. 2015;**2**(2):1018

[144] Wilmore DW et al. Effect of ambient temperature on heat production and heat loss in burn

patients. Journal of Applied Physiology. 1975;**38**(4):593-597

[145] Dries D. Burn Resuscitation: Don't Forget the Feeds. Critical Care Medicine. 2018;**46**(12):2060-2062

[146] Demling RH. Comparison of the anabolic effects and complications of human growth hormone and the testosterone analog, oxandrolone, after severe burn injury. Burns. 1999;**25**(3):215-221

[147] Schäffer M, Barbul A. Lymphocyte function in wound healing and following injury. British Journal of Surgery. 1998;**85**(4):444-460

[148] Clark A et al. Nutrition and metabolism in burn patients. Burns & Trauma. 2017;**5**(1):11

[149] Cochran A, Saffle JR, Graves C. Nutrition support for the burn patient. In: Handbook of Burns. Vienna, Austria: Springer; 2012. pp. 361-379

[150] Evans DC et al. Continuous versus bolus tube feeds: Does the modality affect glycemic variability, tube feeding volume, caloric intake, or insulin utilization? International Journal of Critical Illness and Injury Science. 2016;**6**(1):9

[151] Kirksey TD et al. Gastrointestinal complications in burns. The American Journal of Surgery. 1968;**116**(5):627-633

[152] Sitzmann JV, Pitt HA. P.C.C.o.t.A.G. Association, Statement on guidelines for total parenteral nutrition. Digestive Diseases and Sciences. 1989;**34**(4):489-496

[153] Allard J et al. Validation of a new formula for calculating the energy requirements of burn patients. Journal of Parenteral and Enteral Nutrition. 1990;**14**(2):115-118

[154] Williamson J. Actual burn nutrition care practices: A national survey (part II). The Journal of Burn Care & Rehabilitation. 1989;**10**(2):185-194

[155] Gottschlich MM, Ireton-Jones CS. Classic article: The Curreri formula: A landmark process for estimating the caloric needs of burn patients. Nutrition in Clinical Practice. 2001;**16**(3):172-173

[156] Spanholtz TA et al. Severe burn injuries: acute and long-term treatment. Deutsches Ärzteblatt International. 2009;**106**(38):607

[157] Peck MD, Chang Y. Nutritional support for burn injuries. The Journal of Nutritional Biochemistry. 1999;**10**(7):380-396

[158] Rousseau A-F et al. ESPEN endorsed recommendations: Nutritional therapy in major burns. Clinical Nutrition. 2013;**32**(4):497-502

[159] Barbosa E et al. Supplementation of vitamin E, vitamin C, and zinc attenuates oxidative stress in burned children: a randomized, double-blind, placebo-controlled pilot study. Journal of Burn Care & Research. 2009;**30**(5):859-866

[160] Rizzo JA et al. Vitamin C in burn resuscitation. Critical Care Clinics. 2016;**32**(4):539-546

[161] De-Souza DA, Greene LJ. Pharmacological nutrition after burn injury. The Journal of Nutrition. 1998;**128**(5):797-803

[162] Haberal M, Abali AES, Karakayali H. Fluid management in major burn injuries. Indian Journal of Plastic Surgery: Official Publication of the Association of Plastic Surgeons of India. 2010;**43**(Suppl):S29

[163] Soussi S, et al. Early hemodynamic management of critically Ill burn patients. Anesthesiology. 2018;**129**(3):583-589

[164] Rehou S et al. Acute phase response in critically ill elderly burn patients. Critical Care Medicine. 2019;**47**(2):201-209

[165] Vercruysse G. The rational care of burns. In: Managing Dismounted Complex Blast Injuries in Military & Civilian Settings. Cham, Switzerland: Springer; 2018. pp. 197-208

[166] Kleintjes W et al. An algorithm for responsive fluid resuscitation at the Western Cape Provincial Tertiary Adult Burn Centre. South African Journal of Plastic & Reconstructive Aesthetic Surgery & Burns. 2018;**1**(1):16-18

[167] Soussi S et al. Risk factors for acute mesenteric ischemia in critically ill burns patients—A matched case-control study. Shock. 2019;**51**(2):153-160

[168] Jeschke MG et al. Long-term persistance of the pathophysiologic response to severe burn injury. PLoS One. 2011;**6**(7):e21245

[169] Williams FN et al. Propranolol decreases cardiac work in a dose-dependent manner in severely burned children. Surgery. 2011;**149**(2):231-239

[170] Finnerty CC, Herndon DN. Is propranolol of benefit in pediatric burn patients? Advances in Surgery. 2013;**47**(1):177-197

[171] Pereira C, Murphy K, Herndon D. Outcome measures in burn care: Is mortality dead? Burns. 2004;**30**(8):761-771

[172] Herndon DN et al. Lipolysis in burned patients is stimulated by the β2-receptor for catecholamines. Archives of Surgery. 1994;**129**(12):1301-1305

[173] Vaiva G et al. Immediate treatment with propranolol decreases posttraumatic stress disorder two months after trauma. Biological Psychiatry. 2003;**54**(9):947-949

[174] Wilmore DW et al. Catecholamines: Mediator of the hypermetabolic response to thermal injury. Annals of Surgery. 1974;**180**(4):653

[175] Jeschke MG et al. Burn size determines the inflammatory and hypermetabolic response. Critical Care. 2007;**11**(4):R90

[176] Fram RY et al. Intensive insulin therapy improves insulin sensitivity and mitochondrial function in severely burned children. Critical Care Medicine. 2010;**38**(6). DOI: 10.1097/CCM.0b013e3181de8b9e

[177] Pidcoke HF, Wade CE, Wolf SE. Insulin and the burned patient. Critical Care Medicine. 2007;**35**(9):S524-S530

[178] Ballian N et al. Glucose metabolism in burn patients: The role of insulin and other endocrine hormones. Burns. 2010;**36**(5):599-605

[179] Panda S, Lokesh AB, Sarangi A. Prognostic significance of glycemic control in burn injury patients: A study in Tertiary Care Hospital of Odisha. Apollo Medicine. 2017;**14**(3):160

[180] Stawicki S et al. The glucogram: A new quantitative tool for glycemic analysis in the surgical intensive care unit. International Journal of Critical Illness and Injury Science. 2011;**1**(1):5

[181] Pappada SM et al. Evaluation of a model for glycemic prediction in critically ill surgical patients. PLoS One. 2013;**8**(7):e69475

[182] Van den Berghe G. How does blood glucose control with insulin save lives in intensive care? The Journal of Clinical Investigation. 2004;**114**(9):1187-1195

[183] Becker RA et al. Hypermetabolic Low Triiodothyronine Syndrome of Burn Injury. Fort Sam Houston TX: Army Inst. of Surgical Research; 1982

[184] Becker RA et al. Free T4, Free T3, and Reverse T3 in Critically Ill, Thermally Injured Patients. Fort Sam Houston TX: Army Inst. of Surgical Research; 1980

[185] Dolecek R. Endocrine changes after burn trauma-a review. The Keio Journal of Medicine. 1989;**38**(3):262-276

[186] Børsheim E et al. Pamidronate attenuates muscle loss after pediatric burn injury. Journal of Bone and Mineral Research. 2014;**29**(6):1369-1372

[187] Gosling P et al. Burn and trauma associated proteinuria: The role of lipid peroxidation, renin and myoglobin. Annals of Clinical Biochemistry. 1988;**25**(1):53-59

[188] Gauglitz GG et al. Burns: Where are we standing with propranolol, oxandrolone, rhGH, and the new incretin analogues? Current Opinion in Clinical Nutrition and Metabolic Care. 2011;**14**(2):176

[189] Cancio LC et al. Predicting increased fluid requirements during the resuscitation of thermally injured patients. Journal of Trauma and Acute Care Surgery. 2004;**56**(2):404-414

[190] Endorf FW, Gamelli RL. Inhalation injury, pulmonary perturbations, and fluid resuscitation. Journal of Burn Care & Research. 2007;**28**(1):80-83

[191] Moylan JA. Inhalation injury—A primary determinant of survival following major burns. The Journal of Burn Care & Rehabilitation. 1981;**2**(2):78-84

[192] Gauglitz GG, Herndon DN, Jeschke MG. Emergency treatment of severely burned pediatric patients: Current therapeutic strategies. 2008

[193] Crookshank A, Hughes WB, Hensell DO. Burn critical care. In: Critical Care Study Guide. Springer; 2010. pp. 769-782

[194] Dyer RF, Esch VH. Polyvinyl chloride toxicity in fires: Hydrogen chloride toxicity in fire fighters. Journal of the American Medical Association. 1976;**235**(4):393-397

[195] Walker PF et al. Diagnosis and management of inhalation injury: An updated review. Critical Care. 2015;**19**(1):351

[196] O'Brien DJ et al. Empiric management of cyanide toxicity associated with smoke inhalation. Prehospital and Disaster Medicine. 2011;**26**(5):374-382

[197] Alcorta R et al. Smokc inhalation & acute cyanide poisoning. Hydrogen cyanide poisoning proves increasingly common in smoke-inhalation victims. JEMS. 2004;**29**(8)suppl:6-15

[198] Bagby SK. Acute management of facial burns. Oral and Maxillofacial Surgery Clinics. 2005;**17**(3):267-272

[199] Pruitt BA Jr. Diagnosis and treatment of inhalation injury in burn. Pathophysiology and Treatment of Inhalation Injuries. 1987;**34**:239

[200] Nugent N, Herndon DN. Diagnosis and treatment of inhalation injury. In: Total Burn Care. Vol. 3. Philadelphia, Pennsylvania: Elsevier Saunders; 2007. pp. 262-272

[201] Dries DJ. Key questions in ventilator management of the burn-injured patient (first of two parts). Journal of Burn Care & Research. 2009;**30**(1):128-138

[202] Ishisanya KSA. Occurrence and Early Outcomes of Inhalation Injuries in Burn Injury Patients Admitted to Kenyatta National Hospital; A

Referral Burns Centre in East Africa. 2007. Available online at: http://erepository.uonbi.ac.ke:8080/bitstream/handle/11295/24884/Ishisanya_Occurrence%20and%20early%20outcomes%20of%20inhalation%20burns%20in%20burn%20injury%20patients.pdf?sequence=5 [Last accessed: 24 May 2019]

[203] Pruitt BA Jr, Cioffi WG. Diagnosis and treatment of smoke inhalation. Journal of Intensive Care Medicine. 1995;**10**(3):117-127

[204] Shirani KZ, Pruitt BA Jr, Mason AD Jr. The influence of inhalation injury and pneumonia on burn mortality. Annals of Surgery. 1987;**205**(1):82

[205] Edelman DA et al. Pneumonia after inhalation injury. Journal of Burn Care & Research. 2007;**28**(2):241-246

[206] Rob Cartotto M. High frequency oscillatory ventilation in burn patients. Acta Anaesthesiologica Scandinavica. 2003;**47**(4):495-495

[207] Stawicki S, Goyal M, Sarani B. Analytic reviews: High-frequency oscillatory ventilation (HFOV) and airway pressure release ventilation (APRV): A practical guide. Journal of Intensive Care Medicine. 2009;**24**(4):215-229

[208] Desai MH et al. Early burn wound excision significantly reduces blood loss. Annals of Surgery. 1990;**211**(6):753

[209] Gray DT et al. Early surgical excision versus conventional therapy in patients with 20 to 40 percent burns: A comparative study. The American Journal of Surgery. 1982;**144**(1):76-80

[210] Robins EV. Immunosuppression of the burned patient. Critical Care Nursing Clinics. 1989;**1**(4):767-774

[211] Rennekampff H-O, Tenenhaus M. Debridement of the burn wound. In: Color Atlas of Burn Reconstructive Surgery. Springer; 2010. pp. 10-14

[212] Lamke L-O, Liljedahl S-O. Evaporative water loss from burns, grafts and donor sites. Scandinavian Journal of Plastic and Reconstructive Surgery. 1971;**5**(1):17-22

[213] Lamke L-O. Evaporative water loss from burns under different environmental conditions. Scandinavian Journal of Plastic and Reconstructive Surgery. 1971;**5**(2):77-81

[214] Rosenberg L et al. A novel rapid and selective enzymatic debridement agent for burn wound management: A multi-center RCT. Burns. 2014;**40**(3):466-474

[215] Marzano AV, Borghi A, Cugno M. Adverse drug reactions and organ damage: The skin. European Journal of Internal Medicine. 2016;**28**:17-24

[216] Urbano FL. Nikolsky's sign in autoimmune skin disorders. Hospital Physician. 2001;**37**:23-24

[217] Abe R. Toxic epidermal necrolysis and Stevens–Johnson syndrome: Soluble Fas ligand involvement in the pathomechanisms of these diseases. Journal of Dermatological Science. 2008;**52**(3):151-159

[218] Nadelmann E, Czernik A. Wound Care in Immunobullous Disease. London, England: IntechOpen; 2018

[219] Patel GK, Finlay AY. Staphylococcal scalded skin syndrome. American Journal of Clinical Dermatology. 2003;**4**(3):165-175

[220] Giuliano A et al. Bacteriology of necrotizing fasciitis. The American Journal of Surgery. 1977;**134**(1):52-57

[221] Wong C-H et al. Necrotizing fasciitis: Clinical presentation, microbiology, and determinants of

mortality. Journal of Bone & Joint Surgery. 2003;**85**(8):1454-1460

[222] Green RJ, Dafoe DC, Rajfin TA. Necrotizing fasciitis. Chest. 1996;**110**(1):219-229

[223] Lee JY et al. Extended negative pressure wound therapy-assisted dermatotraction for the closure of large open fasciotomy wounds in necrotizing fasciitis patients. World Journal of Emergency Surgery. 2014;**9**(1):29

[224] Seifert AW et al. Skin shedding and tissue regeneration in African spiny mice (Acomys). Nature. 2012;**489**(7417):561

[225] Tam J et al. Fractional skin harvesting: Autologous skin grafting without donor-site morbidity. Plastic and Reconstructive Surgery Global Open. 2013;**1**(6):e47

[226] Katherine Lincoln D, Paul Liu M, Lee Rogers D. Clinical experience and best practices using epidermal skin grafts on wounds. Wounds. 2015;**27**(11):282-292

[227] Osborne SN, Schmidt MA, Harper JR. An automated and minimally invasive tool for generating autologous viable epidermal micrografts. Advances in Skin & Wound Care. 2016;**29**(2):57

[228] Veliu S, Kröpfl J, Vrbnjak D. CELLUTOME™ epidermal harvesting system. Albanian Journal of Trauma and Emergency Surgery. 2018;**2**(2). DOI: 10.32391/ajtes.v2i2.13

[229] Lantis JC, Paredes JA. Topical wound care treatment and indications for their use. In: The Diabetic Foot. Springer; 2018. pp. 281-304

[230] Osborne SN et al. Epidermal micrografts produced via an automated and minimally invasive tool form at the dermal/epidermal junction and contain proliferative cells that secrete wound healing growth factors. Advances in Skin & Wound Care. 2015;**28**(9):397

[231] Branski LK et al. A review of gene and stem cell therapy in cutaneous wound healing. Burns. 2009;**35**(2):171-180

[232] Khavari P, Rollman O, Vahlquist A. Cutaneous gene transfer for skin and systemic diseases. Journal of Internal Medicine. 2002;**252**(1):1-10

[233] Atiyeh BS, Costagliola M. Cultured epithelial autograft (CEA) in burn treatment: Three decades later. Burns. 2007;**33**(4):405-413

[234] FDA. Summary of Safety and Effectiveness Data (SSED). 2018. Available from: https://www.fda.gov/downloads/BiologicsBloodVaccines/BloodBloodProducts/Approved Products/PremarketApprovalsPMAs/UCM621989.pdf [Accessed: 14 February 2009]

[235] Anderson RR, Parrish JA. Selective photothermolysis: Precise microsurgery by selective absorption of pulsed radiation. Science. 1983;**220**(4596):524-527

[236] Alster TS, Nanni CA. Pulsed dye laser treatment of hypertrophic burn scars. Plastic and Reconstructive Surgery. 1998;**102**:2190-2195

[237] Donelan MB, Parrett BM, Sheridan RL. Pulsed dye laser therapy and z-plasty for facial burn scars: The alternative to excision. Annals of Plastic Surgery. 2008;**60**(5):480-486

[238] Manstein D et al. Fractional photothermolysis: A new concept for cutaneous remodeling using microscopic patterns of thermal injury. Lasers in Surgery and Medicine: The Official Journal of the American Society for Laser Medicine and Surgery. 2004;**34**(5):426-438

[239] Krakowski AC et al. Ablative fractional laser resurfacing helps treat restrictive pediatric scar contractures. Pediatrics. 2014;**134**(6):e1700-1705

[240] Grunewald S et al. In vivo wound healing and dermal matrix remodelling in response to fractional CO_2 laser intervention: Clinicopathological correlation in non-facial skin. International Journal of Hyperthermia. 2011;**27**(8):811-818

[241] Graber EM, Tanzi EL, Alster TS. Side effects and complications of fractional laser photothermolysis: Experience with 961 treatments. Dermatologic Surgery. 2008;**34**(3):301-307

[242] Hantash BM et al. In vivo histological evaluation of a novel ablative fractional resurfacing device. Lasers in Surgery and Medicine: The Official Journal of the American Society for Laser Medicine and Surgery. 2007;**39**(2):96-107

[243] Hunzeker CM, Weiss ET, Geronemus RG. Fractionated CO_2 laser resurfacing: Our experience with more than 2000 treatments. Aesthetic Surgery Journal. 2009;**29**(4):317-322

[244] Ozog DM et al. Evaluation of clinical results, histological architecture, and collagen expression following treatment of mature burn scars with a fractional carbon dioxide laser. JAMA Dermatology. 2013;**149**(1):50-57

[245] Waibel JS, Wulkan AJ, Shumaker PR. Treatment of hypertrophic scars using laser and laser assisted corticosteroid delivery. Lasers in Surgery and Medicine. 2013;**45**(3):135-140

[246] Taylor JA et al. A comprehensive approach: Multidisciplinary management in a burn center. Clinical Pediatrics. 1989;**28**(9):404-407

[247] Yuxiang L et al. Burn patients' experience of pain management: A qualitative study. Burns. 2012;**38**(2):180-186

Chapter 11

Urosepsis: Flow is Life

Nissar Shaikh, Umm-E-Amara, Jazib Hassan, Zeeshan Qazi, Arshad Chanda, Zia Mahemood, Mahommad Zubair, AR Raju Vegensa, Abdul Gafoor M. Tharayil, Adel Ganaw, Ranjan Matthias and Muna Al Musalmani

Abstract

Urosepsis is one of the important etiological factors for community as well as hospital-acquired infections. Accordingly, urosepsis is divided into community-acquired and hospital-acquired urosepsis. Obstruction to the flow of urine is a common risk factor for community-acquired urosepsis, whereas the indwelling urinary catheter is the risk for the hospital-acquired urosepsis. *E. coli* remained the most common bacteria-causing urosepsis. If not treated early and appropriately, urosepsis can complicate into septic shock and multiple organ dysfunction. The cornerstone for the improved outcome of these patients is initial resuscitation and proper antibiotic therapy and restoring the flow of urine or removing the infected urinary catheter. Community-acquired urosepsis can be prevented by removing the obstruction to flow of urine permanently. The hospital-acquired urosepsis can be prevented by strictly following catheter-associated urinary tract infection prevention bundle and removing the catheter as early as possible.

Keywords: *E. coli*, microbiology, sepsis, septic shock, community-acquired and hospital-acquired urosepsis, urine obstruction, urinary catheter

1. Introduction

The mortality from sepsis is reaching higher than prostatic and breast carcinoma; up to 31% of sepsis originated from the urogenital tract organs, and hence it is termed as urosepsis [1]. Urosepsis is a severe infection and 5% lead to severe sepsis, and it is an important aetiology for hospital-acquired infection and accounts for around 40% of the nosocomial infections [2]. About 5% of urosepsis patients complicate in severe sepsis and organ dysfunction; Patients with comorbidities are at a higher risk for urosepsis, severe sepsis and septic shock with a higher morbidity and mortality [3]. Hence, the early diagnosis and management is the key for better outcome. The presence of bacteria in the urogenital tract produces an overwhelming pro-inflammatory reaction involving macrophages and neutrophils by stimulating the cellular immunity, complement system and endothelial cells. the production of nitric oxide is triggered, which leads to a decreased vessel tone resulting in hypotension. This initial phase is followed by a counter regulatory anti-inflammatory response syndrome, leading to an immunosuppressive state, which accounts for the mortality in the longer course of sepsis. The activation of compliment system causes coagulopathy and fibrinolysis leading to microthrombi formation and organ dysfunction [4].

The common aetiology of community-acquired urosepsis is the obstruction to the urine flow, and patient quickly tends to go into septic shock and multi-organ dysfunction due to urinary stagnation and bacterial growth. The obstruction also affects the pharmacokinetics of antibiotics. Relieving the obstruction is the cornerstone for survival of these patients, hence giving the title of the chapter.

We will discuss urosepsis in the following subheadings.

2. Epidemiology

The community acquired urosepsis is rare and commonly occurs due to structural or functional abnormality leading to urinary flow obstruction. It contributes to 5% of total sepsis case, whereas the hospital-acquired urosepsis contributes to 40% of sepsis cases [5]. Occurrence of urosepsis is more frequent in females than in males. For the community-acquired urosepsis, the frequent risk groups are the patients with obstructive uropathy. Hofmann reported that majority of obstruction to the flow of urine was due to urinary calculi (65%), tumours in 21%, gestation in 5%, urinary tract anomalies in 5% and surgical interventions in 4% of their patients [6]. Other risk factors for urosepsis are old age, female gender, immunosuppression, steroid therapy, chronic renal failure and prolonged surgical time [7]. In elderly bedbound patients, the urinary catheter is the foremost cause for urosepsis. Healthcare-associated infection frequency vary according to geographical location of the countries; prevalence of healthcare-associated infections is 4% in the United States of America, 6% in the European countries and 15.5% higher in developing countries [8, 9].

3. Classification

Urosepsis is classified into two categories.

3.1 Community-acquired urosepsis

Community-acquired urosepsis when presents with urosepsis from the community. It accounts for 7% of all sepsis cases. It is more frequent in females and has a shorter ICU stay. Mainly caused by Gram-negative bacteria and 63% had *E. coli* with 41% having bacteraemia. Yang et al. have shown that ESBL-producing *E. coli* and *K. pneumoniae* (ESBL-EK) accounted for 20.7% of the pathogens causing

Community-acquired urosepsis	Hospital-acquired urosepsis
Obstructive uropathy or genitourinary tract abnormalities are common aetiology	Prolonged urinary catheterization is a common aetiology
Gram-negative bacteria in 85% and Gram-positive in 15% [12]	Gram-negative bacteria in 66% and Gram-negative in 21%
Source control by endoscopic stent or image-guided nephrostomy	Removal of urinary catheter is the source control
Board-spectrum antibiotics depend on local antibiogram	Initial antibiotics should cover pseudomonas

Table 1.
Differences between community-acquired urosepsis and hospital-acquired urosepsis.

bacteraemic community-acquired urinary tract infections [10]. The 28-day mortality was higher in the non-HCRI group (29%) [11].

3.2 Hospital-acquired urosepsis

Hospital-acquired urosepsis is one of the healthcare provider-related sepses and acquired during the hospital stay. It was found in 31% of these patients; *E. coli* represents 58% of all isolations with a different resistance profile with resistance to ciprofloxacin, aminoglycosides and co-trimoxazole. The 28-day mortality in hospital-acquired urosepsis was 15% [10]. In contrast the hospital-acquired urosepsis with extended B-lactam enzyme had a significant higher mortality of 41% [10] (**Table 1**).

4. Risk factors

There are risk factors for both community- and hospital-acquired urosepses. Community-acquired urosepsis occurs mainly in patients with obstructive uropathy, genitourinary tract structural abnormalities and carcinoma of the urinary bladder, whereas the hospital-acquired urosepsis occurs in catheterized elderly patients, on immunosuppression therapy [13, 14].

4.1 Age and gender

The combination of age more than 65 and female gender is a significant risk factor for the development of urosepsis. Bacteriuria is frequent in elderly population; more than 50% of geriatric females will have bacteriuria. A multicentre study showed that patients older than 65 years of age admitted with febrile UTIs were nearly 2.5 times more likely to develop bacteraemia than patients under the age of 65 [15].

4.2 Comorbidities

The diabetes, nephrocalcinosis and azotaemia (chronic kidney disease) are related to the increased incidence of urosepsis. van Nieuwkoop et al. reported an association between comorbid disease and urosepsis, where diabetes was significantly associated with an 80% increased risk for urosepsis. In diabetic patients, poor glycaemic control, autonomic neuropathy, higher urinary glucose, immune dysfunction and diabetic microangiopathy facilitate bacterial adherence to uroepithelium [15].

4.3 Obstructive uropathy

The number of factors causing obstruction to the urinary flow increases the risk of urosepsis significantly. The congenital factors causing obstruction to the urinary flow are ureteric or urethral strictures, phimosis, ureterocele and polycystic kidney disease, whereas the acquired aetiological factor leading to urinary flow obstruction are calculi, prostatic hypertrophy, tumours of the urinary tract, trauma, pregnancy and the radiation therapy causing fibrosis [12].

4.4 Environmental and host factors

These are the external factors that contribute to bacterial virulence, transmission of bacteria to host and compromise of host defences. This includes inappropriate and unnecessary antibiotic consumption, limited healthcare facilities and the lack of local surveillance programmes.

4.5 Voiding disabilities

Traumatic spinal injuries, cerebrovascular accidents, neurogenic bladder, cystocele and vesicoureteral reflux due to various aetiologies, either trauma or congenital, lead to increased usage of urinary catheterization and ultimately increased incidence of urosepsis. Urosepsis risks are multiplied due to indwelling long-term catheters and the spread of multidrug-resistant bacterial strains. Richards et al. showed that 23% of all cases of hospital-acquired sepsis were due to UTI and mostly seen in catheterized patients [16].

4.6 Urosurgical interventions

Trauma of urological intervention either diagnostic or therapeutic in the presence of bacteria can lead to the development of urosepsis. Common urological interventions are prostate biopsies, stone interventions and transurethral prostate resections. Urosepsis rate after these surgical interventions are transurethral resection of prostate up to 4% [17] trans rectal prostate biopsies up to 0.8% [18] lithotripsy: 1% [19] ureterostomy for stone treatment up to 9% patients will have severe sepsis [20] percutaneous kidney stone surgery up to 7% will develop sepsis [21] and up to 8% endoscopic urethrotomy patients develops sepsis [22] (**Table 2**).

5. Diagnosis

Typical presentation in community-acquired urosepsis patients is triad of loin pain, fever and leukocytosis. Hospital-acquired urosepsis patients frequently manifest leukocytosis and hypotension. Urosepsis quickly complicats into septic shock with multiple organ dysfunction. One third of these patients will have septic shock with tachycardia and tachypnea and other organ dysfunctions [12].

5.1 Laboratory work-up

Apart from complete blood count (CBC) and electrolyte monitoring, the serum C-reactive protein and procalcitonin (PCT) levels should be obtained. They will tell us the patient deterioration and presence of sepsis and septic shock. Serum lactate will give diagnostic as well as prognostic value [11].

Risk factors	
Age and gender	More than 65 years and female
Comorbidities	Diabetes mellitus, nephrocalcinosis and chronic kidney disease
Obstructive uropathy	Ureteric, urethral strictures, phimosis, ureterocele, polycystic kidney disease, calculi, prostatic hypertrophy, tumours of the urinary tract, trauma, pregnancy and the radiation therapy
Environmental and host factors	Bacterial virulence, transmission of bacteria to host and compromise of host defences
Voiding disabilities	Traumatic spinal injuries, cerebrovascular accidents, neurogenic bladder, cystocele and vesicoureteral reflux
Urosurgical interventions	Prostate biopsies, stone interventions and transurethral prostate resections

Table 2.
Risk factors for urosepsis.

5.2 Urine culture

Urinary culture and sensitivity are important not only in the diagnosis but also equally important in the management of urosepsis. The culture should be done within hours or persevered properly. A positive culture is highly diagnostic, and negative culture will rule out the urinary infections.

5.3 Blood culture

As significant number of urosepsis patients had Gram-negative bacteraemia, which correspond to the severe sepsis and septic shock.

5.4 Imaging studies

Imaging studies will help in diagnosing renal calculi as well as urosepsis aetiology and complications.

5.4.1 Abdominal radiography

Abdominal radiography has a limited value; it shows the presence and extent of calcification and calculi within the renal system. It is of help in monitoring change in position and increase in size or number of renal stones. Intravenous urography gives the anatomical details of the urinary system. It also helps in the diagnosis of reflux nephropathy and papillary necrosis.

5.4.2 Ultrasound scan

Ultrasound is routinely performed in emergency department. It helps in the diagnosis of renal stone, prostate and bladder pathologies. It is one of the common imaging studies for the patients presenting to emergency with loin pain.

5.4.3 CT scan and MRI abdomen

These modalities of imaging studies will accurately diagnose microabscesses in the kidney and other genital organs. It will accurately diagnose the bacterial nephritis, renal microabscesses, perinephric abscesses, hydronephrosis and emphysematous pyelonephritis [12] (**Figure 1**).

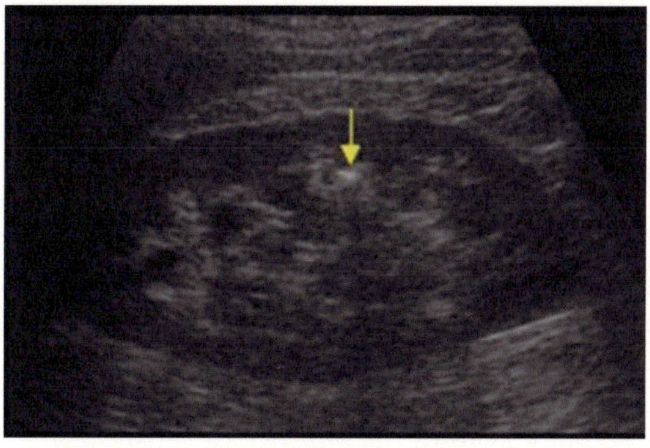

Figure 1.
Renal USG showing calculi.

6. Microbiology and microbial resistance in urosepsis

Urinary culture is not specific for diagnosis, but it rules out the origin of urosepsis if it is negative. It should be obtained at midstream and procedure immediately. Blood cultures must also be taken before administrating the antimicrobial agent, can be ones results are available. Blood cultures can be positive in up to 41% of the cultures [23]. About 93% of the patients admitted with community-acquired urosepsis had *E. coli* growth, whereas 66% of the hospital-acquired urosepsis patients grow *E. coli*. Interesting factor is that the urinary catheter-associated urosepsis is associated with Gram-positive infections. *Candida* infections are common in patients with stents in the urinary tract. In female patients, the *E.coli* urosepsis is common as compared to the male patients (92 and 60%, respectively) [23] (**Table 3**).

Risk factors	Common organism
Community-acquired urosepsis	Gram-positive bacteria 15% Gram-negative bacteria 85%
Hospital-acquired urosepsis	Gram-positive bacteria 21% Gram-negative bacteria (66%) with increased frequency of ESBL, multidrug resistance fluoroquinolone resistance and aminoglycoside resistance
Patients with prolonged and infected ureteric stents	*Candida* species
Patients with diabetes mellitus	*E. coli*, *Klebsiella pneumoniae*, *Proteus* and *Pseudomonas* causing emphysematous pyelonephritis, rarely *Candida* and *Cryptococcus*

Table 3.
Bacteriology of urosepsis.

7. Complications

The main complications of urosepsis are bacteraemia (23%), endotoxemia (34%) and septic shock up to 2.5%. The common organ involved is the kidney [24].

7.1 Post-obstructive acute kidney injury

Up to 10% of acute kidney injury (AKI) episodes are caused by urinary tract obstruction; in the elderly, it will increase to 22% of AKI. The mechanisms in the pathogenesis of obstructive nephropathy lead to renal vasoconstriction and progressive renal fibrosis; while renal vasoconstriction is reversible after the release of obstruction, renal fibrosis may result in irreversible loss of function. Post-obstructive AKI rarely progresses to end-stage renal disease after the release of obstruction, but significant percentage (21%) of these patients have chronic renal impairment. The best time to release urinary obstruction in the setting of post-obstructive AKI is not known; in patients with sepsis, it should be performed as an emergency. The renal outcome inversely correlated with elapsed time from admission to the release of obstruction, which could suggest that the release should be performed as an emergency even in the absence of sepsis [25].

Acute pyelonephritis
Emphysematous pyelonephritis
Renal abscess
Prostatic abscess
Post-obstruction acute kidney injury
Fournier's gangrene
Septic shock with multi-organ dysfunction

Table 4.
Complications of urosepsis.

7.2 Acute pyelonephritis

It can occur with or without urinary obstruction, common in females. If not treated appropriately, it will progress into emphysematous pyelonephritis, papillary necrosis and perinephric and renal abscess.

7.3 Emphysematous pyelonephritis

A life-threatening necrotizing infection of renal parenchyma and perinephric area, if not treated, can be fatal. Common bacteria are *E. coli*, *Klebsiella pneumoniae*, *Proteus* and *Pseudomonas*, and rarely fungi are common in patients with diabetes mellitus. It can be managed by percutaneous drainage and antibiotic and supportive care [26].

7.4 Renal abscess

It is common in patients with diabetes mellitus. The reflux and back pressure of the infected urine is the main aetiology for the renal abscesses. About 75% of renal abscesses is caused by *E. coli*. Treatments are percutaneous drainage, antibiotics and supportive care [12].

7.5 Prostatic abscess

It occurs exclusively in diabetic patients and immunosuppressed patients. Prostatic abscess can rupture into the urethra. Percutaneous drainage is key for better outcome of these patients [27].

7.6 Fournier's gangrene

It is the necrotizing fasciitis of genitalia. Prompt diagnosis and earlier antibiotics and surgical debridement are the essential factors for better outcome [28] (**Table 4**).

8. Management of urosepsis

Septic shock is the most severe complication of urinary tract infection.

8.1 Initial resuscitation

Urosepsis patient will be dehydrated and febrile and may be in shock, hence initially resuscitating with fluid challenges. Fever is usually controlled by paracetamol. If after initial resuscitation, if their hemodynamic parameters is not improving, they should be started early on vasopressors. These uroseptic shock patients should be initially managed following sepsis protocols in the first hour. O_2 supplementation, IV fluid and antibacterial administration and advanced hemodynamic monitoring are useful. With the goal of central venous pressure (CVP) 8–12, intrathoracic blood volume index (ITBV) and global end-diastolic index (GEDVI) within normal range. Cardiac contractility will be monitored by cardiac index (CI), cardiac functional index (CFI) and the isovolumic contraction of the heart (D/P max). Uroseptic shock patients may have respiratory distress, earlier intubation and maintain mixed O_2 or saturation of 70% will improve the outcome [29]. Blood sugar should be maintained around 10 mmol/L. If these urosepsis patients had respiratory distress, they should be immediately intubated and ventilated. As a part of multi-organ dysfunction, these patients may be in disseminated intravenous coagulopathy and should be taken care and resuscitated with blood and blood products.

In antibiotics and bacterial resistance, proper antibiotic administration in septic shock patients improve their outcome [30].

Kumar et al. demonstrated that administration of an effective antimicrobial within the first hour of documented hypotension was associated with a survival rate of 80% [31]. Hence the initial antibiotic in these patients selected on the basis of local antibiogram and as soon as culture are available changed the antimicrobial to the narrow spectrum.

As the common bacteria is *E.coli* in the community-acquired urosepsis, the third generates cephalosporin and fluoroquinolones and combinations are a better choice where as in the hospital-acquired urosepsis, we should add an antipseudomonas antibiotics with combination with amino glucosides or should be initial antimicrobial therapy. Biofilm formation by microorganism is a vital factor in the progress of urosepsis, which is formed in association with urinary catheters, scar tissue and stones, and minimal inhibitory concentrations (MIC) in biofilm are increased up to 100-fold; hence, the high dosages of antibiotics needed in combination with the attempt to remove the biofilm should be considered [32].

Most of these patients' therapy for 2–3 weeks goes parallel with the relief of symptoms and sign with clinical improvement. The cultures should be repeated after 2–4 weeks of cessation of therapy [30].

8.2 Source control

Obstruction to the urinary flow is one of the foremost causes and risks for community-acquired urosepsis. This obstruction should be cleared as soon as possible, either with endoscopic insertion of stent or image-guided percutaneous drainage. The endoscopic stenting is a minimally invasive procedure hence preferred in shock patients with coagulopathy. If the patient has hydronephrosis or renal abscesses, the choice is percutaneous drainage by nephrostomy [33]. In hospital-acquired urosepsis, the indwelling urinary catheter is the frequent cause of urosepsis. In all hospitalised patients with indwelling urinary catheters, catheter-associated urinary tract infection (CAUTI) bundles should be followed strictly. It should be removed as early as possible; if still required the condom catheter can be used, and an antipseudomonal antibiotic should be started [34, 35].

9. Prevention

Community-acquired urosepsis can be prevented up to some extent by relieving the obstruction to the flow of urine or correction of the urinary tract abnormalities, whereas the hospital-acquired urosepsis can be prevented by following the CAUTI bundle, removing urinary catheter and using the condom catheters.

Preventing the urinary tract infection in females, it can be done by following few general principles such as clean genitalia, drinking plenty of water particularly after intercourse, urinating frequently and wiping from front to back.

In elderly patients, the regular use of cranberry juice or capsule may be helpful. In elderly postmenopausal patient, intravaginal oestriol therapy is useful in preventing UTI. In this group of patients, antibiotics highly effective. Other risk factor such as inconsistence, cystocele should be taken care. Elderly man, incontinence of the bladder and enlargement of prostate is risk, so they should be taken care condom catheter or surgical intervention.

Endo-urological procedure such as ureteroscopy involving instrumentation of the genitourinary tract which has a risk for postoperative urosepsis. The urinary tract interventions are more risky in patients with positive preoperative urine cultures or foreign bodies within the urinary tract causing obstruction. It has been demonstrated that perioperative antibiotics reduce urosepsis after uroendoscopy [36–37].

10. Conclusion

Sepsis is a medical emergency; urosepsis is a sepsis originating from the urinary tract. Urosepsis contributes significantly to the overall epidemiology of sepsis. The common and most frequent aetiology of urosepsis is either congenital or acquired obstruction to the flow of urine. The risk factor for urosepsis varies from metabolic diseases to the renal calculi. Based upon the environment in which the patient gets infection, urosepsis is divided into community-acquired urosepsis and hospital-acquired urosepsis. In the diagnosis of urosepsis apart from monitoring blood count, acute-phase proteins and serum lactate and blood and urinary cultures, the imaging studies play an important role. If not treated early and managed properly, urosepsis can progress into pyelonephritis, renal and prostatic abscesses and septic shock.

The cornerstones for the management of urosepsis are initial organ supportive resuscitation, appropriate early antibiotics, relieving obstruction to urinary flow and the source control. Obstruction to the urine flow is the important and most frequent factor for the urosepsis as it facilitates the bacterial growth and repeated sepsis. It is of vital importance to relieve the obstruction and restore the normal flow of urine as soon as possible to reduce the morbidity and mortality.

Prevention of urosepsis starts from well hydration to the clean genitalia, periurological procedure antibiotics, maintaining free flow of urine and strictly following the CAUTI prevention bundle in the hospitalised patients.

Author details

Nissar Shaikh[1*], Umm-E-Amara[2], Jazib Hassan[1], Zeeshan Qazi[1], Arshad Chanda[1], Zia Mahemood[1], Mahommad Zubair[1], AR Raju Vegensa[1], Abdul Gafoor M. Tharayil[1], Adel Ganaw[1], Ranjan Matthias[1] and Muna Al Musalmani[3]

1 Surgical Intensive Care Unit, Hamad Medical Corporation and Weill Cornell Medical College, Doha, Qatar

2 Apollo Institute of Medical Sciences and Research, Hyderabad, India

3 Department of Medicine, Infectious Disease Section, Hamad Medical Corporation and Weill Cornell Medical College, Doha, Qatar

*Address all correspondence to: nissatfirdous99@gmail.com

References

[1] Angus DC. The lingering consequences of sepsis: A hidden public health disaster? The Journal of the American Medical Association. 2010; **304**(16);1833-1834

[2] Wagenlehner FM, Lichtenstern C, Rolfes C. Diagnosis and management for urosepsis. International Journal of Urology. 2013;**20**(10):963-970

[3] Rosser CJ, Bare RL, Meredith JW. Urinary tract infections in the critically ill patient with a urinary catheter. American Journal of Surgery. 1999;**177**: 287-290

[4] Astiz ME, Rackow EC. Septic shock. Lancet. 1998;**351**:1501-1505

[5] Johansen TE, Cek M, Naber K, Stratchounski L, Svendsen M, Tenke P. Prevalence of hospital acquired urinary tract infections in urology departments. European Urology. 2007;**51**:1100-1112

[6] Hofmann W. Urosepsis and uroseptic shock. Zeitschrift für Urologie und Nephrologie. 1990;**83**:317-324

[7] Qiang XH, Yu TO, Li YN, Zhou LX. Prognosis risk of urosepsis in critical care medicine: A prospective observational study. BioMed Research International. 2016;**2016**:5. 9028924. DOI: 10.1155/2016/9028924

[8] Magill SS, Edwards JR, Bamberg W, Beldavs ZG, Dumyati G, Marion A, et al. Multistate point-prevalence survey of health care–associated infections. The New England Journal of Medicine. 2014; **370**:1198-1208

[9] Allegranzi B, Bagheri Nejad S, Combescure C, et al. Burden of endemic health-care-associated infection in developing countries: Systematic review and meta-analysis. Lancet. 2011;**377**: 228-241

[10] Yang YS, Ku CH, Lin JC, Shang ST, Chiu CH, Yeh KM, et al. Impact of extended-spectrum b-lactamase-producing *Escherichia coli* and *Klebsiella pneumoniae* on the outcome of community-onset bacteremic urinary tract infection. Journal of Microbiology, Immunology, and Infection. 2010;**43**: 194e9

[11] Cardoso T, Ribeero O, Costa-Pereira A, Carneiro A. Community acquired and healthcare related urosepsis. A multicentre prospective study. Critical Care. 2008;**12**:8

[12] Karla O, Raizada A. Approach to a patient with urosepsis. Journal of Global Infectious Diseases. 2009;**1**:57-63

[13] Lipsky BA. Urinary tract infection in men. Epidemiology, pathophysiology, diagnosis and treatment. Annals of Internal Medicine. 1989;**110**:138-150

[14] Peach BC, Garvan GJ, Garvan CS, Cimiotti JP. Risk factors for urosepsis in older adults: A systematic review. Gerontology and Geriatric Medicine. 2016;**2**:1-7. Peach et al reviewed the risk factors for urosepsis

[15] van Nieuwkoop C, Bonten TN, van't Wout JW, Kuijper EJ, Groeneveld GH, Becker MJ, et al. Procalcitonin reflects bacteremia and bacterial load in urosepsis syndrome: A prospective observational study. Critical Care. 2010; **14**:R206

[16] Richards MJ, Edwards JR, Culver DH, Gaynes RP. Nosocomial infections in combined medical surgical intensive care units in the United States. Infection Control and Hospital Epidemiology. 2000;**21**:510-515

[17] Colau A, Lucet JC, Rufat P, Botto H, Benoit G, Jardin A. Incidence and risk factors of bacteriuria after transurethral

resection of the prostate. European Urology. 2001;**39**:272-276

[18] Lange D, Zappavigna C, Hamidizadeh R, Goldenberg SL, Paterson RF, Chew BH. Bacterial sepsis after prostate biopsy—A new perspective. Urology. 2009;**74**: 1200-1205

[19] Charton M, Vallancien G, Veillon B, Prapotnich D, Mombet A, Brisset JM. Use of antibiotics in the conjunction with extracorporeal lithotripsy. European Urology. 1990;**17**:134-138

[20] Mariappan P, Loong CW. Midstream urine culture and sensitivity test is a poor predictor of infected urine proximal to the obstructing ureteral stone or infected stones: A prospective clinical study. The Journal of Urology. 2004;**171**:2142-2145

[21] Koras O, Bozkurt IH, Yonguc T, et al. Risk factors for postoperative infectious complications following percutaneous nephrolithotomy: A prospective clinical study. Urolithiasis. 2015;**43**:55-60

[22] Ravichandran S, Nambirajan T, Athmalingam G. Traumatic posterior urethral stricture—A randomized study of core-through urethrotomy and anastomotic urethroplasty [abstract 087]. BJU International-Supplement. 2003;**91**(Suppl S2):20

[23] Chin BS, Kim MS, Han SH, Shin SY, Chris HK, Chae YT, et al. Risk factors of all causes in hospital mortality among Korean bacteraemia urinary tract infection (UTI) patients. Archives of Gerontology and Geriatrics. 2010;**52**: 50-55

[24] Qiang XH, Yu TO, Li YN, Zhau LX. Prognosis risk of urosepsis in critical care medicine, a prospective observational study. Bio Med Research International 2016; 9028924

[25] Hamdi A, Hajage D, Glabeke EV, Belenfant X, Vincent F, Gonzalez F, et al. Severe post-renal acute kidney injury, post-obstructive diuresis and renal recovery. BJU International. 2012: 1027-1034. DOI: 10.1111/j.1464-410X.2012.11193.x

[26] Evanoff GV, Thompson CS, Foley R, Weinman EJ. Spectrum of gas within the kidney. The American Journal of Medicine. 1987;**83**:149-154

[27] Kalra OP, Agarwal NK, Sharma SK, Sakhuja V, Chugh KS. Acute bacterial prostatitis with giant prostatic abscess. Indian Journal of Nephrology. 2002;**12**: 88-89

[28] Shaikh N, Khawaiter J, Al-Thani H. Necrotizing fasciitis: A surgical and medical emergency. Surgical Science. 2012;**3**:518-525

[29] Otero RM, Ngyuyen HB, Huang DT, Gasesk DF, Goyal M, Gunnerson KJ, et al. Early goal directed therapy in severe sepsis and septic shock revisited concepts. Controversies and Contemporary Findings Chest. 2006; **130**:1579-1595

[30] Elhanan G, Sarhat M, Raz R. Empire antibiotics treatment and misuse of culture results and antibiotic sensitivities in patients with community acquired bacteraemia due to urinary tract infections. The Journal of Infection. 1997;**35**:283-288

[31] Kumar A, Roberts D, Wood KE, Light B, Parrillo JE, Sharma S, et al. Duration of hypotension before initiation of effective antimicrobial therapy is the critical determinant of survival in human septic shock. Critical Care Medicine. 2006;**34**:1589-1596

[32] Kumon H. Management of biofilm infections in the urinary tract. World Journal of Surgery. 2000;**24**:1193-1196

[33] Tandigdu Z, Truls E, Johansen B, Bartoletti R, Wagenlehner F. Management of the Urologic Sepsis Syndrome. European Urology Supplements. 2016;**15**:102-111

[34] Urinary Tract Infections in Elderly Persons: Chapter 32: American Society of Nephrology/Geriatric Nephrology Curriculum: Manisha Juthani-Mehta. www.asnonline.org/education/distancelearning/curriculum/geriatism/chapter32.pdf downloaded on 2nd October 2018

[35] Wolf JSJ, Bennett CJ, Dmochowski RR, et al. Urologic surgery antimicrobial prophylaxis best practice policy panel. Best practice policy statement on urologic surgery antimicrobial prophylaxis. The Journal of Urology. 2008;**179**:1379-1390

[36] Chew BH, Flannigan R, Kurtz M, et al. A single dose of intraoperative antibiotics is sufficient to prevent urinary tract infection during ureteroscopy. Journal of Endourology. 2016;**30**:63-68

[37] Scotland KB, Lange D. Prevention and management of urosepsis triggered by ureteroscopy. Research and Reports in Urology. 2018;**10**:43-49